Biomedical Visions Epistemology, Medicine, and Art Practice

Biomedical Visions
Epistemology, Medicine, and Art Practice

Edited by Elizabeth W. Hughes
and Alfred Freeborn

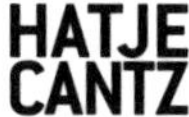

Introduction

Alfred Freeborn

In the spring of 2019, the world-famous singer Ariana Grande shared images of a brain scan on her Instagram feed, joking that they were both "hilarious and terrifying" (Sorto 2019). Grande had been open with the public about her struggle with post-traumatic stress disorder (PTSD) after her concert in Manchester, England, in May 2017 was the target of a suicide bombing attack, which killed twenty-two people, several of them children. Many of Grande's 378 million followers expressed concern at the scans and repeated calls for her to take a break from the media. In response Grande later wrote on her Instagram:

> didn't mean to startle anyone with my brain thingy. It just blew me away. I found it informative and interesting and wanted to encourage y'all to make sure you check on your brain / listen to your bodies / take care of yourselves too. I love science and seeing the physical reality of what's going on in there was incredible to me. I mean I feel it all the time, but seeing it is totally different and super cool ... just know I will continue showing up and giving as much of my energy as I can and do my best even tho my brain looks like the world map. (that's why her hairs so big it's full of trauma ... k ariana, log off) love u. (Sorto 2019)

The scans showed Grande's brain in four different axes, each a disembodied cerebral cloud of fluorescent color. Posted alongside another image comparing scans of a healthy brain to one with PTSD, the scans invite us to discern the patterns of traumatic residue present in Grande's brain. Set free from their technical context at the scanning console, they effortlessly partake in an at once highly personalized and mass-mediated communication. This moment captures well the Janus face of biomedical visualizations as they circulate today. On the one hand, they can legitimize patient experiences and perceptions and can empower patients and convince doctors in the search for a diagnosis, treatment, or cure. But they are also deceptive messengers. Grande's scan most likely came from one of the Amen Clinics, a network of expensive single-photon emission computed tomography (SPECT) clinics established by the controversial celebrity psychiatrist Dr. Daniel Amen, who claims to be able to diagnose PTSD and other disorders with the technology. The reality is, however, that neither Amen nor anyone else can diagnose PTSD with a brain scan and attempts to replicate his claims have been disappointing. The self-evident value placed on the visualization is clearly in tension with its questionable legibility. Visualizations in biomedicine are typically only legible to trained specialists, but these images spread in the public sphere to be interpreted and recontextualized by untrained eyes.

The point for Ariana Grande and her followers is not that the image revealed a new fact about her experience or diagnosis, but that it made what she already felt visible. Grande's Instagram post exemplifies the potent mixture of affect, mediation, and biomedical technology that has begun to transform late-modern experiences of health and sickness. To summarize in a deliberately bold fashion: biomedical technologies increasingly mediate and shape our subjective experiences of illness, but biomedical knowledge cannot satisfy our subjective desires for total control of our bodies and their environments. Biomedical images can validate experiences of illness—they can make them real, they can make them public—but they can also conceal the real extent of our biomedical knowledge. We live in an age of biomedical visions, of promissory technologies and therapies that will render the truth of our bodies, yet behind these visions we find the persistence of epistemic uncertainty, overdiagnosis, unnecessary interventions, and healthcare inequalities. This is not to downplay the amazing successes of biomedicine, but to bear witness to the frictions between a scientific ideology inflated by the expectations of investment capital and its practical realization in increasingly complex areas of human health and sickness.[1]

1 Scientific ideology is used here as defined by Canguilhem. See chapter 1 in Georges Canguilhem (1988).

But how should we approach this scientific ideology and its diverse visual incarnations? The term *biomedicine* has accrued many meanings: as a type of medicine, as a worldview, as a scientific framework. Its first usage in the English language occurs in the first quarter of the twentieth century, where it means the application of the biological sciences to medical problems. It is our contention, however, that it is best grasped not through such a static definition but as a historically specific organization of science, technology, and medicine that fully emerged only in the second half of the twentieth century (Quirke and Gaudillière 2008). While in epistemological terms the project of using laboratory biology to investigate disease can be traced back to the mid-nineteenth century and the age of Claude Bernard and Rudolf Virchow, it is only a century later that we can rightly speak of a living and breathing biomedicine in which information from the lab can be rapidly deployed at the bedside and vice versa (Keuck and Huber 2017). The sociologists Paul Keating and Alberto Cambrosio describe the organization of contemporary biomedicine in terms of "platforms" that involve the regulation and circulation of samples, entities, and techniques between laboratory and clinic: "in contemporary hospitals all sorts of body samples leave the patient to travel routinely and frequently to diagnostic laboratories . . . [returning] to the patient in the form of results that acquire meaning as part of the therapeutic relationship that exists between patients and increasingly complex teams of healthcare professionals" (Keating and Cambrosio 2003, 6–7).

Moreover, while commentators have rightly warned against biomedicalization understood as accelerating the fragmentary and alienating forces of technoscience in modern society, biomedicine in practice also offers multiple possibilities for subjectivization (cf. Clarke et. al. 2009). Genetic tests are worked into a sick individual's identity and brain scans become representations of personal trauma in social media posts. While the body beneath the skin and its mediation through technology threatens to fragment, displace, and alienate an individual's experiences, much work goes into recontextualizing these technical images within the subjective lifeworld and life history of the individual. Of course, this movement between laboratory and lifeworld is not always smooth or linear. Often the therapeutic relationship is infected with biases and prejudices, or the bodily sample fails to return to the clinic with meaningful answers. Patients themselves are increasingly active agents in challenging and articulating the uncertainty, bias, and prejudice that mark the movement of biomedical knowledge. It is in this refracted space between visualized bodies and visions of health and sickness that we begin our discussion.

Biomedical Visions explores a wide range of biomedical themes: personalized medicine, neuroimaging, pathology, genetic counseling, Alzheimer's disease, endometriosis, chronic fatigue, and structural inequalities in healthcare. In addition to this broad selection of topics, the scholarly and artistic methods adopted have both diverse origins and destinations: perspectives from art history, visual studies of science, science and technology studies, sociology, and cultural anthropology converge with watercolor paintings, sculptures, comic strips, advertisements, and infographics. There is, of course, an existing wealth of literature across the history, anthropology, and social studies of biomedicine that has attended to the importance of visualization and visual technologies (e.g., Clarke et al. 2009; Edwards 2010). Building on this rich foundation, our collection examines the interrelation of visual languages and images of sickness and health; it looks at how technical images are painstakingly constructed to give realistic or natural visualizations of the body and its parts; it examines how the human eye (and ear) is trained and learns to perceive the world, but also how human perception is itself studied, contrasted with, and disciplined by mechanical vision; it investigates how visualizations co-construct biomedical imaginaries and futures (Ostherr 2013). While biomedical technologies are foregrounded, there is also attention paid to the clinical encounter and medicine as a social practice. Human beings are complex biopsychosocial systems with individual life histories that are not epistemologically exhausted by quantitative definitions of normality and abnormality. Bodies are more than the abstract objects of biomedicine; they are archives of concrete experience.

This collection of texts is a series of experiments in cross-disciplinary collaboration (with a few exceptions). Each chapter is the product of a unique coming together of two or more different ways of thinking about biomedicine, knowledge, and the visual. There are difficulties in working across disciplines. It is not easy for artists to find scholars who they trust to let them talk about their work. It is not always easy for clinicians to take a step back and see their work from a different perspective. The chapters are arranged in a structure that reflects both the collaboration and the thematic ground covered. The volume begins with a pair of conversations across artistic practice, epistemology, and medicine, which literally stage the opening of a dialogue and an encounter between different perspectives.

In the opening chapter on "Medical Materials in Art," the art historians Virginia Marano, Charlotte Matter, and Laura Valterio carefully guide us through a discussion with the artist Jillian Crochet and the medical historian and physician Vincent Barras on the use of medical materials within different artistic practices. For example, one of Crochet's works, *Primordial Preservation* (2019), involves a plastic bag filled with green-flecked swamp water from southern Louisiana, suspended on an IV stand adorned with a thin snake-like velvet object filled with sand, being steadily aerated via a tube attached to a motor. The work probes anxieties about contamination, environment, and artificial materials or bodies in a particularly personal manner: Crochet spent years trying to find a diagnosis for her disability, which one doctor initially explained as a byproduct of living near farms in the American South where there was heavy use of pesticides like dichlorodiphenyltrichloroethane (DDT), but later proved to be the result of a genetic disease. The uncertainty between genetic and environmental explanations of disease; the substitution of swamp water for vital bodily fluids; the contrast of the metal stand with the ominous snakelike object—all these juxtapositions call into question the material orders that sustain biomedical visions of health as total control of the porous borders between our bodies and the messy environments in which they exist. The question of how medical materials are used by artists reveals not only the polysemic nature of these materials but raises fundamental questions about how medicine creates and is shaped by material orders in its vision of a healthy "normal" body and environment.

Taking materiality in a different direction, "Building Blocks of the Spectrum" explores how specific materials lend themselves to artistic visualizations of biomedical ideologies and, at the same time, how biomedical research makes use of particular visual practices, diagrams, and concepts. The artist Jacob van der Beugel and the historian and philosopher of medicine Lara Keuck converse together on how artistic practice can be a site to reflect on and question the promissory claims of biomedical visions, with particular regard to research into Alzheimer's disease. Anchoring their conversation around van der Beugel's mural *Matter in Grey* (2018) for the Chemistry of Health Department at Cambridge University, a series of spectrums depicting healthy, diseased, and treated brain cells in concrete, they unpack the work of the spectrum concept across biomedicine. As they note, we increasingly conceptualize human differences as existing along a spectrum: we are all unique individuals, but we all have our place on a single continuum that is our common humanity. This image is both aesthetically persuasive and epistemically powerful in resolving complexity. But in the context of biomedicine, hard boundaries rather than continuous dimensions are often needed to guide clinical decision-making, and there is continuous negotiation over how to lump or split disease categories. Their conversation additionally reflects on how artistic practice and the history and philosophy of science both offer a site to step back from these negotiations and explore alternative and competing perspectives on the question of defining disease and the limits of biomedicine.

These opening conversations are followed by two collaborations that explore how bodies and embodied experiences are mediated both through biomedical technologies and visual imaginaries. In "Tangled Tendrils" the historian of science and medicine Jaipreet Virdi recounts her personal journey to receiving a diagnosis of endometriosis, reflecting on the resonances and silences between biomedical visualizations and the experience of a complex and poorly understood disease. Artist Nimisha Bhanot offers a visual response to Virdi's text: her watercolor draws together key aspects of Virdi's journey, while also interweaving her thoughts within Virdi's text as interjections in bold. Biomedicine often differentiates illness from disease, the former being the subjective experience of the patient, the latter an objectively defined entity. Within this framework, the subjective becomes *real* only once a disease has been confirmed by a clinician or a laboratory test. In particular with illnesses of complex and uncertain origin, only once a physical abnormality has been revealed can the pain and suffering be legitimized within the biomedical framework. In contradistinction, this chapter beautifully and passionately argues for the vital importance of making intersubjective moments, relationships, and alliances in which the experience of pain can be made visible in parallel with the work of biomedical technologies. As Virdi puts it, illness experiences and pain can be captured at the meeting point of layered expertise, whereby the making visible of an individual's experience of endometriosis is the work of the multiple epistemic standpoints of surgeon, sufferer, and supporter.

In the following chapter, "Mediating Fatigue," the visual culture scholar Milton Fernando Gonzalez Rodriguez and the historian of science and visual artist Paula Muhr juxtapose two very different visual practices involved in biomedical visions of fatigue: the rhetorical image-making of advertisement and the operational image-making of experimental research. The results of the former circulate in mass publications evoking cultural imaginaries for illness experiences and their medicalization, whereas the latter images are highly context-specific tools for making epistemic objects accessible. In the first half of the chapter, Gonzalez Rodriguez conducts a semiotic analysis of pharmaceutical advertisements published in medical journals in 1960s Latin America. Paying close attention to the imagery and language in these sources, the particular construction of fatigue and its remedy in these visualizations are examined. In the second half, the focus shifts dramatically as Muhr follows the technical production of statistical maps of the brain, what she calls operative images, within experimental neuroimaging research into chronic fatigue syndrome. The contrast reveals precisely how different these two visual practices and contexts are, and how different approaches are required to make sense of them—but both contribute in important ways to the historical construction and evolution of biomedical visions of fatigue.

The following three chapters engage more closely with ways of thinking with images in biomedicine, from the close reading of pathological signs through the microscope to the envisioning of future disease etiologies through infographics.

Tuberculosis, as the historian of medicine Gideon Manning and pathologist Stephen Geller remind us in "Images of Tuberculosis," is a disease as old as mankind itself and one that continues to affect millions worldwide. While the symptoms and experiences of the disease were described in great detail long before the technical developments of the nineteenth century, it was only with microscopic and staining techniques that the bacterial origin of the disease was first made visible to the pathologist. Manning and Geller recount how Robert Koch first made visible through his carefully colored hand drawings of microscopic landscapes the thin rod-shaped bacillus he believed responsible for the disease in the late nineteenth century. They do so not to frame this as a simple achievement of biomedical research, but to contextualize these new insights against other contemporary visualizations of tuberculosis: the descriptions found in the writings of Charlotte Brontë and Edgar Allan Poe and the depictions seen in the portraiture of John Severn and Edvard Munch. Moreover, they emphasize the importance not only of looking down the microscope in this period, but of *listening* to the patient's body. They show how two generations earlier the French physician René-Théophile-Hyacinthe Laennec used macroscopic clinical evidence to develop a method of listening for cavities in the heart and lungs using the stethoscope, legitimizing what the authors call the "auditory eye." While the origins of modern biomedicine in nineteenth-century pathology and clinical medicine involved a careful education of the physician's senses, the increasingly automated and quantitative methods in today's biomedical clinic challenge this aesthetic regime. While the nineteenth-century pathologist was trained to see dynamically and synthesize evidence to depict a total picture of disease, the modern physician is often restricted to standardized tests and diagnostic algorithms. The chapter concludes with a spirited defense of the value and complexity of the trained judgment of the pathologists in contemporary biomedicine.

In "Patterns of Pathology" the historian Flora Lysen elucidates three important points in the evolution of interpreting brain waves for signs of abnormality. First, she shows how the various meanings of "pattern" in early electroencephalography (EEG) are defined by a zigzag dialectic between human and machine, between experience and quantification: patterns are both perceptible forms and imperceptible statistical regularities. Moreover, she shows how the idea of an objective pattern of pathology in brainwaves is continually oversold, with clinical practice still relying on human vision. Nonetheless, it seems that today this may be changing as data scientists and AI produce a new shift in the dialectic between human and machine vision. In dialogue with Lysen's historical investigation, the artist Marlene Bart has produced three tableaux that engage with research into the history of clinical EEG and gender norms embedded in its classificatory project, as well as contemporary questions of artificial intelligence. The duo recounts their dialogue and collaboration in three diaristic vignettes that are spaced throughout the text, revealing in detail the genesis of the two parallel projects, and the fruitful interaction of artistic and scholarly research.

In the last chapter exploring how biomedicine thinks with images, the historians and philosophers of biomedicine Cornelius Borck and Robert Meunier probe the power of visualizations in recent and even future biomedical research with their chapter "Imaginary Imaging." This chapter takes as its focus a single infographic from LifeTime, a Europe-wide biomedical research network, which envisions the possibility of an "interceptive medicine" that intervenes before disease develops rather than waiting to treat it. The particular image in question appears to use the visual languages of molecular biology to show the cellular pathways that result in different forms of disease. However, it was not created by biomedical researchers, but by the freelance designer Johannes Richers in collaboration with the artist Karin Kimel, and as Borck and Meunier show, it makes complex use of different historical traditions of visualization. Through their visual and conceptual analysis, they characterize interceptive medicine as a total bracketing of the sick patient and the cultivation of a hyperreal space, somewhere between science fiction and scientific visualization, in which probabilistic disease trajectories are mapped. Moreover, they enumerate the different risks and blind spots of this particular vision of personalized medicine: overdiagnosis, unbalanced interventionism, and the ongoing commercialization of therapeutics.

The final two chapters switch attention directly to patients and their role in contemporary biomedicine and public health services. Personal decision-making aids (PDAs) deploy infographics and cartoons to communicate with patients and are widely used in genomic medicine. The penultimate chapter, "Building Biosociality," makes apparent the challenges in designing PDAs, which must visualize often incompatible ways of approaching clinical decisions on the road to receiving a diagnosis for a genetic disorder: balancing statistical probabilities calculated from clinical studies with personal fears of potential guilt, surprise, or disappointment in a test's outcome. Through a sociological analysis of the visual strategies in a particular PDA used in Canada (British Columbia), Adam Christianson and Arianne Hanemaayer expose ways of thinking and assumptions that underemphasize patient empowerment. But most importantly, this transdisciplinary collaboration with illustrator Sophia Martineck, media designer Alexandra Hamann, and the medical geneticists Jan M. Friedman and Alison Elliott, takes these insights and works them into a practical tool, a new set of visual strategies, which might increase patient empowerment in the process of deciding whether or not to undergo genetic testing.

The final chapter of the volume, "Seen but Not Heard," is the result of a transdisciplinary project between Awa Naghipour, Golnar Kat Rahmani, and Joana Atemengue Owona that interrogates intersectional discrimination and inequality in the realm of German healthcare. After interviewing individuals who experienced discrimination in the healthcare system, they distilled these encounters with epistemic and social injustice into key phrases that were recorded, musically transcribed, then cast on lead tablets as silent scores. Alongside the artwork, the group produced a leaflet on How Not to Gaslight. Developed through close collaboration, the chapter reflects the authors' diverse backgrounds in medical science, clinical practice, sociopolitical engagement, and the arts. Too often the experiences of people in marginalized groups are silenced in the clinic. This collaboration seeks to make visible the multilayered reality of those who are seen but not heard and opens up conversations for tackling structural inequalities in German healthcare.

Finally, in an epilogue, the art historian Cat Dawson picks out various threads developed within the volume and reflects critically on one of the volume's central themes: images are a primary way of knowing the body, yet they inevitably promise too much and disappoint us in our pursuit of corporeal self-control. Together, these diverse contributions show how biomedical technologies and social orders have been coproduced, either through certain visual practices or within a specific biomedical imaginary. They elucidate how biomedical knowledge is coded and mediated through technical images and specific visual styles and explore artistic practices as a method of closing the gap between embodied experiences of illness and technoscientific visualizations of diseased bodies. In our highly polarized era in which biomedical practices are increasingly politicized, this volume raises questions and new discussions in the spirit of thinking together across disciplinary and professional divides. *Biomedical Visions* draws together different perspectives on epistemology, medicine, and artistic practice to make sense both of how biomedicine *looks* and how we might *look differently* at biomedicine, in the past, and in the future.

C

Canguilhem, Georges (1988) *Ideology and Rationality in the History of the Life Sciences*. Translated by Arthur Goldhammer. Cambridge, MA: MIT Press.

Clarke, Adele E., Laura Mamo, Jennifer Ruth Fosket, Jennifer R. Fishman, and Janet K. Shim (2009) *Biomedicalization: Technoscience, Health, and Illness in the U.S.* Durham, NC: Duke University Press.

E

Edwards, Jeanette, ed. (2010) *Technologized Images, Technologized Bodies*. New York: Berghahn.

H

Huber, Lara, and Lara Keuck (2017) "Philosophie der biomedizinischen Wissenschaften." In *Grundriss Wissenschaftsphilosophie: Die Philosophien der Einzelwissenschaften*, edited by Simon Lohse and Thomas Reydon. Hamburg. Meiner, F.

K

Keating, Peter, and Alberto Cambrosio (2003) *Biomedical Platforms: Realigning the Normal and the Pathological in Late-Twentieth-Century Medicine*. Cambridge, MA: MIT Press.

O

Ostherr, Kirsten (2013) *Medical Visions: Producing the Patient through Film, Television, and Imaging Technologies*. Oxford: Oxford University Press.

Q

Quirke, Viviane, and Jean-Paul Gaudillière (2008) "The Era of Biomedicine: Science, Medicine, and Public Health in Britain and France after the Second World War." *Medical History* 52 (4): 441–52.

S

Sorto, Gabrielle. "Ariana Grande Shares Brain Scan and Opens Up about PTSD." CNN Entertainment, April 12, 2019. https://edition.cnn.com/2019/04/12/entertainment/ariana-grande-ptsd-brain-scan-instagram-trnd/index.html.

On the Use, Reuse, and Misuse of Medical Materials in Art: A Conversation with Vincent Barras and Jillian Crochet

Virginia Marano,
Charlotte Matter, and Laura Valterio

1 Porous Relations: Materials between Medicine and Art

LAURA VALTERIO The purpose of this conversation is to reflect on the use, reuse, and "misuse" of medical materials in art. We are grateful for the opportunity to explore this topic from different methodological positions in exchanging our perspectives as art historians with yours, Jillian, as an artist, and yours, Vincent, as a historian of medicine and trained physician. We have chosen four works of art from different periods and contexts, each addressing a distinct facet of the subject.
We would like to discuss with you: What do these artifacts tell us from the points of view of art making, art history, and the history of medicine? What kind of status can we assign to these multilayered creations? We are particularly interested in how their aesthetic and functional dimensions interact and coexist, sometimes in conflict. The first example we would like to discuss is a work by Jillian, titled *Primordial Preservation* (2019). FIG. 1

JILLIAN CROCHET This work is composed of a metal pole for intravenous infusion, also called an IV stand, and a plastic

FIG. 1 Jillian Crochet, *Primordial Preservation*, 2019, algae, copper tube, IV bag, plastic tubing, air pump, IV stand, sand, silk velvet, dimensions variable. Courtesy of the artist
FIG. 2 Detail of Jillian Crochet, *Grieving Organism*, 2018, held by two people
FIG. 3 Jillian Crochet, *Grieving Organism*, 2018, velvet, sand, fur, dimensions variable. Courtesy of the artist

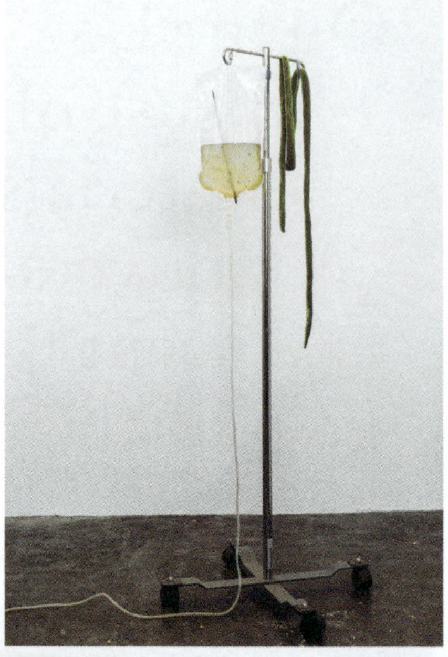

FIG. 1

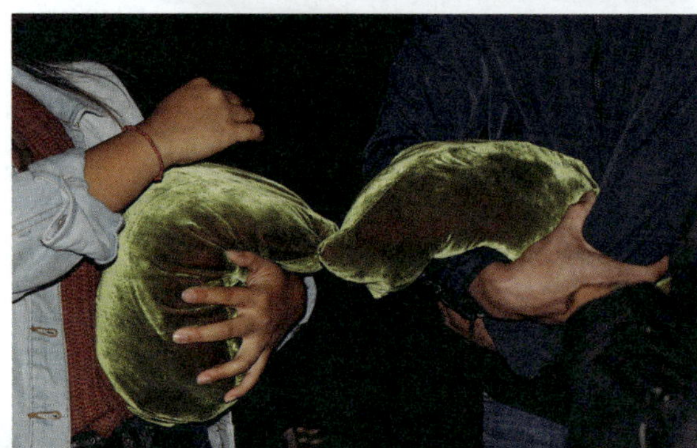

FIG. 2

FIG. 3

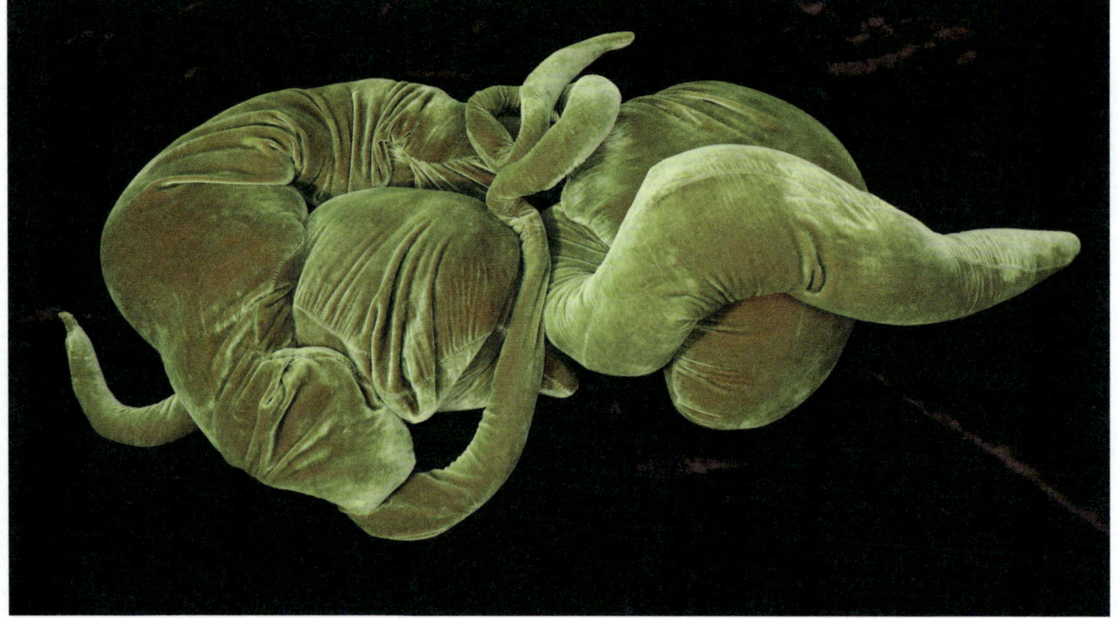

fluid bag filled with algae water that I collected from the swampy bayou in southern Louisiana, where my family is from. There is a copper tube inside the bag that acts as an air release. A plastic tube connects the IV bag to a motor, which acts like an aerator, as it forces air up the tube and into the bag, making this soothing bubbling sound. Hanging on the other side of the IV stand is a thin, snakelike green velvet object filled with sand. It is heavier than it looks. I have a disability that is a genetic disease, and I spent a decade just trying to figure out the diagnosis. Different doctors suspected that it could be genetic, but one of the first doctors I saw from Louisiana just shrugged it off as a byproduct of the pesticides my family was exposed to. Coming from the South and growing up near farms, my family and I were around heavy pesticide usage like dichlorodiphenyl-trichloroethane (DDT). There is no way to know what DDT and other chemicals can cause on a long-term basis to you and your children. So, when I was thinking about using the swamp water, I thought about how it and I share a kind of genetic and epigenetic history—memories of a sort. DDT and other kinds of chemicals were developed in wartime, as were a lot of medical treatments and testing still in use nowadays, which feel antiquated at times. For example, the kinds of tests I have received for nerve conditions involved being shocked over and over again. All of this was on my mind when thinking about the history of medicine, but also when I was creating this work.

CHARLOTTE MATTER Could you tell us more about the velvety snakelike object, which is akin to some of your other works, such as *Grieving Organism* (2018)? FIG. 2 AND 3

These are tactile sculptures made to be touched, which question normative subject/object relationships centered on visuality and address notions of care (cf. Crochet et al. 2022). I would also be curious to know more about the title itself, *Primordial Preservation*.

JILLIAN CROCHET Regarding the title, I was thinking about preservation and lifesaving means. By preservation, I mean both ecological preservation and the preservation of my own, and other, bodies. Many medical apparatuses that are used for various interventions involve a lot of plastic. Although one might assume that something like algae could not survive in a plastic IV bag, it can actually live for quite a long time. As for the term *primordial*, this came from thinking about the primordial soup—one theory for evolution is that life generated out of small porous cyanobacteria bumping into each other and sharing DNA. Regarding the velvet structure, it could be read as a snake, but to me, it's more of a vine. In southern Louisiana, both the plants and bugs tend to be ginormous and luscious. There are all sorts of both native and non-native vines, like kudzu, which is an invasive plant species taking over the landscape in the Southern states very fast. The velvet structure has this weird, creepy, lush green that looks unnatural, although it can be found in nature. This vinelike thing is filled with sand and can be touched and held. When one holds it, it can provide comfort from the weight of it and by caressing it, through stimming. But, of course, you don't need comfort unless you're in pain already—so I was thinking about pain and comfort and trying to expand them to allow for these contradictory things to exist together.

VINCENT BARRAS When I look at this work, what strikes me is that it includes one of the most familiar and common items found in many hospitals around the world. The IV stand, which holds the fluids that are infused into a person's veins, therefore immediately evokes something rather primordial in that sense too. In a hospital, it is more likely to be handled by nursing staff than by doctors; this object thus also speaks of hierarchies within medicalized care. Caregivers suspend a fluid bag and connect it to the veins of the patient, which is then connected to the fluid. In this understanding of medicine and care, the patient's body is conceived as an envelope enclosing bodily fluid, which is undergoing a pathological condition. Additional fluid, such as blood or other types of physiological fluids, must be added to this bodily envelope in order to supplement or strengthen the body. As a device, the IV stand reflects a very specific conception of the body, which is quite different, for instance, from that of traditional Chinese medicine, where the

body is thought of more in terms of energies and points of puncture, rather than tubes and fluids. When I consider *Primordial Preservation* from the point of view of a historian or anthropologist of medicine, this work immediately suggests something that is connected to a specific body in a specific space. I also interpreted the green velvet shape as a snake. Beyond its rather obvious symbolism related to the medical world, it further evokes the animal world in general. In a certain sense, it acts as a kind of counterpart to the IV stand signaling "health," since the snake can present a danger. If the snake were to bite me, its venom would enter my blood and make me sick. In that sense, this object seems very ambiguous, as it oscillates between health and toxicity. It also fluctuates between the animal and human world, the technical and the natural.
JILLIAN CROCHET It is interesting what you say about the ambiguity of the work, since dirty water is not what one would want pumped into their body at the hospital. Typically, an IV fluid would be sterilized, kept separate from the body, and handled with gloves and masks in a sterile environment. Obviously, the algae water is not sterile at all. A family member caught a flesh-eating disease from falling into the swamp water. Concerning the animal world versus the human world, it is interesting that we as humans are also an animal but think that animals are completely separated from us (Taylor 2017).[1] Similarly, the distinction between clean versus dirty is not as clear-cut as we may think.
CHARLOTTE MATTER I was intrigued when you mentioned the materiality of plastic, especially in combination with water. The liquid in *Primordial Preservation* appears contaminated because it is not pristine but tinted, and because the caption informs us that it contains algae. FIG. 4

But then there is also the fact that plastic, the container's material, itself contaminates water by cluttering up oceans and leaching endocrine disruptors that enter and modify our bodies without us even realizing. "Plastics and their chemicals," as Max Liboiron observes, "defy containment, a hallmark approach to industrial waste management, as they blow, flow,

1 In light of the discussed ambiguities between the animal and human worlds, and the concepts of cleanliness versus contamination, Sunaura Taylor's *Beasts of Burden: Animal and Disability Liberation* provides a critical perspective. This text challenges the rigid separations between humans and animals, and the abled and disabled, advocating for a more inclusive understanding of interspecies solidarity.

FIG. 4 Detail of Jillian Crochet, *Primordial Preservation*, 2019, yellow-green algae liquid in the IV bag

FIG. 4

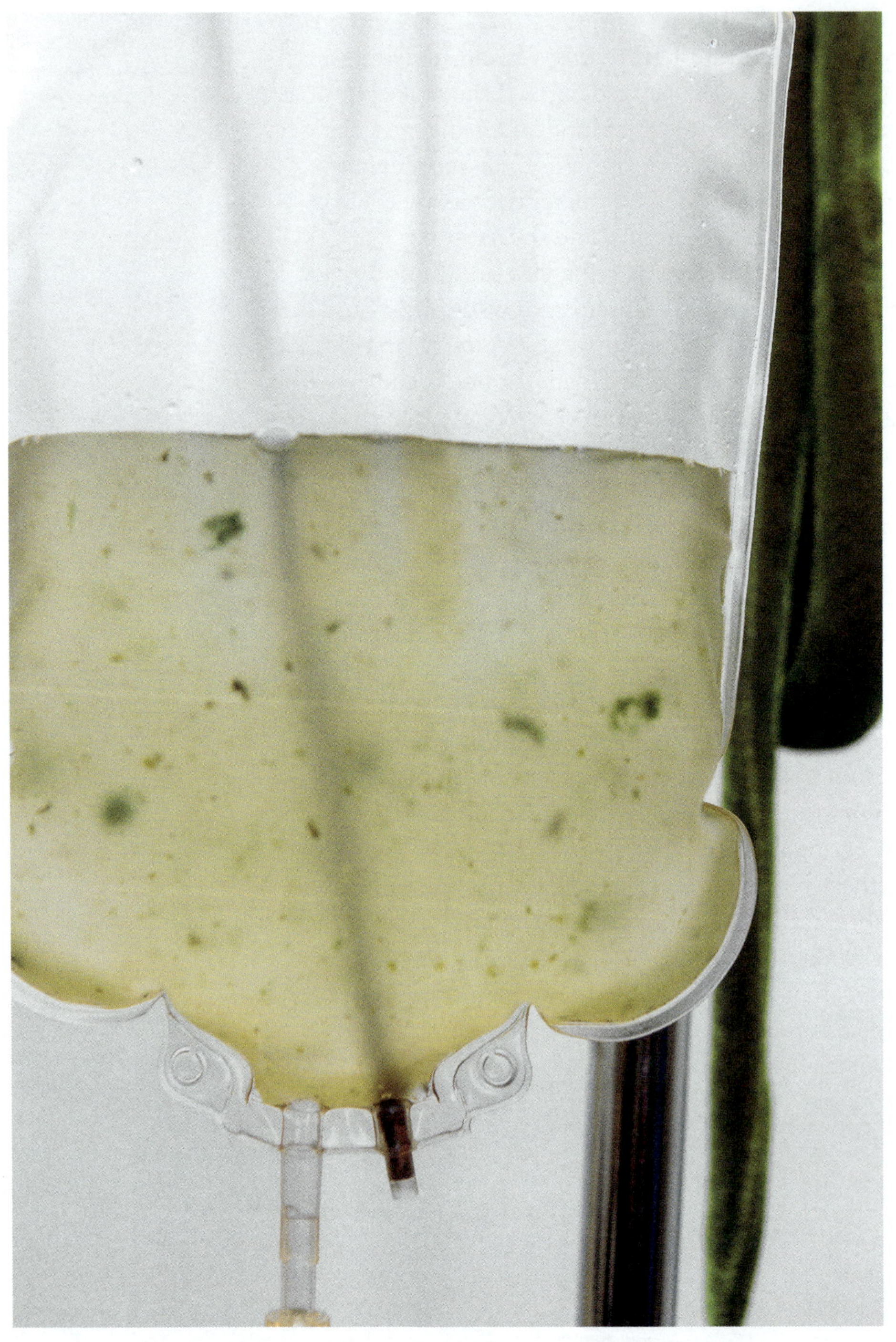

and off-gas so that their pollutants are ubiquitous in every environment tested" (2021, 17). This creates a tension between the visibility and non-visibility of toxicity.[2] Returning to the notion of human and more-than-human worlds, you could almost say that plastic has a kind of agency in the microcosm of this work—for better or worse. It's as if you're inviting more porous definitions of these different entities. I also found it interesting how Vincent responded to the velvet object as something menacing, whereas you were suggesting that it could have a soothing effect.

2 On the question of the (in)visibility of industrial contamination, see also Ofrias (2017).

JILLIAN CROCHET I enjoy dealing with dichotomies and mixing things up because nothing is black and white, and everything is living in discordance. My doctor was talking the other day about the beneficial impact of certain foods and changing one's diet, but she also pointed out that a number of chemotherapies are based on toxic plants.

LAURA VALTERIO There is an interesting ambiguity in your work between what heals us and what harms us. Vincent read the velvet object as a threatening, snakelike form; however, in Western culture, snakes have historically also symbolized the process of healing. The serpent entwined around a rod was a traditional attribute of the Greco-Roman god of medicine, Asclepius, and is still used today as a symbol by medical institutions, hospitals, and pharmacies. This semantic ambiguity is deeply rooted in the Greek term *pharmakon* and the Latin *medicamentum*, which carry the double meaning of "poison" and "medicine." This polysemy, famously explored by the French philosopher Jacques Derrida (1981, 61–171) in his essay "Plato's Pharmacy," locates toxicity not in the substances themselves but in their use.

2
The Body Reclaimed: Contending with Medical Representation and Objectification

CHARLOTTE MATTER Speaking of indeterminacy in terms of remedy and poison, let us consider the use of X-rays in art with a series of works from the 1970s by Italian artist Ketty La Rocca

(1938–1976). La Rocca had been mostly working with collages, combining text and images, and had also experimented with video, sculpture, and performance when she began using X-rays in the early 1970s. By then, she had been diagnosed with cancer and would later die of a brain tumor. In a series called *Craniologie* (1973), La Rocca superimposed X-rays of her own skull with photographed hands and handwritten text. FIG. 5A, 5B, 5C

She traced new lines on top of the X-ray, reading "you you you you you," repeated like a mantra on top of her cranium. La Rocca thus appropriated and indeed reclaimed the medical display of her body. The medical image is overwritten and thereby transformed by the artist's own handwriting; it is further overlaid with photographs of a hand. Depending on the gesture, the hand appears in some works like an intruding element, evoking a kind of sexual penetration, while in other works it suggests a thing that has grown and nested inside the body, an embryo, perhaps, or a tumor. The hand is external, like a scolding finger or a groping hand, but it has also been internalized, literally and metaphorically. Both the word "you" and the X-ray serve a similar purpose, which is to signify a kind of oppressive violence through a self-portrait that reproduces an image of oneself imposed from the outside and informed by normative conventions—be they linguistic or medical. In a text titled "You, You" (1972–1973), La Rocca explained her repetitive invocation of the second person pronoun as such: "'you, you' tries to hamper the visual and mental process / and to reduce the language to a simple bit of information / and to make immediately clear the asymptote of alienation" (La Rocca 1974). The process of "alienation" described by La Rocca is tied to the experience of a gendered and medicalized body. In her *Craniologie*, however, the ascription of what it means to be a woman, and more specifically a *sick* woman—the "you" forcefully assigned by medical imagery and societal expectations—is disrupted by a radical subjectivity. The last aspect I want to mention is that La Rocca used to work as an assistant radiologist in the late 1950s, before turning to art, which means that the technique was known to her. In more than one way, she had an

FIG. 5A Ketty La Rocca, *Craniologia 1*, 1973, lightbox, 2 parts overlapped, X-ray and handwriting on plexiglass, 70 × 50 × 15 cm. Courtesy of Archive Ketty La Rocca | Michelangelo Vasta and Kadel Willborn, Düsseldorf

FIG. 5B Ketty La Rocca, *Craniologia 5*, 1973, lightbox, 2 parts overlapped, X-ray and handwriting on plexiglass, 70 × 50 × 15 cm. Courtesy of Archive Ketty La Rocca | Michelangelo Vasta and Kadel Willborn, Düsseldorf

FIG. 5C Ketty La Rocca, *Craniologia 12*, 1973, lightbox, handwriting on X-ray, 70 × 50 × 15 cm. Courtesy of Archive Ketty La Rocca | Michelangelo Vasta and Kadel Willborn, Düsseldorf

FIG. 5A

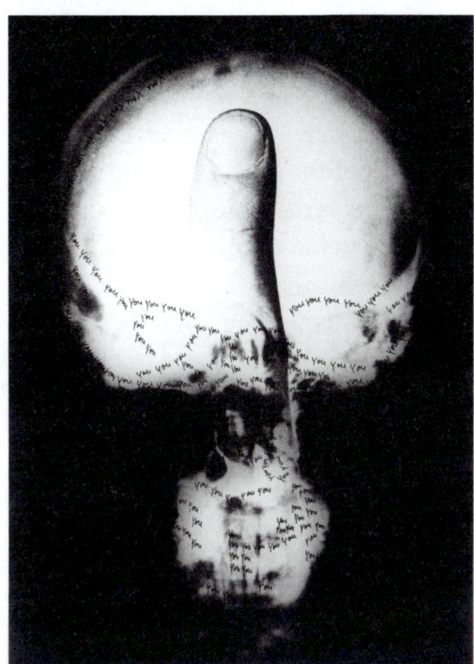

FIG. 5B

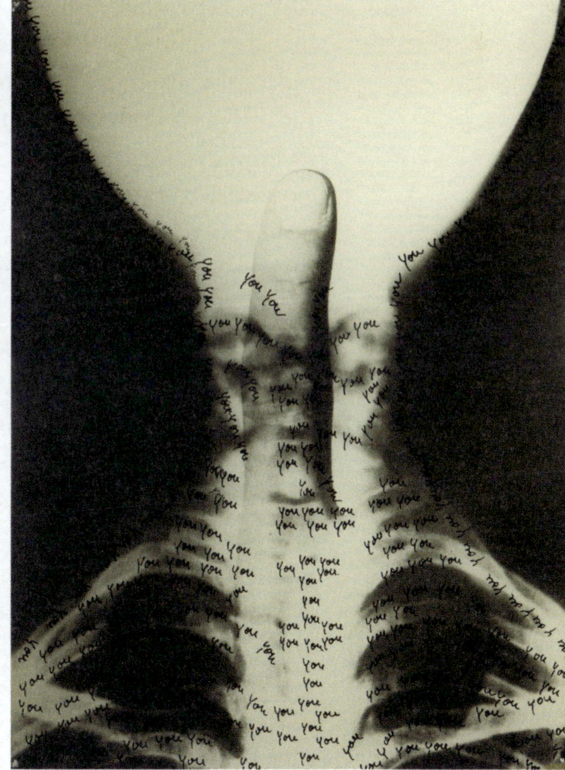

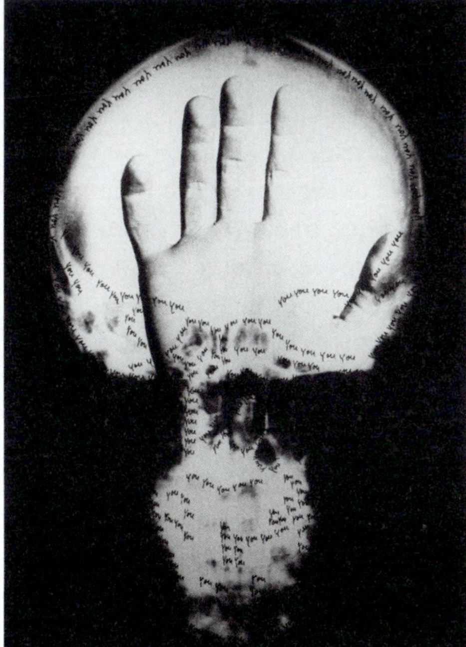

FIG. 5C

intimate, embodied relation to these images: they related to her past, to questions of labor and financial livelihood, to caregiving, as well as to her present and insecure future in light of her illness. Some have also speculated that her cancer may have been related to her exposure to radiation from her work with X-rays.

VINCENT BARRAS This work was shown five years ago in an exhibition titled *Sublimi anatomie* (Sublime Anatomies) at the Palazzo delle Esposizioni in Rome.[3] I also participated in this exhibition with a performance-lecture that lasted a couple of hours, during which I talked about everything we can imagine, know, and say about the body—in fact, "The Whole Body" was the title of my performance. I remember that many artists exhibited works that showed views of the body, but also their views of the body. La Rocca's multilayered object, made up of X-ray, plexiglass, and ink, contains so many biographical layers but also technical, historical, and medical aspects. Oncology and radiology are indeed deeply intertwined; many of the first radiologists at the end of the nineteenth century and the early twentieth century almost all died of cancer because of their exposure to radiation. Technology and safety precautions have now evolved, so we know more about how to prevent this type of exposure for radiologists and technicians, but it remains a very dangerous workplace. On the other hand, these technologies obviously help to save many lives. If you discover a tumor early enough, you can save a patient's life. Even today, the most efficient way to do so remains working with X-rays or advanced techniques of radiology like MRI or CT scans that help locate hidden tumors. So again, these images of medicine are very ambiguous, as they can save lives, but at the same time X-rays are carcinogenic and may have caused La Rocca's cancer. We can reasonably suspect that she was affected by radiology when working as a technician. The skull in her works also functions as a *vanitas*, a reminder of our mortality. In fact, this relates to the materiality of the work too, since we can observe a material decay in old X-rays. You can't find the plastic films that La Rocca used anymore. In the archives of the hospital where I work as a historian, tons and tons of this old material are now

3 The Museum of Veterinary Anatomy's (MAVet) *Sublime Anatomies* exhibition at the Palazzo delle Esposizioni, Rome (October 22, 2019–January 6, 2020), showcased the interplay between art and medicine through nineteenth-century ceroplastic models, highlighting the detailed anatomical study within a historical and contemporary dialogue.

disintegrating. In this way, the materiality of these images is very interesting because the material is disappearing on its own.
JILLIAN CROCHET The question of material dissolution, or dematerialization, is also intriguing because most of these image procedures are nowadays digitalized, which is not to say they are not material, but they have a different physical presence. I must get a lot of MRIs and the more you expose yourself, the more dangerous it is in potentially causing cancer. It can affect you, but you need it in order to be treated or to make sure that you do not die from some other reason.
A potentially dangerous diagnostic tool is an ambiguous and troubling thing. When I see an X-ray of my body, it looks very foreign—almost unnatural—it is a part of your body, but it is not recognizable. It skews your perception of self and identity. Thinking about the medical field where the patient is kind of objectified, this objectification steps further and further away from the self. You're a thing to be studied and experimented on. One doctor will only look at your arm, but the other doctor will only look at your brain, so I think maybe that separation of the whole—the self—is what's happening with the superimposition of the skull with the hand.
CHARLOTTE MATTER When considering the artistic interest in X-rays, it is indicative to note that these images were conceived and perceived in aesthetic terms from the outset.[4] The technique of X-ray images, which Wilhelm Röntgen purposefully did not patent, was almost immediately experimented with as an artistic medium. La Rocca's *Craniologie* must thus be considered in light of a larger history of the use of X-rays in art, which still needs to be written, with numerous artists having explored their materiality and meaning, both before La Rocca and after, including Meret Oppenheim (*X-Ray of My Skull*, 1964), Barbara Hammer (*Sanctus*, 1990), and Donald Rodney (*The House That Jack Built*, 1987; *Britannia Hospital*, 1988), who addressed questions of race, diaspora, vulnerability, and chronic illness, drawing from his own experience of sickle cell anemia (see Hutchinson 2018; Chambers 2003; Das 2019; Marano, Matter, and Valterio, 2024).

4 For an excellent study of the cultural history of X-rays and the impact of medical discourse and imaging technologies on twentieth-century architecture, see Colomina (2019).

3
Do Not / Fit into the Mold: The Politics of Care and the Subversion of Bodily Norms

LAURA VALTERIO Let us now discuss another material related to the world of medicine and art, namely plaster. Between 1950 and 1951, Mexican artist Frida Kahlo painted some orthopedic plaster corsets that she wore during an extended period of hospitalization. Kahlo's youth was marked by a traumatic accident that left her with a broken spine, pelvis and foot injuries, and later affected her mobility and reproductive life. Throughout her life, she relied on corsets of various shapes and materials to support her body, some of which are now on display in the Museo Frida Kahlo in Mexico City. Interestingly, Kahlo staged the working of the plaster corsets in a series of photographs that show her lying on a hospital bed while painting the surface with the aid of a mirror, as she could not directly see the traces of the brush. FIG. 6

These images challenge the association between the horizontal body and unproductivity, reframing painting from a predominantly visual art to a form of movement, just as the artist's body was in a state of immobility. One of the corsets bears the image of an unborn child at its center underneath a red hammer and sickle, the symbol of the Communist Party, of which Kahlo was a member. The painted corset stands out as a critical stance on the artist's lived experience of hospitalization and disability, addressing her dependence on medical care. The image of the unborn child is derived from an anatomy book (Kraus 2010, 57). After experiencing her first miscarriage, it seems that Kahlo was not allowed to see the fetus she had lost, so she apparently began to dive into anatomical treatises to gain the knowledge that she had been denied (Ankori 2005, 34). By painting the anatomical image of an unborn child on the corset, she reminds us of the deep gap that exists between anatomical representations and the lived body, which encompasses pain, emotions, and the richness of experience. Of course, there is also a gendered dimension to the corset. After its introduction in the early modern period (cf. Leoty 1983), this item served both orthopedic and aesthetic purposes, but it soon became a staple element of women's fashion (see McFadden 2024). It flattened the bust and accentuated the breasts and hips, sculpting the classic hourglass figure that dictated standards of feminine beauty and sexualized the female body as a reproductive body (Bordo 1993, 162). Corsets restricted physical mobility and helped confining female bodies to traditional gender roles. In a sense they immobilized women socially, evolving into a symbol of patriarchal oppression (Bordo 1993, 181). The materiality of Kahlo's corset is also interesting because plaster was used for centuries by sculptors to replicate classical statues, helping to spread Western ideals of physical beauty and health around the world. As a cheaper alternative to precious white marble, it facilitated the dissemination of an aesthetic associated with whiteness, perpetuating constructions of race, hygiene, and physical perfection. The depiction of the red hammer and sickle expresses Kahlo's belief in the power of political principles to liberate bodies from pain and suffering. This was a core idea for the artist, who also depicted herself in a painting titled *Marxism Will Give Health to the Sick* (1954), where she wears a leather corset and holds the red book of the *Communist Manifesto* in her hand. She has let go of her mobility aids and is held only by the two colossal hands of Marxism, while Karl Marx's robust hand strangles the US capitalist eagle. FIG. 7 Through this detail, Kahlo aligns herself with the anti-imperialist position of Mexican nationalism, rejecting a colonial dependence on a North America perceived as technologically and medically superior. By painting the red hammer and sickle on her corset, the artist presents us with a utopian vision of a politics that heals bodies and cares for them, inviting us to reflect on the intersections of medical and political support. FIG. 8

JILLIAN CROCHET Marxism is an interesting lens to think through the value of the disabled body in capitalism.
The collapse of the healthcare industry today in the US is a terrible predicament that is partly related to Covid-19 and mostly due to capitalism. Over one million[5] people have died from the virus in the US since the beginning of the pandemic.

5 According to a study published in *Nature*, approximately one million people died from the virus in the US between February 2020 and May 2022 (Silva, Goosby, and Reid 2023).

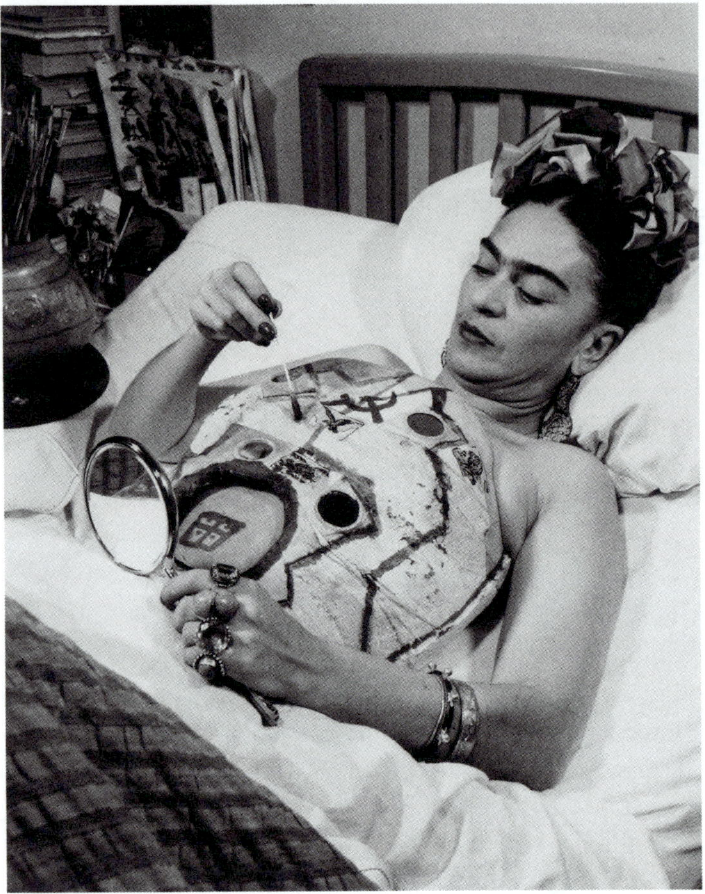

FIG. 6

FIG. 7

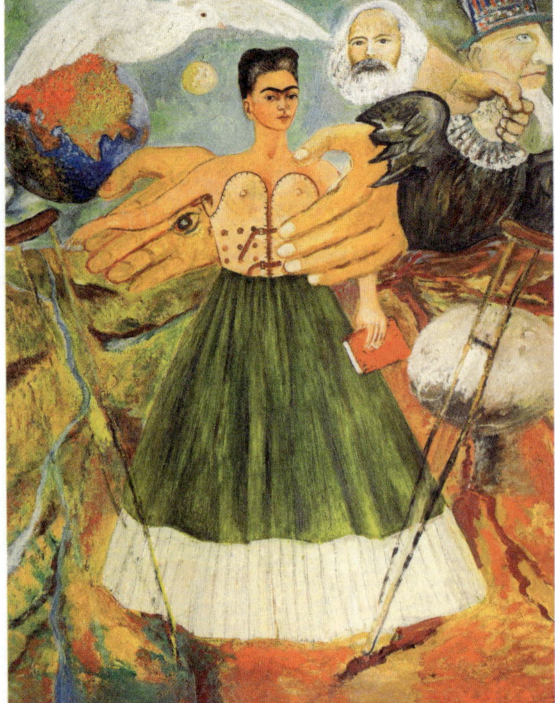

FIG. 6 Juan Guzmán, *Frida Kahlo in Hospital Painting Cast*, 1950s, gelatin silver print, 23.5 × 18.4 cm, Copyright Phillips Auctioneers LLC

FIG. 7 Frida Kahlo, *Marxism Will Give Health to the Sick* (original title: *Peace on Earth So That Marxist Science May Save the Sick and Those Oppressed by Criminal Yankee Capitalism*), 1954, oil on Masonite, 60 × 76 cm, Mexico City, Museo Frida Kahlo

The practice of wearing masks has been abandoned at the expense of disabled people, vulnerable people, and the elderly. Reflecting on Marxism, I am thinking about the value of taking care of each other and the community—or a kind of collective equalization in the most idealistic sense of communism. Returning to the corset painted on by Kahlo, I am struck by how it must have been quite disorienting to be immobilized and painting with a mirror. In a way, this separates you from your body but also reflects it back to yourself, in a cycle or act of connection.

LAURA VALTERIO The corset is a medical device that Kahlo would wear as a personal item, but it is now exhibited in museum spaces. Though it may not have been initially conceived as a work of art, it is certainly treated as such now. Given the relevance of display practices in the history of medicine, how can we think the status of artifacts that straddle the realms of art and medicine? And what are the ethical issues at stake in displaying artifacts that bear witness to personal, lived experiences of illness and hospitalization as art in a public context?

VINCENT BARRAS When a medical object has been used, it is either discarded or becomes a cultural object that is given a lot of respect. At the Institut des humanités en médecine (Institute for Medical Humanities) in Lausanne, where we collect such items, as well as in other similar institutions, it is impossible to touch any object without gloves. Each of them is handled with the utmost care, as if it were an original and unique artwork. This is because these items, which used to be plentifully around some decades ago, have all been thrown away and only a few remain today. Through their preservation, their status changes; they become a cultural item, gaining high value. I find it quite amusing how the status of certain objects can change so drastically over time. My other reaction to Kahlo's work with plaster, in relation to Laura's comment on the use of plaster in art, is that the material dimension of plaster is also very present in medicine, since it is still used today—although it is increasingly being replaced by other plastic materials like resin. The corset painted by Kahlo is made from plaster, but such devices could also be made with iron and very hard materials. Importantly, these devices are supposed to correct the body, so the idea of body normativity is also very present in these kinds of objects. They become a way to observe how much a society does or does not accept nonnormative bodies. When you have a body that does not adhere to the norm, you are expected to conform with the majority, literally to "fit into the mold" (in French we say *entrer dans le moule*). The question of what is considered a "normal" body, how your body fits into what kind of standards, and when you are outside of such norms, is very political. When I see this kind of plaster corset, I thus immediately perceive the political dimension of the body.

LAURA VALTERIO This is an important aspect that reminds us that hospitals are also spaces in which bodies are formed. It has been suggested that the image of the unborn child on the corset may be a reference not only to Kahlo's complex reproductive life but also to her own body. After her accident, she was apparently immobilized in a hospital for nine months, during which the corset was intended to shape her body as a sort of maternal uterus (Burrus 2005, 201). When used in art for reproductive purposes, the mold is also technically referred to by the term of Latin origin *matrix*, which means both "mother" and "womb." The hollow form of the plaster corset is an indexical negative trace of the absent body and could be used to recast its form many times. The notion of normativity addressed by Vincent also informs the multiplication of certain body images and types. But Kahlo's corset seems to explore this reproductivity through its negation, because the form of the body was not meant to be replicated, but to stand in as its uniqueness. And I think that the image of the unborn child connects this dimension to her personal reproductive experience.

JILLIAN CROCHET Talking about the normative and nonnormative body, in disability justice we are trying to politically reframe disability against its misconception as something abnormal: disability is "normal," because each body is different. The way that people view disability as a problem that needs to be solved, or the idea that a body needs to fit into a

FIG. 8 Frida Kahlo, plaster corset with fetus, hammer, and sickle, ca. 1950–1951. Mexico City, Collection Javier Lumbreras. Courtesy of Artemundi Global Fund

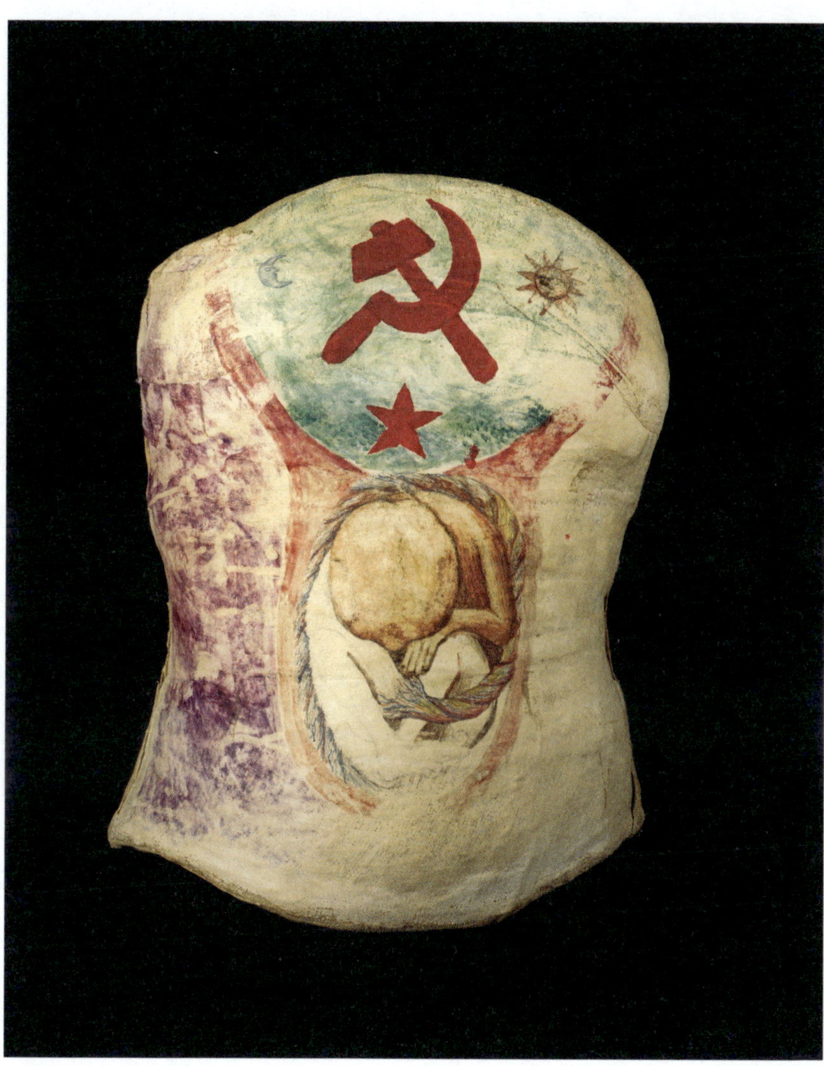

FIG. 8

FIG. 9 Lorenza Böttner, *Untitled*, 1993, markers on a sanitary napkin. Private collection. Exhibition view *Lorenza Böttner: Requiem for the Norm*, April 15–August 14, 2022, Leslie-Lohman Museum of Art, New York. Photo: Virginia Marano

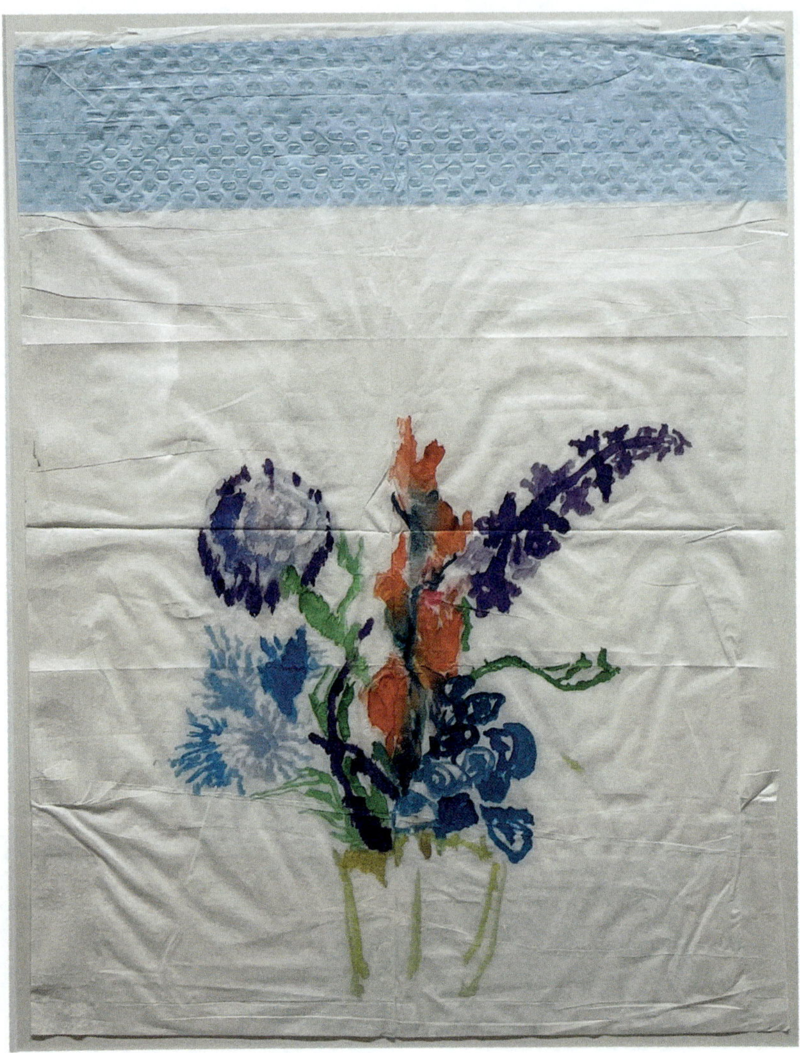

FIG. 9

standardized, idealized mold, is not helpful. We need to broaden our perspective to accept that all bodies simply exist—there are no "good" or "bad" bodies. This shift in thinking acknowledges the natural diversity among us.

4
Precarious Lines: Images of Death and Decay and Sensory Perception

VIRGINIA MARANO Taking this idea further, let us consider another example of the use of medical materials in art with a work by Lorenza Böttner (see Preciado 2023). Born in Punta Arenas, Chile, Böttner lost both arms in an accident at the age of eight. She and her mother relocated to Germany for treatment, where she was placed in various rehabilitation centers alongside the so-called thalidomide children, and where she rejected prosthetics and eventually abandoned "disability education" to dedicate her time to painting and performance. In 1978, she was accepted into the Kunsthochschule Kassel (School of Art and Design Kassel). There, exposed to dance, performance, and conceptual art, she began a multidisciplinary practice focused on the experimental construction of self. Her primary media were performance as well as drawing and painting, which she realized using her mouth and feet. She graduated in 1984 with a thesis titled *Behindert?* (Disabled?). In it, she investigated the notion of disability and examined the lineage of mouth-and-foot painters, exploring diverse methodologies of creating art and reflecting on her own embodied experience. This defies established narratives of art history as a history of the use of hands, while concurrently redefining visual codes that constitute a body as human. Böttner's work articulates a critique of the construction of disability and the concomitant processes of de-sexualization, internment, and invisibilization to which transgender and functionally diverse bodies have been historically subjected. As the artist approached an untimely death in 1994 due to AIDS-related complications, she drew a bouquet of colorful flowers on a medical napkin, most likely using her mouth. FIG. 9

The napkin is made of white plastic with a broad blue strip at the top. Its surface is textured, adding depth to the simple depiction of the bouquet—orange leaves, purple ferns, blue starburst petals, a purple dandelion, green foliage, and stems in shades of yellow-green. Drawn with felt-tip markers, the colors bleed into the napkin's fabric. The juxtaposition of the flowers, symbolizing life and its fleeting nature, with the backdrop of a sanitary pad—a medium rarely seen in art—offers a thought-provoking dimension to her exploration of identity and the body's materiality.

VINCENT BARRAS I was immediately struck by the material and its interplay with the drawing. It is an image of flowers, which is a common motif in art. Then again, the material clearly suggests the materiality of the hospital or medical world—the world of illness, health, and recovery. The interplay between these two worlds is very striking for me. The blue strip is also reminiscent of the surgical mask we wore during the pandemic. Everybody had to enter into direct contact with this unfamiliar materiality, putting it onto their nose and mouth, in close contact to the skin. The materiality of the mask is something many people are uncomfortable with, because it reminds them of something artificial—with its plastic material and synthetic, blue color. Böttner's work is really interesting in juxtaposing this artificiality with a representation of flowers, which connote the idea of nature.

JILLIAN CROCHET The materiality is quite noisy—not in the sense of its making sound but from my experience of these pads. Then there are these flowers and the idea of what is natural and unnatural. Plastic, at this point, may as well be considered natural. At the same time, the flowers are also a reminder of mortality, given their seasonal life cycles. It's interesting what you brought up, Vincent, because when people see any kind of medical equipment, or a disabled person in a wheelchair, or something that reminds them of their own mortality, they are often uncomfortable with that. So people avoid the "other"—disabled people, especially visually disabled people—because their presence reminds them of the precarity of their own life, of death, of illness and all these inevitable things that our society is trying to avoid.

CHARLOTTE MATTER I love how you described this work in auditory terms, Jillian. I have another immediate sensory response to it, which concerns the olfactory dimension. On the one hand, this napkin would typically be used to absorb bodily fluids, such as blood, urine, and feces, so it would potentially involve a vast array of odors, some of them conventionally connoted as unpleasant. Then again, the flowers drawn onto the napkin codify smells that are typically perceived as pleasant and commercialized as such by the perfume and cleaning industry. This brings us back to notions of cleanliness and dirt, and all related value judgments. Böttner's work thus creates an interesting tension by evoking supposedly contrasting odors, calling into question normative conceptions thereof. Which smells do we find pleasant, and why? Of course, this has to do with personal memories and experiences, but also with social conventions. Precisely because the napkin relates to care, it further recalls intimate and embodied relations to smell. This work also reminds me of two recent works. One is Jesse Darling's *Untitled (Still Life)* (2018–ongoing), which consists of fresh flower bouquets enclosed in vitrines that gradually decay over the course of an exhibition and address the labor of care. FIG. 10 I recently saw this work at the Migros Museum für Gegenwartskunst in Zurich, but even before, whenever I would only see pictures of it, the rotting flowers provoked in me this visceral, olfactory response just by way of an image. The other work I'm reminded of is *Support System (for Tina, Park, and Bob)* (2016) by Carolyn Lazard. For this durational performance, visitors brought a bouquet of flowers as an entrance fee and in return spent half an hour with the artist, so the work consisted of shared time, but also of a kind of evolving sculptural work with bouquets being added. FIG. 11 Flowers are a recurring motif in art, as Vincent previously observed, but they also relate to the medical world, because they are such a common presence in hospitals in this very conventionalized way of showing your care and support to someone.

VINCENT BARRAS . . . and this causes many problems in hospitals since everybody brings flowers when visiting a patient, but the first thing that a nurse will do is store them away in a safe environment because they may carry microbes. This is quite contradictory because in many hospitals you will also find a florist; it's a whole business and very much related to healthcare institutions. In terms of all the senses that you mentioned, Charlotte, a hospital really is a microcosm of the whole world. Smells, colors, and touch are exacerbated but at the same time also annihilated. If you go to a hospital and listen, for instance, you can experience it as a huge factory of sounds of every kind, machines, people, bodies, interactions, words. It's a very active sound machine. Then you have the odors: flowers, but also urine, feces, sweat, and products of chemistry—all of which smells very strong. This sensory world, however, is in constant tension with the scope of medicine, which tries to avoid anything that smells because it could mean that it carries microbes from the outside world and may thus be dangerous. This work really plays with the tension between these two worlds.

JILLIAN CROCHET This tension between sensory overload and the attempt to nullify and/or sanitize in seeking to preserve life really is a chaotic microcosm of our efforts, and inevitable failure, to escape disability and death—a natural fate. Even though I reject a purely medicalized understanding of disability, I still engage with the medical-industrial complex to try and heal what I can and stave off further deterioration of my body and muscles. It's hard to live in the reality of cognitive dissonance wherein multiple opposing realities are true, but it's something disability cannot escape. It is often ignored or denied, such as the mass denial of the deadly effects of Covid-19. In some ways it would be much simpler for us all to just wear masks, so we could protect each other, everyone, but people don't want to face what reminds them of their proximity to death and disability. Therefore, many disabled people have to risk their lives to exist within society. Böttner's work reminds me of this complicated coexistence in which disabled

FIG. 10 Jesse Darling, *Untitled (Still Life)*, 2018–ongoing, flowers, vases, water, vitrines. Exhibition view *Interdependencies: Perspectives on Care and Resilience*, 2023–2024, Migros Museum für Gegenwartskunst, Zurich. Photo: Stefan Altenburger Photography, Zurich. Courtesy of Jesse Darling and Arcadia Missa, London
FIG. 11 Carolyn Lazard, *Support System (for Park, Tina, and Bob)*, 2016, 24 gifted bouquets, documentation of performance and collectively produced sculpture, dimensions variable. Courtesy of Carolyn Lazard

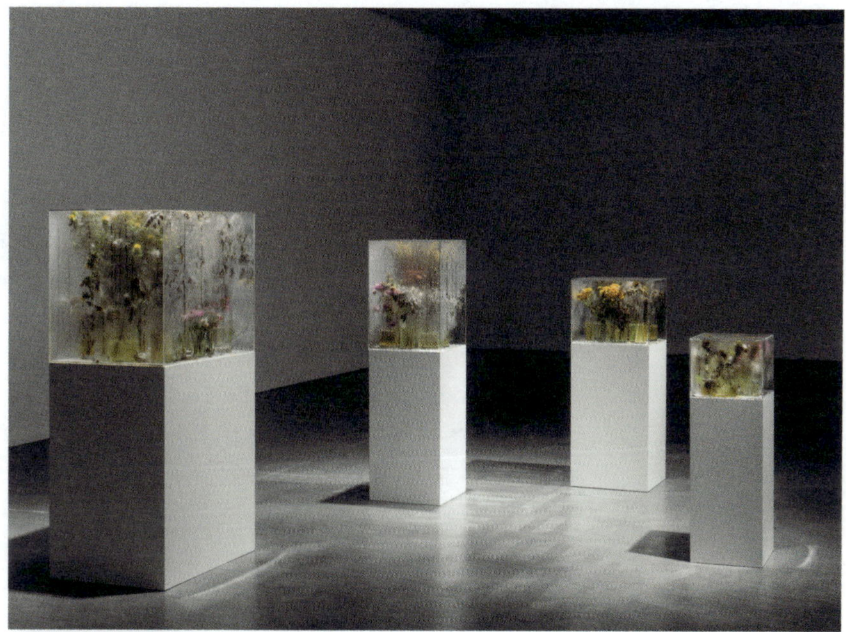

FIG. 10

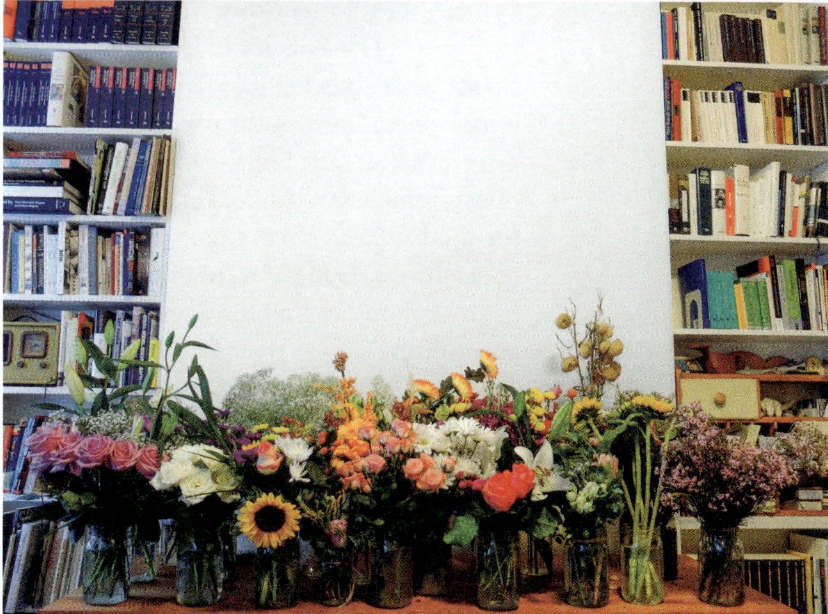

FIG. 11

bodies have to exist, wearing masks to be out in the world and experience pleasure in community, or to do necessary things like grocery shopping. I also love the dark humor Darling and Lazard are pointing to in these rituals in hospitals and funerals, often used in futile attempts to cover up the "gross" smell of death, or to "beautify" the "ugly." People often say things like "I brought some beautiful flowers to 'liven up' the place," but those flowers will imminently die, and are actually apt metaphors for the cycle of life.

LAURA VALTERIO Another interesting aspect in Böttner's work regards the artist's bodily posture, since this napkin was likely painted with the mouth, in close proximity with the material. This idea brings us back to the notion of encountering the artistic material differently, though from the perspective of the artist. Like in La Rocca's and Kahlo's case, Böttner's artistic manipulation of a medical device is a way of asserting ownership and personalizing a standardized tool, by imbuing it with the traces of lived experience. And as Jillian was previously saying about flowers as an image of precarity, if we think about the traditional role of flowers in the pictorial genre of the still life—which, in Spanish, is called *naturaleza muerta*—this motif speaks again to the idea of how closely intertwined the realms of art and medicine are. In this sense, I find your observation about La Rocca's radiographs and the notion of the *vanitas* really striking, Vincent.

5
Repurposing Medical Materials in Art: The Politics of Discard and Revaluation

CHARLOTTE MATTER To conclude, I want to return to our initial questioning of the use, reuse, and "misuse" of medical materials in art, and relate it to the matter of value. The notion of use, which Sara Ahmed explores so eloquently in her *What's the Use? On the Uses of Use* (2019), is intricately tied to value conceptions. And value, in turn, has a fraught relation to the history of bodies that have been considered as useful or not, and accordingly exploited and/or marginalized. There's a troubling relation between the use and value of the materials we have been looking at, and the question of how certain bodies—sick and disabled bodies, but also more generally nonnormative bodies—are valued. On the other hand, these works also open up the possibility to reconsider conceptions of use and value through strategies of reuse and "misuse." Picking up on what Virginia was previously alluding to, when she observed that a sanitary napkin is an unusual artistic medium, I was thinking about how this relates to what you, Laura and Vincent, mentioned while discussing Kahlo's work and how plaster is an affordable material. Underlying these observations is the fact that we are dealing with materials that have a lot of use value but little exchange value, to use Marxian terms. The question then becomes: How can we think about value and class relations in terms of materials from the realm of medicine as they become appropriated in art? Donald Rodney (1988, 33) for instance was using X-rays as an artistic medium not only because they held specific meaning to him as a chronically ill artist, but also because they were affordable and easily accessible. He used to buy them in bulk, for one British pound per kilogram. As we are looking at these different works, we might consider material hierarchies, both in terms of art-historical conventions, but also in relation to the previously addressed hierarchies of certain bodies and notions of health. So how can we make sense of the use and value of these materials?

VINCENT BARRAS I think that's really the throughline of all these works. The value of materials can also be very political and crude because medicine is very expensive. Even the smallest item, like the napkin, can be very expensive when used in the medical world, because the production process has to be strictly controlled and there are huge businesses surrounding all these materials. So when I see this humble napkin, or when I think about how an artist would buy kilos of X-rays because they were cheap, I think about how for each medical material, there are different registers of value. For instance, the "cheap" masks many of us used during the pandemic actually represent a billion-dollar industry, with some countries having the resources to produce them and others not, so some will have to buy them and some will profit from them. For each material used in these works of art, there is a whole economy of production behind.

LAURA VALTERIO Then again, the value of these works of art seems to derive less from the materials themselves and more from the way in which they are used. Even if certain materials stand for a big industry, once they are used for medical purposes, they seem to be somewhat devalued, and eventually they are discarded. Yet, in the case of the artworks we have discussed, the same medical materials are reinvested with significance through an artistic intervention which gives them new meaning. Another throughline in these works is therefore the potential of reusing and revaluing as a political act.

JILLIAN CROCHET Yes, definitely, insisting that these materials that make life possible and our disabled bodies are valuable, and reclaiming them is a political act. As it pertains to value, the disabled body is often not valued or seen as important and worthy of safety—as if it were discardable. On the other hand, the medical industry makes billions of dollars to avoid death and disability. The disabled body is both devalued in a certain sense, but also very expensive and profitable, used to turn a huge profit, with extreme price gauging by insurance companies and medical equipment companies. Our bodies and these works are beautiful—valuable—because they are fragile, complicated, and layered.

VIRGINIA MARANO Through the artistic transformation of medical objects and spaces into art interventions, we observe a shift both in their aesthetics and function. In this conversation, we considered the works of Ketty La Rocca, Frida Kahlo, and Lorenza Böttner, along with those of Jillian Crochet. These different practices defy normative categorizations, embodying a radical form of artistic expression that transcends traditional boundaries. They bring to the forefront intersectional perspectives on the topic, discussing the role of gender, disability, and class. Such dialogues between art and medicine, as we have explored here, open a space for critical engagement with medicalization practices from the point of view of different methodologies and highlight the essential role of creative practices in questioning and expanding our understanding of the material world. They call for a broader, more inclusive approach to the ways in which objects, bodies, and spaces are perceived and interacted with. Through this lens, the intersection of art and medicine becomes a vital space for reimagining and enriching the concepts of object, function, and norm, emphasizing the critical need to defy a system that aims to categorize human experience into normative experiences of health and illness, ability and disability.

A

Ahmed, Sara (2019) *What's the Use? On the Uses of Use*. Durham, NC: Duke University Press.

Ankori, Gannit (2005) "Frida Kahlo: The Fabric of Her Art." In *Frida Kahlo*, edited by Emma Dexter and Tanya Barson. Exhibition catalogue, Tate Modern, London, June 9–October 9. London: Westerham Press Limited.

B

Bordo, Susan (1993) *Unbearable Weight: Feminism, Western Culture, and the Body*. Berkeley: University of California Press.

Burrus, Christine (2005) "The Life of Frida Kahlo." In *Frida Kahlo*, edited by Emma Dexter and Tanya Barson. Exhibition catalogue, Tate Modern, London, June 9–October 9. London: Westerham Press Limited.

C

Chambers, Eddie (2003) "The Art of Donald Rodney." In *Donald Rodney: Doublethink*, edited by Richard Hylton. London: Autograph.

Colomina, Beatriz (2019) *X-Ray Architecture*. Zurich: Lars Müller Publishers.

Crochet, Jillian, Carmen Papalia, Whitney Mashburn, and Georgina Kleege (2022) "Handle with Care: Art and Touch." Conversation on Zoom, organized by the Contemporary Jewish Museum, San Francisco, December 15. https://www.thecjm.org/learn_resources/889 (Accessed: March 10, 2024).

D

Das, Jareh (2019) "Illness as Metaphor: Donald Rodney's X-Ray Photographs." *Nka: Journal of Contemporary African Art*, no. 45 (November).

Derrida, Jacques (1981) "Plato's Pharmacy." In *Dissemination*, edited by Barbara Johnson, 61–171. Chicago: University of Chicago Press.

H

Hutchinson, Ishion (2018) "In the Archive: Donald Rodney's 'Splash Crowns.'" *Tate Papers*, no. 43. https://www.tate.org.uk/tate-etc/issue-43-summer-2018/archive-donald-rodney-sketchbooks-splash-crowns-ishion-hutchinson (Accessed: March 14, 2024).

K

Kraus, Arnoldo (2010) "Frida Kahlo: das Leben, ein Schmerz." In *Frida Kahlo Retrospektive*. Exhibition catalogue, Martin-Gropius-Bau, April 30–August 9. Munich: Prestel.

L

La Rocca, Ketty (1974) "You, You." In *Il corpo come linguaggio: La "Body-art" e storie simili*, edited by Lea Vergine, bilingual text. Milan: Giampaolo Prearo Editore.

Leoty, Ernest (1893) *Le Corset à travers les Âges*. Paris: Paul Ollendorff.

Liboiron, Max (2021) *Pollution Is Colonialism*. Durham, NC: Duke University Press.

M

Marano, Virginia, Charlotte Matter, and Laura Valterio (2024) "Bodily Matter and Complex Embodiment in the Art of Donald Rodney." *RACAR: Revue d'art canadienne / Canadian Art Review*, special issue "Cripping Visual Cultures," no. 2 (Fall).

McFadden, Elizabeth (2024) "Revealing the Iron Corset." Wellcome Collection. See at: https://wellcomecollection.org/articles/X8eq-xIAACUAjiaN (Accessed: March 13, 2024).

O

Ofrias, Lindsay (2017) "Invisible Harms, Invisible Profits: A Theory of the Incentive to Contaminate." *Culture, Theory and Critique* 58, no. 4: 435–56.

P

Preciado, Paul B., ed. (2023) *Lorenza Böttner: Requiem for the Norm*. Leipzig: Spector Books.

R

Rodney, Donald (1988) *Sketchbook No. 14*. Page 33. Tate Archive, London.

S

Silva, S., E. Goosby, E. and M. J. A. Reid (2023) "Assessing the Impact of One Million COVID-19 Deaths in America: Economic and Life Expectancy Losses." *Scientific Reports* 13, 3065.

T

Taylor, Sunaura (2017) *Beasts of Burden: Animal and Disability Liberation*. New York: The New Press.

Building Blocks of the Spectrum

Jacob van der Beugel and Lara Keuck

This chapter takes the shape of a dialogue between the artist Jacob van der Beugel (JVDB) and the historian and philosopher of medicine Lara Keuck (LK). They discuss how JVDB's artworks engage with medical knowledge about health and disease and can be put in conversation with critical reflections about the conditions and assumptions of biomedicine. The point of departure of their conversation is JVDB's mural *Matter in Grey* (2018), which reflects contemporary research into the gradual course of Alzheimer's disease from protein aggregation to death. This work is used to explore the ways in which we can question the aesthetic and epistemological appeal of the continuum and gradualist approaches to health and disease: Why is a spectrum so convincing? When do aesthetic metaphors break down? How can their making and disruption highlight inadequacies and disconnects between realities and aspirations? And what are the similarities and differences in the epistemic situations of scientists, humanities scholars, and artists?

Accordingly, the contribution draws on two meanings of the term "converse": first, as the dialogue between the two authors, and second, as the transposition or shape-shifting of one form of reflecting knowledge into another, in this case between art and history and philosophy of medicine. The process of creating this edited conversation[1] shows not only similarities to academic practices of writing and revising, but also to JVDB's artistic practices of prototyping, mixing materials, creating agglomerated blocks of concrete with diverse insertions of other (recycled) materials, cutting, polishing, and arranging them as a mural.

The resulting text is thus structured in five sections that individually zoom in on particular aspects of building and

1 The text grew out of a recorded and transcribed conversation about JVDB's work *Matter in Grey* and its resonances with LK's work on gradualist approaches to disease generally, and specifically Alzheimer's. After presenting the project at the September 2023 authors' workshop in Berlin, the authors edited, cut, rearranged, and added text, structured it along the section headings, and included photographs of JVDB's works. This draft was presented at a second virtual authors' workshop. Following helpful comments, in particular by Gideon Manning, Alfred Freeborn, and Elizabeth Hughes, the authors included some excerpts of LK's work, expanded sections, and polished the draft. Footnotes were added but kept to a minimum; they are not intended to represent the academic state of research in history and philosophy of medicine or art history, but simply to provide references to work that is mentioned in the dialogue or to former work of LK and JVDB to which their statements implicitly refer.

inquiring into a spectrum: (1) imaginations of the gradual course from health to disease; (2) the artificiality of the spectrum; (3) backgrounding and foregrounding; (4) polishing the aesthetic, polishing the concrete; and (5) art as a mode of inquiry. When looked at as a whole, the sections—and the open questions—create room for thought about the possibilities, conditions, and limitations of depicting health and disease along a spectrum.

1 Imaginations of the Gradual Course from Health to Disease

LK Your work *Matter in Grey* FIG. 1 reflects the gradual change in appearance of the brains of people with progressive Alzheimer's disease. Can you say a bit more about the context of the work, and why you came up with this piece of art?

JvdB I was tasked to create a piece for the Cambridge Chemistry of Health Department, which specifically researches neurodegenerative diseases. I spoke to one of the lead researchers, Prof. Michele Vendruscolo. We discussed many facets of his work over the ensuing weeks so I could get a broader insight into the purpose of the building and the department's general ethos. And he explained to me that there's a common public misperception that Alzheimer's is regarded as a form of aging; that they go hand in hand. Obviously, it's slightly more complicated because they are interrelated. But he wanted to disentangle this notion of Alzheimer's so that the public perceive it as a disease that needs to be tackled in certain ways.[2] My strategy was to split the ambitions of the institute into four rows of concrete slides of a spectrum or a continuum. The top row as natural aging, if there is such a thing. And then the second row as a progression of Alzheimer's disease. Then the third row is a progression or a spectrum of treated Alzheimer's. Finally, the fourth one is a spectrum of prevented Alzheimer's, which is ultimately the main ideological task of the institute.

So, I prized apart the institute in four rows, really. Now whether that is a realistic way of picking apart an institute,

2 See, for instance, these works from Vendruscolo's lab: Freer et al. (2016) and Rosie Freer et al. (2019). See also: http://www.vendruscolo.ch.cam.ac.uk/research.html (Accessed: May 6, 2024).

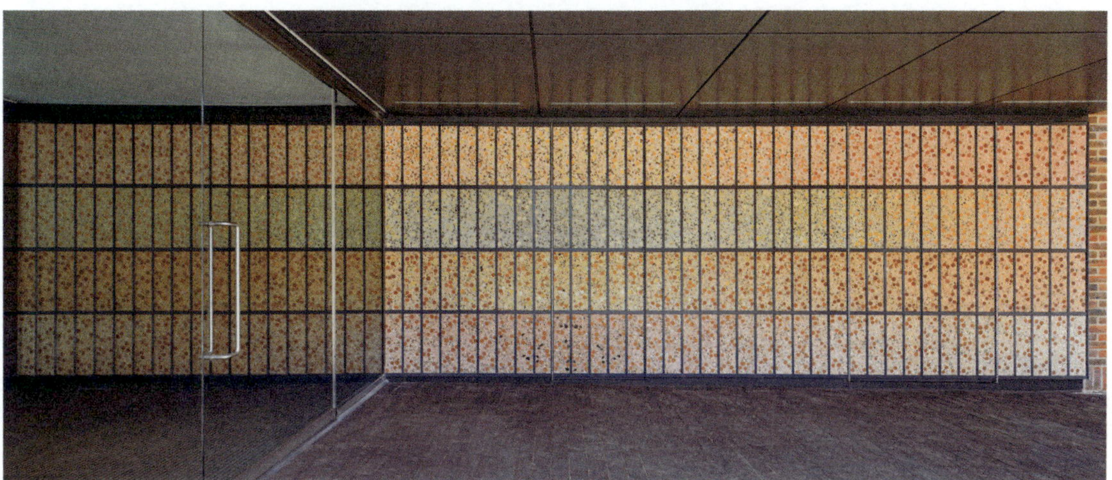

FIG. 1

FIG. 1 Jacob van der Beugel, *Matter in Grey*, 2018, self-healing concrete, ceramics, and mixed recycled aggregates, 10 × 2.5 m. Chemistry of Health Department, Cambridge University, UK. Photo: Paul Riddle

I don't know. It's quite a nice narrative to highlight what happens within the actual building to a broader audience. Looking back at this approach, it feels problematic. But interesting to do nonetheless.

LK What do you think of now as problematic?

JvdB I think the more I learn about anything, the more I realize that you can't really deconstruct it in that way, in a convincing, ideological way. However, actually pulling it apart serves a purpose for treating a disease or making the task of treating and research more manageable. Maybe for that reason it was a good way of dealing with the art commission. But I'm not sure how I would go about doing it now, to be honest. Maybe the naivety was good.

LK Well, the interesting thing about art is that, even if it's a commissioned piece of art, you can always read different things into it, right? The description that you're giving now is that the piece of art does not depict the natural reality of what Alzheimer's disease is, what aging is, what prevention, and what treatment means. Saying that it represents the ideology that drives the research at this institute is giving a different kind of perspective. I don't mean that cynically. I just think that it is important to reflect on the ways in which the conditions and limitations of biomedical research methods shape our knowledge about disease. It is important to make visible that scientific knowledge is conditional and mediated. In this respect, you could say that you have been taking the presentations of the theory of disease by these researchers quite literally, and worked with their metaphors and translated them into working materials for your work of art.

I am stressing that this is not cynical, because I am convinced that this reflective mode is an important epistemic practice and in fact not unknown to medical researchers themselves. To give an example from my historical research: the neuropathologist Alois Alzheimer, after whom Alzheimer's disease was later named, taught his students in the early 1900s that "many examinations have dealt with determining in what fashion and direction the single [staining and fixation] solutions impact the tissue. But pathological anatomy cannot wait until this difficult question is solved. In the meantime, it has to deal with pictures of equivalence, that is to say, it has to compare the pathological tissue with normal tissue that have both been subject to the same chemicals in the same way" (Alzheimer n.d., 1; trans. Keuck 2017, 26). That notion of pictures of equivalence really struck me. It did so not only because of its epistemological underpinnings for understanding the anatomy of mental disorders but also because it shows how much the establishment of the "normal" and the "pathological" was a materially guided, practical issue.

In your work, the relationship between the appeal of metaphors and the practical issues surrounding materiality seems to play an important role. Can you tell me more about your choice to work with concrete blocks?

JvdB Materiality is central to all the projects that I do. My overarching belief is to use materials we are intuitively familiar with, clay and concrete for example, so that complex scientific advances can be anchored physically. Perversely, the more durable the material, the better the anchoring, as Daniel Miller (2005) has observed.

I had completed an epidemiological art commission that looked into blood cancers. In it I had used concrete and the metaphor of concrete cancer, which is when concrete degrades due to water ingress, rust, and structural failure, etc., as a way of depicting blood cancers and people's pathways. It dawned on me that concrete is formed from aggregates: all sorts of different stones, sands, and cements ranging in grading and scale, so that the interlocking matrix acts as a human-engineered glued stone. When I had discussions with Vendruscolo, he talked about misfolding proteins and the aggregation of these misfolding proteins as being central to the progression of Alzheimer's. These discussions about aggregating proteins triggered an idea that centered on building a language around aggregates and using the aggregates in different ways to intimate progression and decline. So that was the starting point for the commission. It then fell to me to work out a visually coherent way of

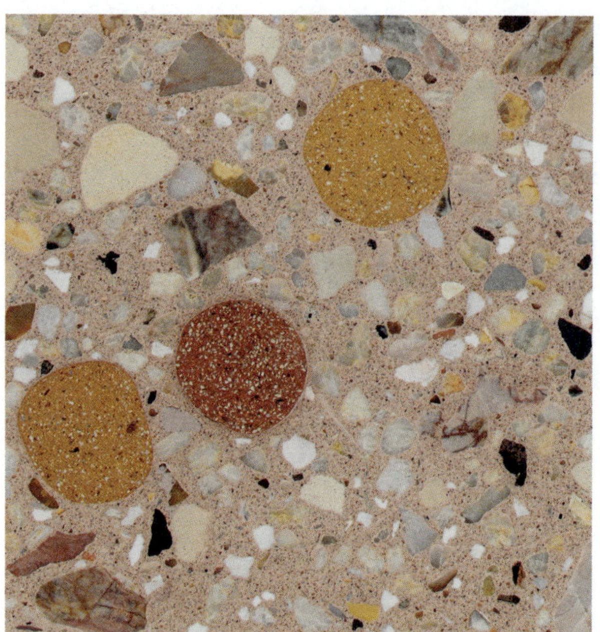

FIG. 2

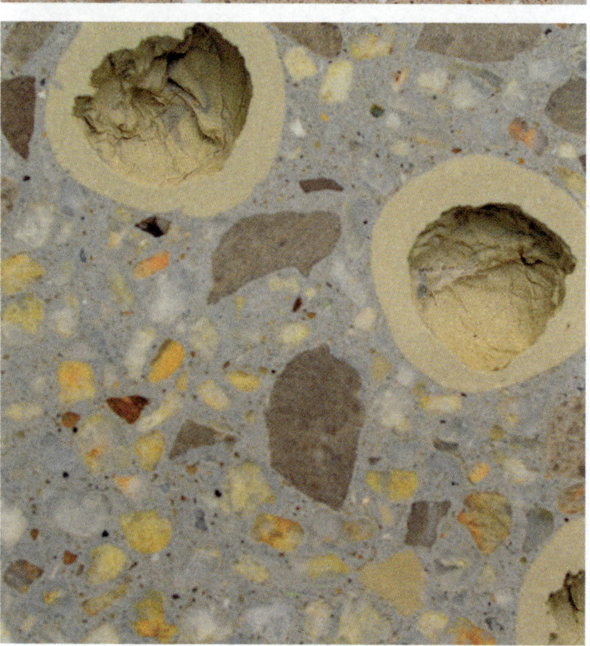

FIG. 3

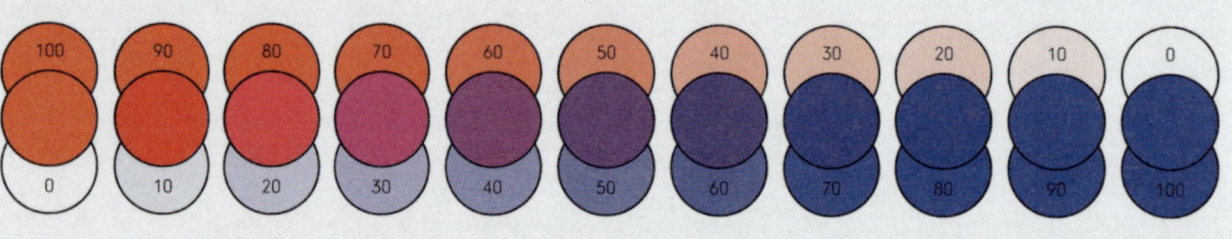

FIG. 4

FIG. 2 *Matter in Grey* panel detail from the middle of the natural aging spectrum. Photo: Jacob van der Beugel

FIG. 3 *Matter in Grey* panel detail from the end of the untreated Alzheimer's spectrum. Photo: Jacob van der Beugel

FIG. 4 Eleven-step line blend with red and blue for ceramic glazes (Au 2015)

describing this decline as a continuum. One of the ways I did this was to start with a panel that represents a normal person's spectrum of health FIG. 2 that then starts to visually age, if there is such a thing as a standard model of aging or health decline.

I then created the end panel with holes, gray in hue, empty. FIG. 3 Then I mixed increments of the normal panel with the Alzheimer's panel in order to get different gradations to that point, very much like line blending in ceramic glaze practices. FIG. 4 It brings to mind the continuum fallacy or the Sorites paradox: When does one thing become the other? This was an aesthetically pleasing way of depicting a spectrum.

The gradation is one of color, aggregates, and then also other kinds of ceramics with holes in them that suggest a cellular decline. So you go from the fleshy pink color, which we usually associate with good health, to a gray endpoint, which has holes and is symbolic of decline. I used the same material spectrum for the Alzheimer's row, but with the starting point already slightly grayer, and then ended with more holes and a quicker deterioration of those ceramic cells or ceramic neurons. Then I applied the same logic to the treated spectrum and prevented spectrum. In the treated row there was an element of degradation, but that decline was much, much slower. I added self-healing concrete in the form of expanded clay particles that contain bacteria that precipitate calcite under the right conditions. As the condition becomes increasingly difficult to treat, the medication (the self-healing particles) starts to overwhelm the concrete matrix. FIG. 5 I find the use of self-healing concrete metaphorically intriguing. Part anthropomorphization, part physical process. This regenerative metaphor is akin to the elixir of life, the holy grail of medicine. Yet, in the context of this piece, it becomes another element that overwhelms.

In the prevented spectrum, I encased the cells of the neurons in a protective clay. FIG. 6 So each cell is surrounded by an impenetrable barrier, suggesting that it is protected from the consequences of aggregation.

3 For the argument that the initial classification of Alzheimer's disease was exploratory, see Keuck (2018).

The process for casting the panels also became symbolic. I poured the concrete, containing the correct proportions of aggregates, into a mold about 50 centimeters long and about 40 millimeters thick. Once it had cured, I sawed through the concrete along its thin side with an enormous stone saw. This was done in a stonemason's yard who cuts funereal tombstones—quite apt really. It's almost like an autopsy of the brain. You slice it open, and you have a doubling of very fragile panels.

LK Autopsy has played a vital role in diagnosing Alzheimer's disease. It really formed the diagnosis as an exploratory category.[3] It was the goal of Alois Alzheimer's research program to show that pathological anatomy could help to better the clinical diagnosis in psychiatry. Patients whose clinical diagnosis had proven difficult were tracked down, and after their deaths he had their brains sent to his laboratory to fix, slice, stain, and examine them under the microscope. He was convinced that the identification of characteristic alterations in their brains could indicate how clinical cases could be ordered into more fitting categories. Publications that would become known as first descriptions of Alzheimer's disease feature descriptions of clinical courses alongside descriptions or drawings of microscopic plaques and tangles in the deceased patients' brains. FIG. 8 Drawings that indeed show striking similarities to your made-up aggregates in the blocks of concrete.

You were saying the more you learn, the more critical you get. I would be interested in knowing more about how this learning process is tied to your own artistic work, to your practices of translating biomedical theories and metaphors into blocks of concrete. Would you say that you take scientific ideas and techniques literally, or how would you describe your own stance?

JvdB I usually recoil at the idea of thinking that I'm a kind of conduit for a researcher's perspective. Because ultimately that's not why I'm doing this. But for this commission . . . I think it's one of the few pieces—or the only piece—I've ever done where I didn't have my own ideological angle from the outset. Once I'd finished the piece, I didn't feel like I had added anything to

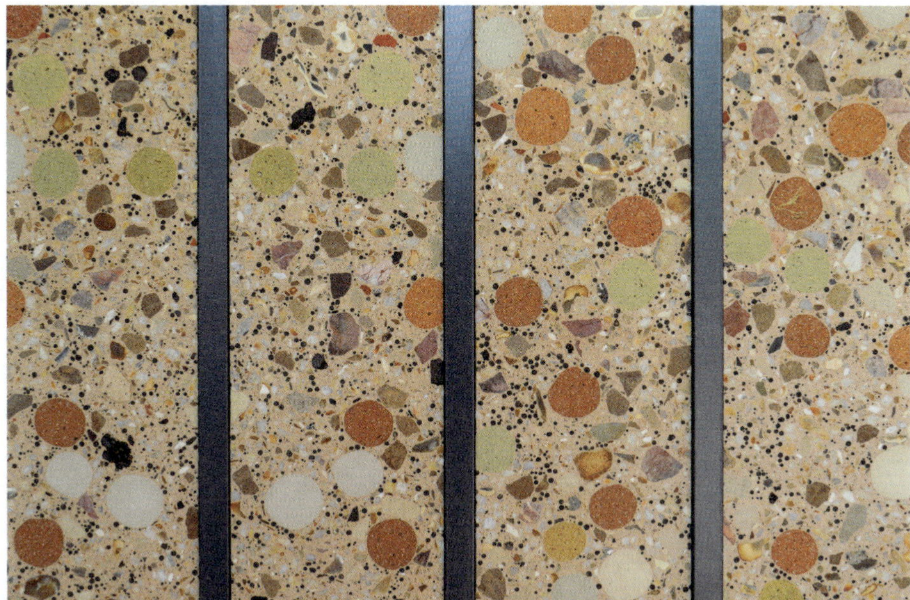

FIG. 5

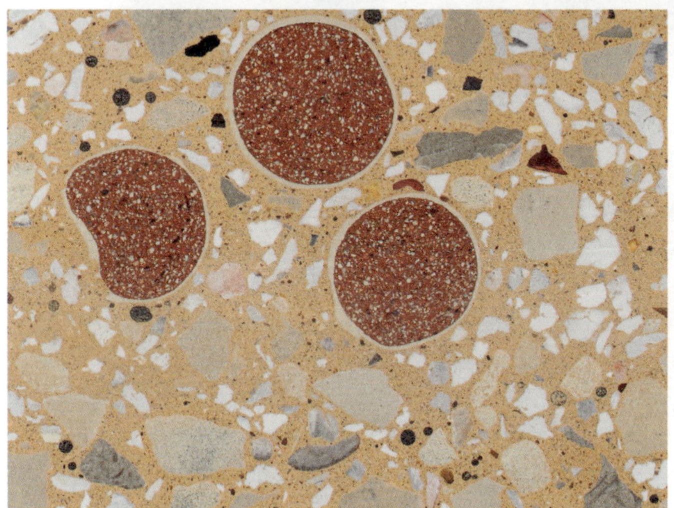

FIG. 6

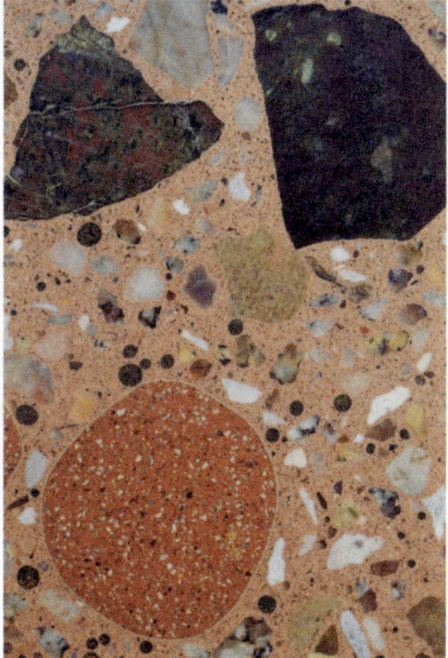

FIG. 7

FIG. 5 *Matter in Grey* treatment panel detail. The small black particles represent self-healing capsules. Photo: Jacob van der Beugel

FIG. 6 Detail of the first panel in the prevented spectrum of *Matter in Grey*. Photo: Jacob van der Beugel

FIG. 7 Detail of the last panel in the prevented spectrum of *Matter in Grey*. Photo: Jacob van der Beugel

FIG. 8 Hand-drawn microscopic image of a stained slice of the brain of a deceased patient who had suffered from severe symptoms of dementia. P indicates a plaque (Alzheimer 1911, table IV, fig. 1).

FIG. 8

the debate. And yet, it still endures as an artwork. By the end I thought, "Is Alzheimer's really preventable or just, at best, treatable as a chronic condition? Isn't prevention illusory?" However, in retrospect, I created the spectrum of prevention with cells that had these protective bands around it. Initially the bands are thick, robust, and impervious. Moving across the spectrum, the protection—or the encapsulations—become thinner until they're delicate to the point that they could break down entirely. This was a way of introducing the idea of entropy—things are always on a spectrum of decline. At the very last moment there is an introduction of an aggressive black aggregate of red serpentine stone (also highly symbolic) to suggest that there would always be something else—the specter of unintended consequences. FIG. 7 So maybe I do myself a disservice in saying there wasn't a conceptual slant from my perspective!

LK How did the researchers react to that?

JvdB Oh, I never told them. Artist's prerogative!

2
The Artificiality of the Spectrum

LK When describing how you crafted a spectrum, you mentioned the Sorites paradox, which is an ancient paradox about a heap of sand. The question of the paradox is: How many grains of sand can you take away before it is no longer a heap? One single grain of sand doesn't make a difference, but there are of course times when there is a heap of sand and times where there is not enough sand to form a heap.

In the original paradox, the grains of sand are seen as interchangeable. In contrast, you are working with quite heterogeneous materials and you show how complex your blocks of concrete can be. To my mind, this makes them much more akin to diseases that exhibit not only vagueness of degree (like in the Sorites paradox) but also combinatorial vagueness, meaning that it is unclear which features necessarily have to be assessed (in other words, questioning whether there is a clear universal meaning of a heap).[4] What did your material choices

4 On the application of theories of vagueness to gradualist approaches to health and disease, see Keil, Keuck, and Hauswald (2016a).

add to the idea of a spectrum? How did they help you visualize not only the problem of the tipping point of vagueness of degree between health and disease but also, more fundamentally, the combinatorial vagueness of what is at stake. What did your practice teach you about the paradox? Put differently: What did you need to do to *create* a convincing spectrum?
JvdB That's the core of this discussion. I think about this an awful lot, probably too much! Because everything I do seems to actually be about creating a visual and textural spectrum. With this piece, I needed to break down the installation into manageable parts. So there are 58 panels in one row, but actually it's a spectrum of 29 because it mirrors onto the other side; a result of cleaving open one concrete block into two panels. I needed to, in essence, find a convincing way of breaking the spectrum down into component parts. And the question was how many component parts do I break it down into in order to cover the space—the physical architecture of the building? But if there are too many parts, which of course produces a more visually convincing spectrum because each step becomes more imperceptible, it becomes unmanageable as a piece. You would also get very narrow panels that wouldn't actually be visually attractive. And where do you stop? That's the continuum fallacy. So the goal was to find a practical breakdown of the space into manageable parts that were still able to depict a convincing visual textural spectrum. And so, there was a balance between what I could technically do whilst remaining appealing to the eye.

I found all sorts of interesting other things along the way, because when I placed panels next to each other without a break, you could very clearly see a difference in color and texture. FIG. 9

This felt unsatisfactory. But I realized that if you insert a border in between them, the spectrum starts to look incredibly convincing because there's a visual break; the brain fills in the gaps. FIG. 10 And that was a fascinating lesson. Ironically, it sets up an amazing analogy for disease progression and classification. Diagnosing or situating the disease within a disease spectrum is categorizing on a continuum.

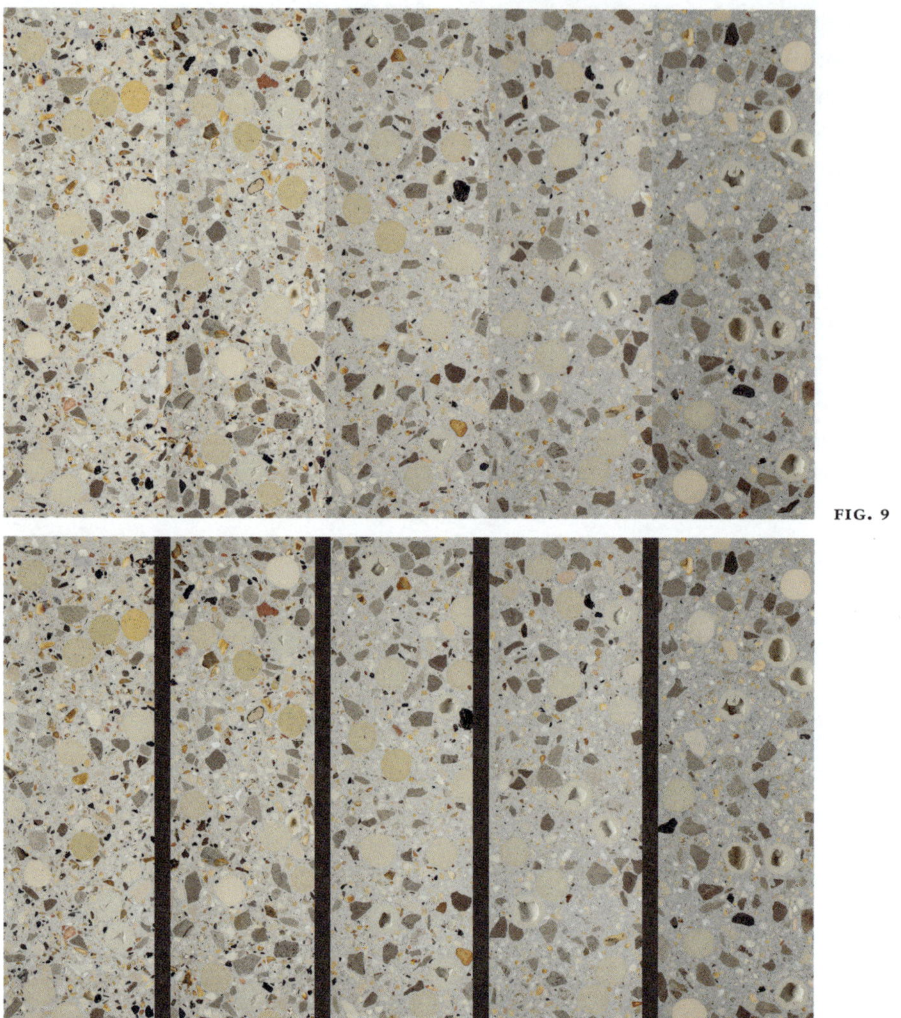

FIG. 9

FIG. 10

FIG. 9 *Matter in Grey* without bars makes the spectrum appear less convincing. Photo: Jacob van der Beugel
FIG. 10 *Matter in Grey* with bars placed between the blocks of concrete creates a more appealing spectrum by introducing visual breaks. Photo: Jacob van der Beugel

LK So would you say that these artistic experiences undermine the difference between a spectrum and categories? Or how would you formulate the question that these insights pose to our thinking about and acting with categorial or gradualist concepts of disease?

JvdB There is a question of the resolution: Are there specific resolutions that make different disease states appear to be on a spectrum and others that make it appear more categorial?

What is the aim of diagnosticians? Do they prefer rigid boundaries to guide their actions or not? Do they imagine the disease to be on a spectrum or categorial? Depending on their beliefs they will find different resolutions more convincing or not.

LK From my historical and philosophical perspective, I would very much agree. One important source of the vagueness is that the definition of reference standards for setting looser or stricter boundaries is interest-relative.[5] In modern medicine, negotiations about the right granularity of grouping cases, and the reasons for lumping or splitting categories, for advocating a spectrum or clear-cut boundaries, are commonplace.

Your work can help a person reflect on the limitations of imagining an ideal continuity. On the one hand, the idea and the aesthetics of a spectrum have something that is instantly appealing; on the other hand, this might disguise some of the dangers that come with that. Because of course there are some implications when boundaries are drawn but also if you imagine there to be a borderless continuity. Classifications guide actions. If the continuity between severe, eventually lethal, symptoms of disease and ever milder, potentially at-risk but potentially also reversible states is stressed, then this claim of continuity might help researchers get funding and expand markets for diagnostics and therapeutics. It could, however, also cause severe stress to not-yet-patients and the allocation of resources in health systems.[6]

Boundaries matter, but so does the lack of boundaries. There might be something deeply unsettling about it. Your work demonstrates that a spectrum can be just as artificial as

5 On interest-relative vagueness in the context of disease classification, see Hauswald and Keuck (2016).

6 On the critique regarding the expansion of contemporary psychiatric classification, see Keuck and Frances (2016). On the expansion of the definition of Alzheimer's to include people without clinical symptoms, see Keuck (2020) and Daly and Keuck (2024).

categories. You have shown me, for instance, your experiments with colored ceramic blocks; if blocks of the same color are doubled up, the spectrum becomes less convincing and the eye sees more boundaries.[FIG. 11 AND 12] Why is this insight so important to you?

JvdB It's a good question. I think my answer centers around the need to pull back the veil on some very human traits, in the hope that we can build on them. I would always prefer to build on something fallible, knowing that it is prone to quakes, as opposed to believing in its infallibility. Boiling it down into layman's terms, "If it sounds too good to be true, it is." This is the case when dealing with spectrums. Ultimately, they are stunning human creations, regardless of how well these models mirror the real world.

3
Backgrounding—Foregrounding

LK I would like to come back to the question of your stance or position as an artist. I see some parallels between your artistic approach and the philosophy of science. In philosophical work about scientific research there is a value in being close to scientific practice in order to get real insight into how the scientists are thinking, what their assumptions are, how they design their experiments, how they conduct them. One part of that approach is trying to find the language to describe these processes. This raises a question about your own agency in this process. As a philosopher of science, are you just reproducing their ideology or do you have a more distant approach to it? If you're too distant, this might mean that you can say something really interesting about your actors, but they might not identify with it at all. So it might change your audience a lot, for the better or the worse.

JvdB Exactly. There is a synergy here to artist residencies in scientific institutes. I've done various artist residencies where you embed yourself into an organization, much in the same way as you describe your research. You have to wrestle with their research and their modus operandi. The trap for

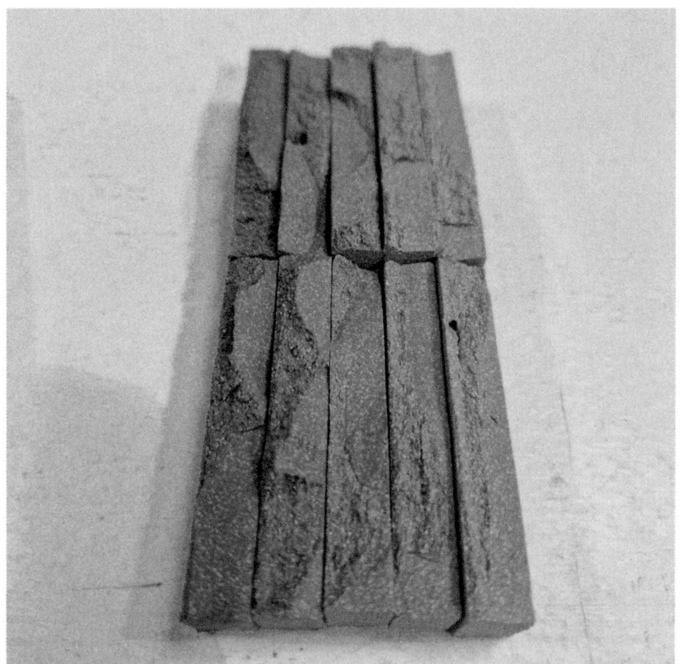

FIG. 11

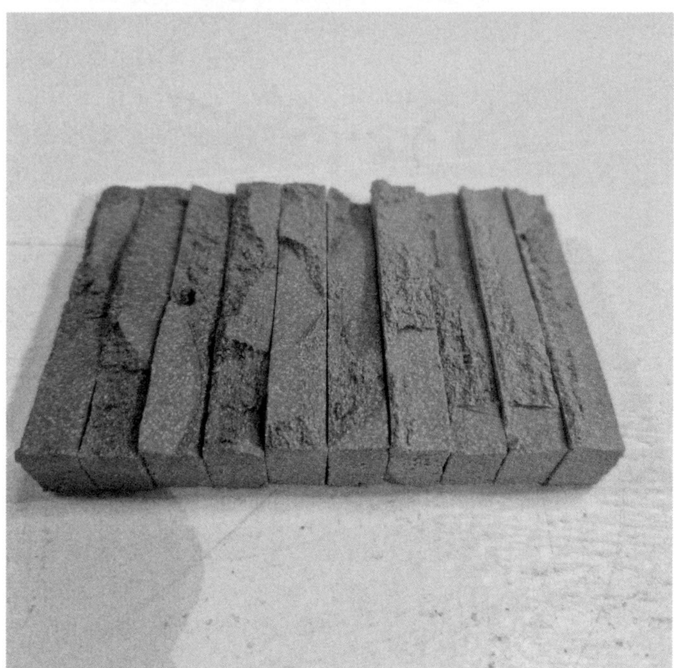

FIG. 12

FIG. 11 A blue-gray spectrum of single-colored ceramic blocks. Photo: Jacob van der Beugel
FIG. 12 A less convincing spectrum using two blocks of each color, another example of the spectrum illusion collapse. Photo: Jacob van der Beugel

artists—and you'll have to answer whether it's the same for you—is to resist becoming dazzled by the science, scientists, and the institutes. For an outsider, it's all really impressive. To retain a shred of neutrality is challenging, yet really important. You can feel seduced and slip into their perspective, especially when you talk to the leads of these institutes. They're the most articulate mouthpiece. So you very rapidly find yourself becoming, not indoctrinated, but much more comfortable with their perspective than with any other kind of opposing perspective. Do you suffer from this? Well, no, probably not. Ultimately you have a perspective that you want to articulate ... tell me about that. How easy do you find it to not fall into this trap?

LK I think it is a to-and-fro. It's always a performative process that you need to achieve, every time in a new way. At least it's that way with the kind of approach I'm adopting. I think it might be different if you have a very rigid, fixed, methodological approach where you say, this is always the perspective that I take on something. Then you can keep more distance. But what I'm really interested in is understanding how different people think, what they understand as knowledge, how they create it, and revise it, and so on. So I need to have a quite dialogical approach. I need to have all this openness. It's a balance between keeping your distance and being open. Because if you are too distant, then perhaps you won't get some really interesting details that you need to understand their perspective. I think understanding in that sense is also that you can slip into the perspective of your interlocutors.

JvdB Have you ever felt like your research has been used in a way that you didn't intend it to be, on purpose or not, or maybe the opposite, where you've been prejudiced prior to doing the research?

LK I guess both. The way I try to work with that is to be—try to be—very explicit about the level on which I am operating. And mostly I have different levels in one paper. On the one hand, I'm trying to describe what others think, but then on the other, I want to make explicit my view on a process. And also make explicit my own positionality, because of course I, too, am changing over time. If I look at some things that I've written in the past, I might later see how at certain points in time I've been situated in debates—not just scientific debates but also historical and philosophical debates that informed me as well. That's the point. You never stand outside. You can stand somewhere else, but there's no point of nowhere. That's my understanding of my positioning. I like to be challenged, to change my perspective on something. Maybe this is also why I like to coauthor papers, though it is sometimes really challenging. However, being open is not well-hedged position. I try to make up for that by always trying to also take a meta perspective on what I am doing. But of course, I cannot see everything. I have my own blind spots.

JvdB That's so interesting, isn't it? But in terms of wanting to remain neutral in order to understand an organization or a disease, from my perspective, neutrality is quite important. It might not be the most ideologically dynamic artwork or piece, but the neutrality is almost a pointer toward an openness to something else. I find it really interesting how there are artworks that are ideologically incredibly assertive. There is a very immediate and probably quite visceral response to that; it's almost like the viewer hasn't done the heavy lifting in order to get into a certain ideological position. So, a vagueness and a neutrality to subject matter that takes in lots of different perspectives, I ultimately find a more convincing approach.

LK And can you say how you understand vagueness in this respect?

JvdB I see vagueness as an openness and not an obfuscation. A vagueness that allows for latency and dynamism, where there is an opportunity to journey to a viewpoint, and backtrack if necessary.

LK That reminds me of the Wittgensteinian idea that sometimes it's more helpful to have blurred boundaries (Wittgenstein 1953, esp. §71).[7] Wittgenstein's example says pointing toward a space doesn't describe a concrete bordered place, an exact spot, but just somewhere out there, and that vagueness

7 For a discussion of this point related to the value of vagueness in medicine and psychiatry, see Keil, Keuck, and Hauswald (2016b).

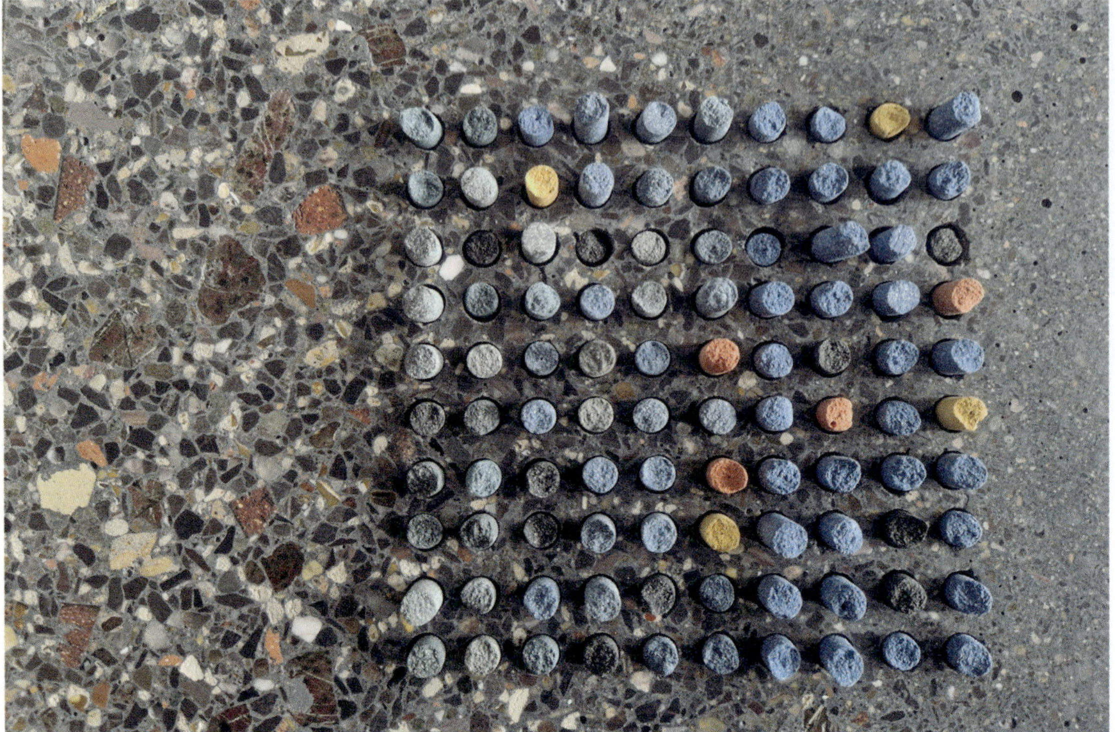

FIG. 13

FIG. 13 Jacob van der Beugel, *Microarray* (prototype), 2023, concrete and mixed aggregates, 30 × 20 × 2.5 cm. Photo: Jacob van der Beugel might be more meaningful. And so, that's maybe what you connect with the openness, right? At first sight, it seems to be the clear task of art or also critical humanities to be the aggressive counter discourse, but that can also be a false cliché in a way. Just as there might be a false precision if you try to point somewhere in that region, and you are misunderstood as referring to an exact place. The exact place seems more precise, but it is just not right. The precise would not be better in that case, because it's not fitting for what you intend to show. Sometimes you can grasp the kernel of a problem better, if you are not setting up two conflicting sides from the beginning, but instead you have an openness that is not so strict about where your boundaries end and where the boundaries of another person or another discipline begin. You are also dealing with this issue in your artwork. How are you making this epistemic situation aesthetically apprehensible?

JvdB By overtly structuring the installation as a literal translation of the objectives of the institute, something we touched upon earlier, there is an ironic position that the art adopts. I think that is the best way to describe it aesthetically. It is ironic because it describes the ambitions that also describe its limitations. It isn't in-your-face irony, rather it quietly points towards a more nuanced perspective. I am intrigued by how you feel it is achieved.

LK I certainly read it that way! But as you said, it is not in-your-face irony, and I think that is fair enough. Because why should we be so sure that one or the other is better? How do we know which of the ambitions exactly will fail?

JvdB It has been said that the sciences have a tendency towards reductionism and materialism. I intuitively empathize with this inclination. It seems entirely logical to keep going one degree deeper with ever increasing granularity. I created some prototype works for a piece yet to be completed that explores this phenomenon. [FIG. 13] I must add that I have worked with cancer epidemiologists who seem to embrace the opposite, which was very refreshing indeed. These works take the shape of mini-microarrays, akin to arrays for gene expressions.

8 Borrowed from the 2022 film of the same name.

I wanted to create a spectrum of clarity. The left side of the little panel is a gray cocktail of aggregates with assortments of color. This was created using recycled aggregates: crushed bricks, road planings, plastics, anything and everything that can be reused for creating a substructure in construction. Protruding from the background are little circular inserts. (In the array these would be wells opposed to protrusions.) As the array moves across, it loses its agglomeration and becomes a monoculture of color, whilst the protrusions become more intense in color. To me, this represents the amazing quality of reducing and refining until there is a distillation; a clarity in one's research, let's say. Yet there is also the converse, a loss of the meta-grounding or background. Clarity is only achieved through filtering and moving through levels of resolution. Meta-perspectives are only visible when the granularity is blended.

LK I love your descriptions of meta-grounding and monocultures of color. Your zooming-in on the background and dealing with its components and incoherencies before and after what you call the filtering process is, to me, the engagement with the methods and assumptions of historiography and philosophy. I don't just want to apply a universal, mono-colored background to the scientific phenomena that I am trying to understand. The background, the mixing, testing, and reflecting on methods, is my field of experimentation. Distancing and disentangling bring epistemic profit, like clarity, but there is also an epistemic cost to these filtering processes. While the methods might differ, I think this Janus-faced epistemic situation is shared in the sciences and humanities.

JvdB Paradoxically you might only be able to achieve a meta-perspective because you are building a larger picture with detailed resolution, perhaps like the Human Brain Project or the Human Genome Project. Yet, I still feel like the metaphor is apt, because in building these large-scale maps you need to make increasingly large assumptions. The more I entangle myself in this subject matter, the more I am unable to disentangle anything. How can one ever have both at the same time, everything, everywhere, all at once![8] Help me, Lara!

LK I am not sure that it is desirable to have it all at once. The interesting moment is when the perspective shifts, when you become aware of foregrounding and backgrounding, of knowing the ambivalence without reducing it to a single way of seeing. However, even if you evoke shifts in perspective, you won't have the full picture. If you think back to our starting point, *Matter in Grey*, we were just looking at different ways of understanding the scientific representations of the course of Alzheimer's disease. There are so many other highly heterogeneous perspectives that can form and inform how and what we do and don't see: the perspectives of people who get such a diagnosis, of people who suffer from symptoms of dementia, the relatives who care for those patients, the sociocultural imagination of people with Alzheimer's who have lost their autonomy, the economic exploitation of the associated fears . . . Even the most integrated, multi-perspectival approach to a phenomenon won't be complete, won't be able to accommodate every possible experience and aspect. To me, these limitations, which have been a key subject of philosophical discourse, imply both the necessity of modesty and the possibility of creativity.

JvdB That is so beautifully put and it answers your "why" question from earlier as well; finding or being mindful of fallibility is a form of modesty that allows for a space in which to create. This tussle between foreground and background is also the subject of a piece I completed for a recent show, called *Wherever the Two Shall Meet.* FIG. 14

This piece describes, broadly, how we haven't finished our evolutionary journey, and that our culture can impact the ways we adapt. The genes I depict in the work are from two different groups of people who both have adapted to increase their ability to absorb oxygen: one due to living in higher altitudes, the other due to deep sea diving. The format of the piece is derived directly from an older Sanger-style genetic sequencing technique that required a more analog and manual procedural technique that conceptually aligns with my way of constructing a piece. FIG. 15 On the surface the title asks,

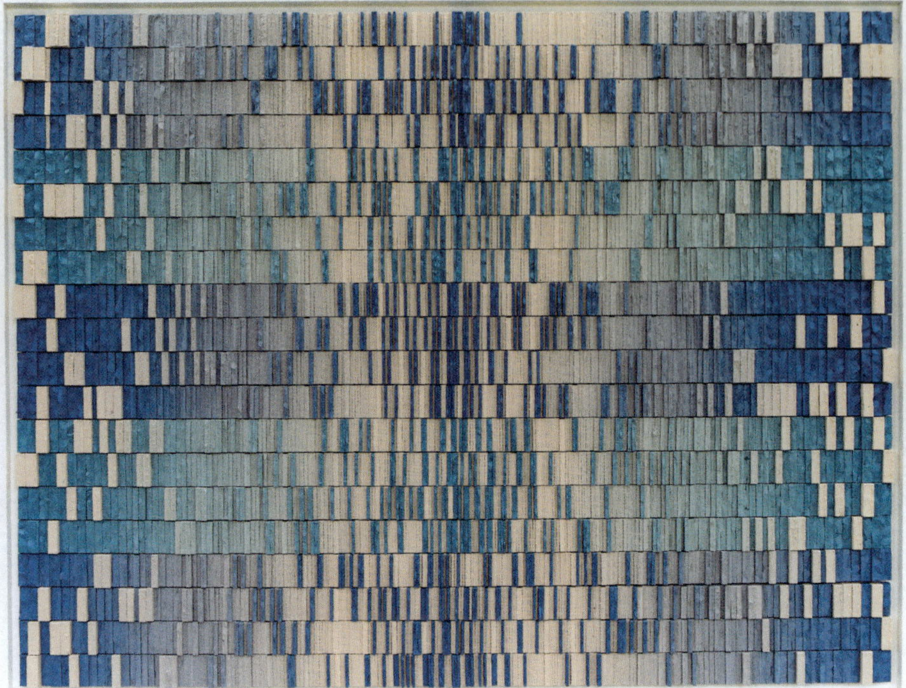

FIG. 14

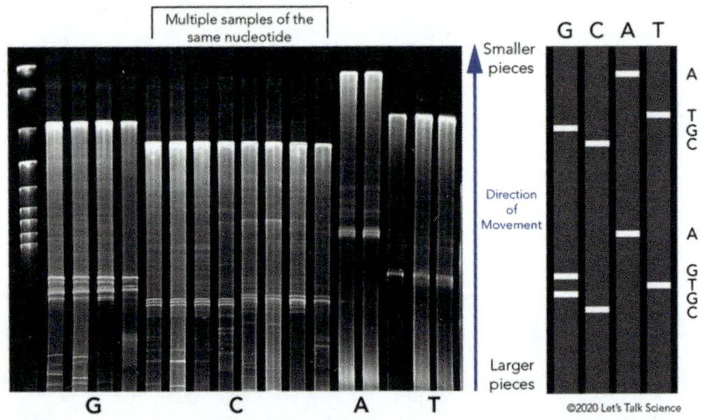

FIG. 15

FIG. 14 Jacob van der Beugel, *Wherever the Two Shall Meet*, 2023, ceramics, 1.8 × 1.3 m. Private collection, United States. Photo: New Art Centre
FIG. 15 Sanger sequencing technique that enables nucleotide visualization. "Sanger Sequencing – Let's Talk Science," August 17, 2020, https://letstalkscience.ca/educational-resources/backgrounders/sanger-sequencing (Accessed: October 30, 2024)

"Where will we find ourselves on this spectrum?" But there is something else going on as well. Foreground and background cross over each other due to their color gradation, almost to the point where they are indistinguishable from each other. Whilst this is me physically recreating the debate about nature/nurture and suggesting the impossibility of teasing them apart, it also highlights the gray areas once again. Where things fall apart and lose clarity. This is the meeting point the title alludes to. It is the area that needs more resolution, more research: the interesting area. In effect you have multiple spectrums colliding and overlapping. There are areas in the work where elements are visually compelling and easy on the eye and then the messy confusing parts, where the colors double up and are unresolved. To me now, this work has become about the nature of working with spectrums.

LK You are absolutely right that we see an increasing interest from the biomedical sciences in taking more factors into account. The gray areas are not necessarily the marginal, they are key fields of research. And the spectrum is probably the icon of this research paradigm.

4
Polishing the Aesthetic, Polishing the Concrete

LK Let's return to the concrete. You mentioned the similarity between your artistic practice of slicing up blocks of concrete and the medical practice of autopsy—slicing up a dead person to examine their bodily structures. Is it just a nice coincidence that the English word "concrete" has different meanings that relate, for one, to your material and, for another, to the concrete in contrast to the abstract, or does this polysemy of "concrete" have a deeper impact on your artwork?

JvdB I love the dualism that comes from presenting something in concrete. Because the word "concrete" brings to mind the factual, a concrete reality, whilst life is so nuanced and so contextually different. We like to see things presented to us as concrete facts: easily digestible, compartmentalized, convincing.

Reality is anything but. In *Matter in Grey* there is an extra level of irony. Not only is its materiality synonymous with the factual and assertively definitive, but the whole layout lends itself to being read in this way due to its seductive construct of the abstract.

LK There's another interesting point about working with concrete in artworks on scientific representations of disease, because there's this abstract idea of a "disease entity." You were referring to that in the beginning: Is there a "normal person"? Are there instances that prototypically represent the course of Alzheimer's disease, normal aging, an ideal course after treatment? If we think that there are instances of this, then it's clear that they have to be concrete people. We have concreteness again. We have individuals in their concrete context-rich life in which so many other things beyond their disease or illness happen as well. Things happen in the physicality of their specific bodies, in the environments that they inhabit. I think in putting the concreteness up front, this can also be understood as a comment on the tension between the specific and the general, the concrete and abstract, the individual person, and general theories of disease, aging, progression, etc. You have the concreteness that is simply there. And then you have some categories or theories, and there needs to be some connection between the specific and the general. If you did the exact same piece again, of course it would look different.

JvdB Exactly. As a person, you have to be able to relate to someone else's model, when you get shoved into that sausage factory. Theirs is the model or process that you will be put in relation to and that will be used on you. And yet, invariably, you fall through its cracks. You probably exist within its boundaries, but still that is the model that gets used. Is that what you were alluding to? But that's just using the word concrete and riffing off it, isn't it. Concrete is amazing. And yet it is also used for things that kind of destroy meaning or have no meaning, for example, in war memorials where it seems to obliterate meaning. It's justifiably got a bad reputation in terms of its environmental footprint, which I think is interesting in itself by the way. That's why I love to use it, because one can't escape our imprint upon the world. I get quite riled by people who say, "well, you shouldn't be using that material because it's bad." That's an incredibly simplistic perspective, because it is one of the materials that is totemic in terms of our footprint on the planet. So perhaps, when discussing the human condition, the use of concrete is incredibly apt.

LK Absolutely. I actually think that concrete encapsulates this idea or underlying emotion, that you can create through your artwork, which shows how you cannot have pure things. You cannot have art that is just beautiful. Something comes with it, which you might not want to have. And the same is true with the striving for perfect health. I mean, what should that be? So it's . . .

JvdB . . . the trade-offs.

LK I think it's even more complicated than a trade-off because you cannot even think of one thing without the other. You can upcycle aggregates of construction work like you have done in *Microarray*, you can make an aesthetically appealing mural out of it, but you cannot do away with the ambivalence that you just outlined so pointedly: the ugly, devastating, destructive side of concrete, and thus of past and present human action.

You are a trained potter, so you have a lot of experience working with clay. How do the different material properties of concrete and clay influence your artistic practice?

JvdB I used to feel that they were similar materials when I first started using concrete. I felt they were materials that were about permanence in stone. This was very naive. There are many things that are different. To me, clay now has an element of freezing human action and then baking it into permanence. There is a unity of movement and immobility. Both things all at once. As a potter you learn to work on the inside and outside of an object simultaneously; this doesn't really happen with other materials. Concrete, by contrast, struggles with this movement but excels in its metaphorical prowess. The aggregates resonate with nature, locality, and cultural associations, but also have a way of hiding, destroying, and obfuscating them. It all depends on what you reveal as an artist. I feel it is most resonant when its inertness is embraced. It isn't alive (although the self-healing component throws this into question). It is an artificially engineered stone. And perhaps this is why using it for *Matter in Grey* serves as a way of highlighting the artifice. The artifice of a spectrum. Our concept of Alzheimer's at this moment is also a snapshot in time—a material construct.

There is also a considerable amount of editing and refining these materials. With a pot, for example, you turn it and trim excess clay to lighten it, to make it more functional and more visually appealing. This also occurs with concrete. When I cleaved open the two panels there was a roughness, an unsatisfactory quality. I put each panel through a process of polishing, a very arduous and physical process. FIG. 16 In the end, the panels retained a sheen and glasslike texture. Here, I like to think that I am making even more visible, what is already present, giving more visual clarity but also imbuing the panels with more luster and appeal. It is difficult to know whether I am acquiescing to my innate desire to create beautiful objects or suggesting the illusory sheen of spectrums. They both serve the same ends!

LK Again, I can't help but see the similarities to scientific practices: to create histological slides of the brains, you stain dead brain tissue to display a pathological process; to understand and examine the living. The corporeality has material properties that limit what can and cannot become visible, but the way you treat it likewise allows for different sorts of resistance to be perceivable or not.

JvdB It might be interesting at this point to discuss the constraints of using spectrums and how this could relate to a wider practical application. I would refer this question back to how I relate it to my own art practice. There is no doubt that using spectrums or gradations has had a massive impact on how I work. I see most things in life and in my art as a process from one to the other, or as being situated within a spectrum of choice or transition. On the surface, this is quite a liberating perspective since it visualizes or conceptualizes subjects with a degree of quiddity. It has an integrity that I like. Conversely, I also regard it as a formal constraint. The ideal way for me to portray something would be on multiple, perhaps even infinite spectrums concurrently—I haven't quite worked out how to do this! Once you really acknowledge spectrums you also have to resign yourself to not being able to depict them: perhaps only a snapshot within one, amongst many. But how does this perspective relate to action in art and diagnoses in disease pathology? In terms of creativity in art, and maybe, Lara, you can elucidate if this chimes with your academic experience, I have this strong sense that these formal constraints act as creative pressure points that force you to continually expand within these boundaries. And whilst these frameworks may eventually crumble under the weight of novelty, something positive happens for me when there are restrictions. It might seem trite or random to think of traditional Japanese craft in respect to this idea, but having been schooled in the pottery tradition, it is a pertinent comparison. Given the rigid scope and aesthetic practice of these crafts, some exceptional leaps have occurred that seem to inhabit novelty and tradition all at once, pushing the craft deeper into itself but to a new depth. In this respect, it is like evolutionary biology: a pressure point seems to push an organism onto a novel pathway, even with the aforementioned constraint intact. The original form is still there in essence, but something feels new. My understanding of spectrums is similar to these creative pressure points. The formal structuring of these spectrums enables points of arrival and departure. There is a truth to them but also the possibility to go deeper into them or beyond. When turning to disease taxonomy and other issues we have discussed I have a sense that there is a synergy with this perspective. The spectrum allows for pressure points to exist, which allow for entry into the disease, but also emergency exits! Perhaps it creates a feeling of not quite getting the diagnosis right and, that this is a tacit understanding of the illusory nature of the constructed spectrum, allowing a small opening for further research/ practical actions.

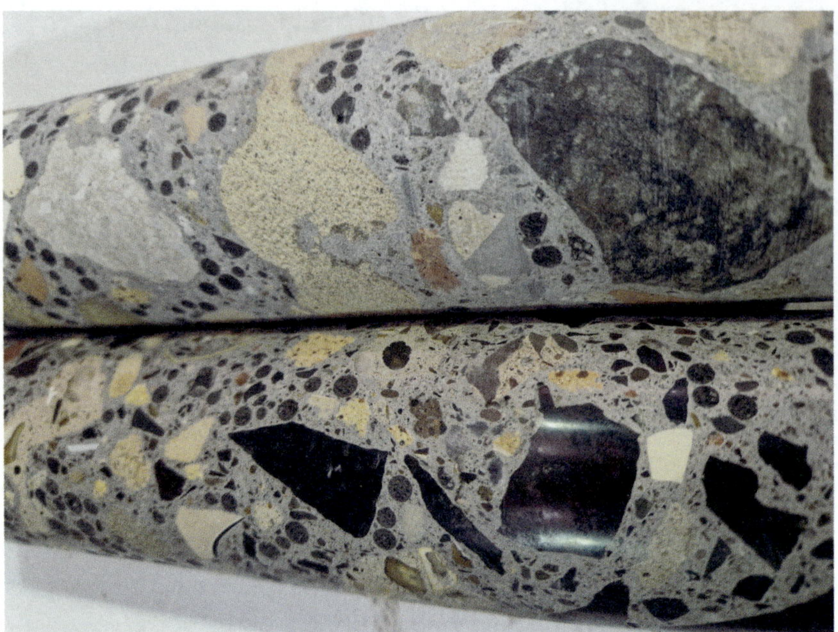

FIG. 16

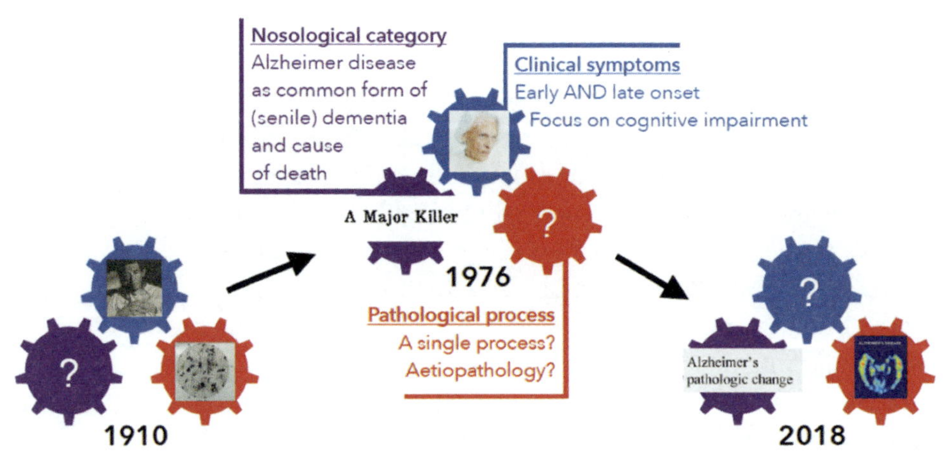

FIG. 17

FIG. 16 Unpolished and polished concrete cores. Photo: Jacob van der Beugel
FIG. 17 Graphical conceptual frameworks of classifying Alzheimer's disease. Adapted from Keuck (2020).

LK I like the expression of pressure points and the productive nature of uncertainty that you stress. But with regards to medicine, we also need to ask: Who can bear the uncertainty? I am acutely aware that it's quite a privileged standpoint that I am taking when I praise—as you do—the reflexive knowledge created by the feeling of doubt. In practice, for patients or relatives waiting for a diagnosis, and also for doctors, in particular young doctors who are not yet confident in their knowledge and skills, doubt can be a very unpleasant, unsettling feeling. For me, this is one of the major challenges when writing about medicine and especially when teaching medical students: taking this unpleasantness seriously while trying to show how it can lead to reflexive knowledge, and how this again can be a resource for dealing with and living through uncertainty. Do you encounter this dilemma in your artistic practice or in the way people react to your artwork?

JvdB You are right to shift the focus to the perspective of doctors and patients and, in my case, viewers. My instinct is telling me it is slightly different. People can afford to test out uncertainties in the arena that art superficially creates, perhaps softening the unsettling transition to a more uncertain perspective. This is the magic of art: the creation of a world that is experimental but at the same time still firmly rooted in the real world. People are able to dip their toes into new waters. Sometimes the temperature is more jarring, other times it allows for a gradual acclimatization. In the situation you describe, people are not afforded such a speculative luxury.

There is also another element to your question, which is people's relationship with uncertainty and doubt. I would love to know if we, as a whole, are less capable of dealing with unpleasantness in general. Again, this is just a gut instinct and perhaps I am blinkered by the current polarization pandemic that eviscerates the middle ground: gray, opaque, and uncertain. I have a sense that we are less well adjusted to the gray and that we have inadvertently found ways to reaffirm certainty and paper over the cracks of doubt. So that, when it inevitably bursts through the dams we have created, it is all the more unsettling.

9 On different understandings of health and disease that are reflected in contemporary debates on Alzheimer's disease, see Keuck and Freeborn (2020) and Daly and Keuck (2024).

5
Art as Mode of Inquiry

LK When I give lectures on history and philosophy of medicine, I often face a dilemma of visualization. If I refer to scientific representations and illustrations, I often get questions that seem to me to address the scientific content itself rather than the reflection upon this scientific content. If I don't show pictures, however, many people find it much more difficult to follow. I have tried to address this problem in creating my own illustrations that focus on the meta-level issue that I am addressing. For instance, I came up with a schematic representation of historical reconfigurations in the classification of Alzheimer's disease. FIG. 17 I noted that this worked particularly well when communicating with scientists. Perhaps because my amateur graphics resemble illustrations in scientific papers.

However, I always felt a bit uncomfortable when showing this schematic to historians, who could easily see this as an overly simplistic representation of a much more complex history. Recently, I have also started to show artwork in my presentations, for instance, in order to illustrate epistemic situations. I find this helpful and inspiring. Yet I also have the feeling that I am to some degree instrumentalizing artwork for my purposes, which might be problematic in its own way. In the course of our conversation, I sometimes had the same impression. On the one hand, your artwork can be regarded as a mode of inquiry; I think it can be very nicely used to illustrate some important elements of how scientific knowledge is made and how it can be challenged. For instance, your artistic representation of the scientific framing of the course of Alzheimer's disease makes the human activity in creating scientific knowledge palpable. This, again, allows us to render the scientific infrastructures, actors, and theories into objects of analysis, thereby opening up the possibility that they are debatable, fallible, and adjustable. What are decisions that have been made, how are they shaping our understanding of health and disease, and what would alternatives look like?[9] *Matter in Grey* can, in this respect, be seen as an entry point for opening up a metascape, in which such questions about conditions, contingencies, assumptions, and alternatives can be addressed. However, I am also aware—and you emphasized this several times—that your main purpose is to create aesthetically compelling artwork. How do you see the relationship of art and its uses outside of art contexts?

JvdB Talk about saving the most difficult till the end! To answer this partially I think beauty needs to be considered, just for a second. This is often maligned in the art world, perhaps for good reason, and I note you stated "aesthetically compelling" as a circumvention. It is such a fragile and elusive quality, and there is a balance between individual responses and more universal traits. I have always been captivated by this property. I suspect it is a very normal thing to engage with, nothing new here. What I can say is that the effects of this quality, in my experience, do a couple of things. It can provide a neutral arena to engage with subject matter in a nonthreatening way. One is seduced into engaging with the subject matter that is depicted. On reflection perhaps seduction isn't so neutral after all, but the allure enables a comfort or receptivity. Most interesting of all, is that for something to be truly visually engaging or beautiful there needs to be a small degree of disharmony within the harmony, something minute that sows the seed of imbalance. There are countless examples from art history of this; my favorite is Japanese Raku ware, where tea bowls can be repaired with gold leaf, called *kintsugi*; the accidental immortalized. Perhaps, the black serpentine stone aggregate that is ever so slightly disruptive in the prevented row in *Matter in Grey* FIG. 18 is this disharmony. To conclude, the "visually appealing" is a fragile balance of harmony, with some degree of dissonance. This is why I mention beauty, because it specifically relates to spectrums but also to wider applications.

To be able to comment on the relationship of art and external uses, one needs to distill many different viewpoints into a homogeneous whole—not something I am prepared or able to do. I do not position myself as a disruptor with highly ideological narratives. If anything, I feel like the artworks hold

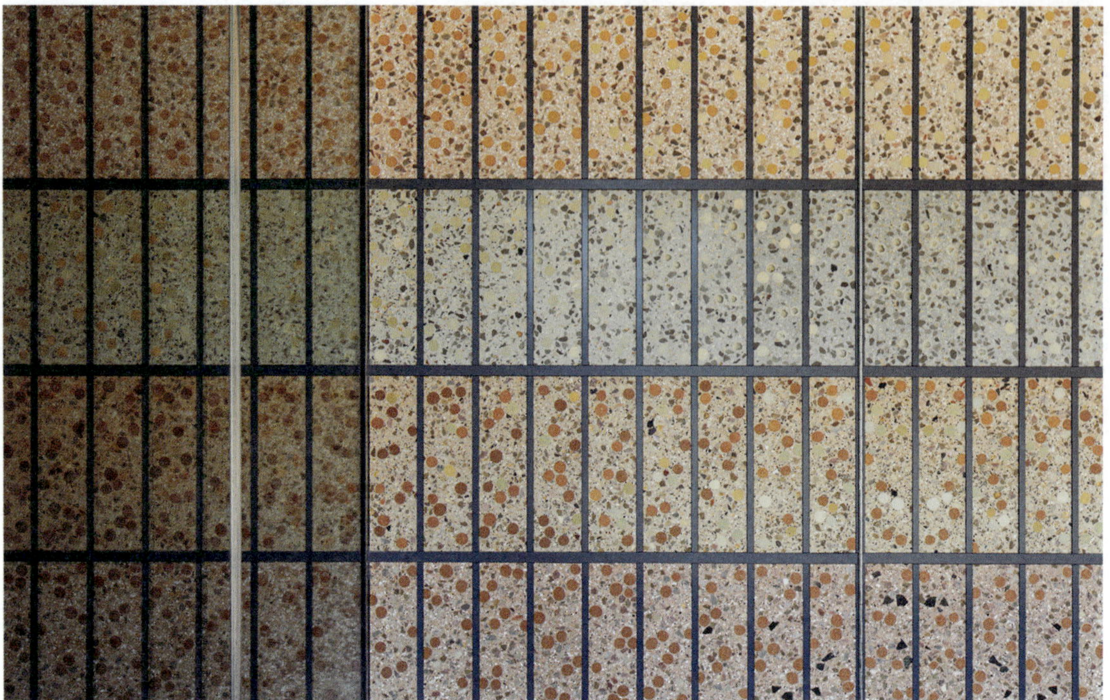

FIG. 18

FIG. 18 Detail from *Matter in Grey*. The black serpentine stone disrupts the preventative spectrum in the bottom row. Photo: Paul Riddle up a "material mirror," in the words of Daniel Miller (2005, 8), to a wider audience or to the researchers who practice within the buildings. I do this in the hope that we can take just a slow second to contemplate things, to create a fissure or bardo where we can reassess what we thought we knew, through a mirror that I have tried to artistically tinge as little as possible.

If you are asking whether art should be used for more illustrative purposes, then this changes the nature of the debate. There are countless examples of this being extremely fertile ground. I love Waddington's valley illustration (see Borck and Meunier in this volume, figure **2B**), and its subsequent contemporary reinventions. Obviously not for its accuracy but for the fact that it cast new light and created a new way of seeing. My answer would be that every artwork comes with its own insights, idiosyncrasies, limitations, and suppositions, which can serve research but also highlight its problems. I dare say *Matter in Grey* will suffer the same fate. So use them at your own peril!

LK What a literally beautiful reflection to end with. Thank you, Jacob.

A

Alzheimer, Alois (1911) "Über eigenartige Krankheitsfälle des späteren Alters." *Zeitschrift für die gesamte Neurologie und Psychiatrie* 4 (1): 356–85. https://doi.org/10.1007/BF02866241.

Alzheimer, Alois. n.d. MPIP-DFA 9/1 (Nachlass Alzheimer), Max Planck Institute of Psychiatry, Munich.

Au, Derek (2015) "Triaxial Testing." Derek Philip Au. May 3, 2015. https://www.derekau.net/blog/2015/05/03/triaxial-testing (Accessed: August 16, 2024).

D

Daly, Timothy, and Lara Keuck (2024) "Alzheimer's Disease: Engaging with an Unstable Category." In *Handbook of Philosophy of Medicine*. Dordrecht: Springer Nature. https://doi.org/10.1007/978-94-017-8706-2_113-1 (Accessed: April 22, 2024).

F

Freer, Rosie, Pietro Sormanni, Prajwal Ciryam, Burkhard Rammner, Silvio O. Rizzoli, Christopher M. Dobson, and Michele Vendruscolo (2019) "Supersaturated Proteins Are Enriched at Synapses and Underlie Cell and Tissue Vulnerability in Alzheimer's Disease." *Heliyon* 5 (11): e02589. https://doi.org/10.1016/j.heliyon.2019.e02589 (Accessed: April 22, 2024).

Freer, Rosie, Pietro Sormanni, Giulia Vecchi, Prajwal Ciryam, Christopher M. Dobson, and Michele Vendruscolo (2016) "A Protein Homeostasis Signature in Healthy Brains Recapitulates Tissue Vulnerability to Alzheimer's Disease." *Science Advances* 2 (8): e1600947. https://doi.org/10.1126/sciadv.1600947 (Accessed: April 22, 2024).

H

Hauswald, Rico, and Lara Keuck (2016) "Indeterminacy in Medical Classification: On Continuity, Uncertainty, and Vagueness." In *Vagueness in Psychiatry*, edited by Geert Keil, Lara Keuck, and Rico Hauswald 93–116. New York: Oxford University Press. https://doi.org/10.1093/med/9780198722373.003.0005 (Accessed: April 22, 2024).

K

Keil, Geert, Lara Keuck, and Rico Hauswald, eds. (2016a) *Vagueness in Psychiatry*. New York: Oxford University Press.

Keil, Geert, Lara Keuck, and Rico Hauswald, eds. (2016b) "Vagueness in Psychiatry: An Overview." In *Vagueness in Psychiatry*, edited by Geert Keil, Lara Keuck, and Rico Hauswald, 3–23. New York: Oxford University Press.

Keuck, Lara (2017) "Slicing the Cortex to Study Mental Illness: Alois Alzheimer's Pictures of Equivalence." In *Vital Models: The Making and Use of Models in the Brain Sciences*, edited by Tara Mahfoud, Sam McLean, and Nikolas Rose, 233: 25–51. London: Progress in Brain Research.

Keuck, Lara (2018) "Diagnosing Alzheimer's Disease in Kraepelin's Clinic, 1909–1912." *History of the Human Sciences* 31 (2): 42–64. https://doi.org/10.1177/0952695118758879 (Accessed: April 22, 2024).

Keuck, Lara (2020) "A Window to Act? Revisiting the Conceptual Foundations of Alzheimer's Disease in Dementia Prevention." In *Preventing Dementia?*, edited by Annette Leibing and Silke Schicktanz, 19–39. New York: Berghahn Books. https://doi.org/10.1515/9781800734982-003.

Keuck, Lara, and Allen Frances (2016) "Reflections on What Is Normal, What Is Not, and Fuzzy Boundaries in Psychiatric Classifications." In *Vagueness in Psychiatry*, edited by Geert Keil, Lara Keuck, and Rico Hauswald, 152–68. Oxford: Oxford University Press. https://doi.org/10.1093/med/9780198722373.003.0008 (Accessed: April 22, 2024).

Keuck, Lara, and Alfred Freeborn (2020) "The Limits of Biomarkers: Contemporary Re-Phrasings of Canguilhem." In *Vital Norms: Canguilhem's "The Normal and the Pathological" in the Twenty-First Century*, edited by P.-O. Méthot, 346–67. Paris: Hermann Philosophie.

Kraus, Arnoldo (2010) "Frida Kahlo: das Leben, ein Schmerz." In *Frida Kahlo Retrospektive*. Exhibition catalogue, Martin-Gropius-Bau, April 30–August 9. Munich: Prestel.

M

Miller, Daniel. 2005. "Materiality: An Introduction." In *Materiality*, edited by Daniel Miller, 1–50. Durham, NC: Duke University Press. https://doi.org/10.1215/9780822386711-001 (Accessed: April 22, 2024).

W

Wittgenstein, Ludwig (1953) *Philosophical Investigations*. Translated by G. E. M. Anscombe. Oxford: Basil Blackwell.

Seeing the Tangled Tendrils Within: Feeling/Seeing Endometriosis beyond Invisibility

Jaipreet Virdi and Nimisha Bhanot

Artist Statement

This composition was created using images Jai deposited in a shared Google Drive folder, images that she captured to keep her family and friends updated on multiple health crises. They document her day-to-day experiences juggling a work/life balance with endometriosis.

Through the images, themes of beauty, pain, and resilience emerge, especially in the selfies she took of herself dressed up just days after a laparoscopy.

The top two quadrants of this composition utilize images of Jai in dresses, concealing the bandages and compresses that helped keep her upright and "together" so she could work. The patterns of the dresses (yellow and blue floral/paisley and maroon with white dots) bleed into other parts of her experience, acting as a layer of concealment within the composition. Layered behind the yellow dress is an image of her desk in preparation for a virtual event held three days after a laparoscopy.

In the middle of the image is her bed and the involuntary shedding of her hair on a paisley pillowcase, layered beside an image of her in a hospital gown and mask. The top left and bottom right corners feature Jai and her partner, Geoff, in the process of waiting. The bottom left quadrant shows the pillowcase and the other side of involuntary hair loss by depicting a close-up view of her scalp, layered over an image of a pelvic ultrasound.

These layers capture different parts of her journey with endometriosis. The murkiness of the aesthetics hints at the possibility of there being more beneath the surface of this composition than is directly accessible to the viewer. The way the layers blend into one another and their irregular order also hint at the impact chronic pain has on one's memory and perception of time.

Nimisha Bhanot

FIG. 1 Nimisha Bhanot, *Tangled Tendrils*, 2024, watercolor and acrylic, 20.5 × 27 cm. Courtesy of the artist

FIG. 1

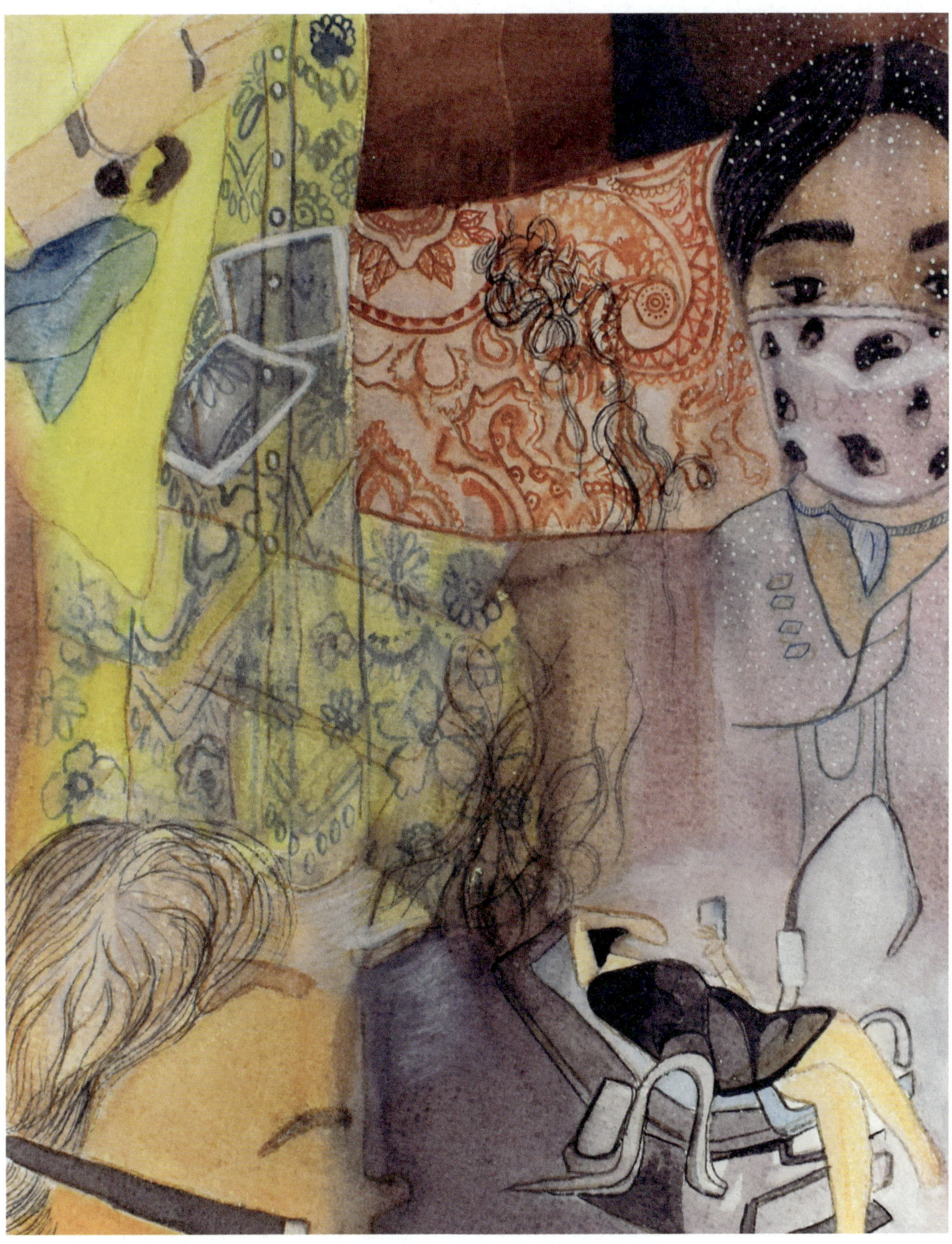

We began our collaboration with a shared kinship through my youngest sister, but I had long followed Nimisha's art on Instagram and other profiles. Her *Badass Desi Pinups* regularly appear on my feed, their bold and rebellious features challenging traditional perceptions of South Asian culture and sexuality (Bhanot 2015). The overly powerful part of these series, I find, is the confrontation of shame and their insistence for us to look beyond our cultural familiarity. It seemed natural to me to invite her for a collaboration that mixes our shared experiences of community, culture, and invisible pain through layers of words and images.

Our method depended on an open and honest exchange of vulnerability. Sharing one's private medical experiences, especially traumatic ones, leads to an exposure of the self that can invite judgment, misunderstanding, and ableism; but at the same time, the very nature of this collaborative essay, one in which artist and writer bring forth their own lived experiences of health issues, requires such openness. To help Nimisha understand the extent of my bodily pain and medical crises, I shared photographs and screening images that I had kept over the years. Some of these were for my distant family, to keep them updated on what was happening; others were kept for my own archive—and, I suppose, health record, to convince skeptical medical practitioners of the extent to which my symptoms affected my daily life. Our coproduction of visuality—words and paint—come together in an affirmed state of trust where words and experiences are believed, where the subjective holds value, and where art has the emotional pressure and baggage to visualize, recreate, and readdress the lack of agency often felt in clinical spaces.

We interrupt this essay at multiple junctures: I take the reader away from the text into the depths of my mind (soul) where trauma resides, and Nimisha guides us momentarily to her studio to witness her adoption of my words to the canvas. **I have created a watercolor painting using various images from Jai's personal digital archive. These images range from diagnostic imaging, to documentation of her medical journey, to her persisting through a day-to-day work/life**

balance. During our Zoom meetings, Nimisha gives me prompts for sharing information—all of which we've kept in a Google Drive folder—that could assert additional visuality for her artistic references. **These references, when considered alongside the essay, invite us into a subjective experience through the language of vulnerability reminding us that the body is an archive.**

Oh, I love that phrase. "The body is an archive." What better way to begin this essay?

1
Envision

I looked up to see the nurse holding the door open as a technician rolled in a desktop station toward my bed. The doctor followed behind in her dark scrubs, her sneakers quiet against the clattering of the station's castor wheels. As my husband, Geoff, took my hand, we all exchanged pleasant greetings, rehearsing what we were trained to say in proper social etiquette. *How are you? I'm fine*. **Social etiquette, smiling through the pain.** Lying on the bed, with wires on various parts of my body hooked to monitors, pain emitting from every muscle and bone, head cloudy from medication, skin gray and rough from lack of care, I was anything but fine. But that's what we say when someone asks how you are. *I'm fine.*

The doctor turned on the vertical monitor to show us the MRI scans we had waited weeks for. A grayscale picture appeared, outlining my entire abdomen—organs, fat, bone, there it all was, in this one picture. Geoff and I stared at the picture intensely, nodding our heads as the doctor explained the reality that I had long felt. Yes, the mass was there, exactly where I had said it was. All the doctors responsible for my care and who had viewed the image were surprised at how large the mass was (*anywhere between six to nine centimeters*), confirming that the questionable nodules were fibroids or likely endometrial masses, but further verification would be made with surgery. It was a mess. **Overwhelming.** Endometriosis was everywhere.[1]

1 "The cause of endometriosis is unknown. There is no known way to prevent endometriosis" (World Health Organization 2023).

We kept staring at the picture, trying to make sense of the words we were hearing to match them to the visuals in front of us. The MRI allowed for a reconfiguration of my body through the medical gaze, producing information to be cross-referenced for the diagnostic process (Prasad 2005, 293; Foucault 1975). The resulting images become "highly mediated representations that are influenced by decisions and values during all aspects of the production process"—that is, they do not *reveal* the inner body, but instead *produce* the body (Joyce 2005, 437–38). **Representation versus reality.** Geoff and I have both taken biology classes before and are familiar with human anatomy. And as a professor in the history of medicine, I knew what I was supposed to be seeing. Still, in this moment, our knowledge was lacking, because we could not see what we were supposed to be seeing; we lacked the trained judgment embedded in the technical expertise for reading these scans (Daston and Galison 2007). It's one thing to feel the mass and pinpoint its location, but a whole other thing to match the feeling to the image produced from the MRI examination.[2] One is invisible, the other visible. One subjective, the other objective. Only one is believed.

Where is it? I asked, staring at the scan, certain that I was looking in the right direction. Is the MRI telling the correct story, the most accurate—even magical—expression of its visual power? Does it behave with full agency, as "one who creates authoritative knowledge and provides access to unseen parts of the body," stripping the human perspective away, as Kelly Joyce (2005, 443) observes? The doctor pointed to a shapeless section in the lower left of the scan. It was nearly completely opaque, and much bigger than I had ever imagined it to be. A gasp escaped my throat, as she continued to explain the results of the MRI. I kept staring at the mass. Here was validation of the pain I'd long complained about, validation of its existence after years of denial in every clinician's office, every hospital bed. It was nearly double the size of my stomach, completely overshadowed my uterus, and—somewhat grotesquely—took up residence in nearly every space of my pelvic region.

2 As Joyce points out, "Medical images allow us 'to know' ourselves in a manner that is portrayed as new and important," even though the examination itself is a constructed artifact (2005, 441).

Here it is in all its glory, this mass of searing agony. I see it and so do they, and it cannot be denied. It is invisible pain materialized, reframed in clinical terminology, "the shadowy unknowable finally exposed by the light of the clinical gaze," as Travis Chi Wing Lau (2020) describes. It is a cry of the flesh manifested, the reason for my erosion of corporeal autonomy (Carel 2008). I have no questions. I am quiet. Shocked at first, then angry. How dare they not see what I have long felt? Seven months later, the mass would be surgically removed, along with multiple adhesions and endometrial lesions. By that time, my body had contorted from the growth, affecting my left hip and leg to the point I could scarcely stand up straight. I had gotten accustomed to wearing clothes with deep pockets should I need to insert my hand and push the weight of the mass upward; it was the only way to stand in front of a class full of students and teach without feeling the need to collapse. The pathological secrets were revealed, confirmed by the objective diagnostics of multiple scans and images, but still, still I had to wait, wait and try hormonal treatment options first, before surgery could be scheduled. *Get it out of me*, I silently screamed daily, feeling the tendrils of the mass slowly slithering around my bowels, bladder, and ribs. *How are you even standing*, the surgeon asked the day of my operation. *You must be suffering.*

How do we picture pain? We are familiar with expressions of agony, the contortions of the body, the winces and gasps that escape from the lips. We can recognize subtle differences as well as anguished screams, but why is it when patients narrate their unseen pain, the one that they have long managed to bear with minimal expressions—both to live in this chronicity and to reduce ableist scorn—why is it they are not believed? In her eloquent meditations, Elaine Scarry (1987) argues that pain destroys language and erodes the bonds of sociality. Perhaps we cannot believe a patient's unseen pain through a medical gaze, because scientific medicine is dependent on verification. For pain to be objectively analyzed and understood, especially for a diagnosis, it needs to be measured, quantified, and captured in an image. There's certainly a tension here between merely describing the condition to the clinical gaze, with the realities of lived experience; one cannot always neatly be translated into the other, especially when the tensions are rooted in epistemic violence and injustice. Still, we need the experience validated, even through another's interpretation of scans and through objectivity, because pain needs to exist outside of the body to be believed.

Our histories prove otherwise. Suzannah Biernoff (2021, 194) points out that social, literary, and iconographic chronicles of pain and suffering show "that pain is as much a cultural phenomenon as a physiological one," an interpretation that is "a compound of body, mind and culture" and constantly negotiated socially.[3] I wonder, then, how do we reconcile what we see with what we understand? That is, how does the consistent throbbing, stabbing, burning sensation I feel inside my abdomen and pelvic region translate to a two-dimensional image that is embedded with the credibility that my words lack? **The haunting memory of an invisible pain, of neglect by the medical gaze, of the blurring of inside and outside, work, home, public . . . all contribute to the archive of the body and a knowledge that is more "true" than the written word set aside for consignment.**

I've had multiple laparoscopic surgeries to remove endometrial adhesions, the remains of the procedure leaving dark, jagged scars on several points across my lower abdomen. Studies have shown that laparoscopic excision—sometimes causally referred to as "clean up" in gynecological clinics—improves the quality of life for endo sufferers: "the silverly tube of the laser is seen cutting, burning, and separating out the malignant tissues, shooting waters to rinse away the blood, and finally vacuuming away the unwanted matter. Abnormal tissue and tubal obstructions are vaporized; the smoke is suctioned out" (Shohat 1998, 259). To date, laparoscopy remains one of the most effective treatments for the disease, though the costs and access of care can be out of reach (if not outrightly denied) for many endo sufferers. One study examined 235 women with chronic pelvic pain from

3 "The implications of this for clinical practice and medical humanities are profound. As well as asking about the severity of a patient's pain, or its precise character (in order to make a diagnosis or offer appropriate pain relief) one would want to know how an individual's pain was negotiated socially (in hospital, at home or in the workplace) and what their pain meant to them" (Biernoff 2021, 194).

endometriosis who underwent laparoscopy, finding that of the 135 who were available for follow-up after two to five years, significant improvements in health were observed: the women showed significant reductions in pain scores, non-menstrual pelvic pain, dyspareunia, and dyschezia. Quality of life and sexual function with pleasure were increased, and discomfort during sex decreased (Abbott et al. 2003). Yet as a treatment "gold standard," it wasn't enough for these women; one-third required further surgeries, and 68 percent experienced a return of endometriosis. For a moment there, I know they believed it was over, this pain and suffering they had become accustomed to, only to face the disappointment over its return. Recurrence of endometriosis meant another go on the healthcare-merry-go-round.

If medical photographs act as "mediating spaces navigating" between the surgeon who takes the photos via laparoscopy and the person whose pained body is being photographed, then can the two perspectives be relational (Padfield 2021, 148)? The images capture the physicality of pain—the bleeding, the adhesions, the nodes—but they are captured in conjunction with the surgeon's expertise. The laparoscope is a telescopic rod lens connected to a video camera and a fiber-optic light source (either halogen or xenon) that relays images to a television monitor above the operating table (Saorsa and Phillips 2019, 113). During a laparoscopic excision, an assistant positions the laparoscope for the surgeon, who is then guided by the visuals to perform the operation through small incisions. As Jac Saorsa and Rebecca Phillips explain, this is an *indirect* procedure "in the sense that, while she is working from images on the screen, the surgeon is not actually looking at the real patient lying on the table, nor does she see the real, physical part of the patient's body that she is operating on, because the incisions are only made large enough to accommodate the slender instruments she is using" (2019, 113). There certainly is a disconnect here, between the surgeon's gaze and the physicality of the anesthetized patient's pain in this scenario, one that seems to hinder shared dialogue.

4 See also Howell (1995).

When the Paris clinicopathological system was accepted in the nineteenth century as a new method for correlating patient's symptoms with pathology lesions found in cadavers, the idea was that any visible symptom had an underlying cause. Essentially, if you presented with pain in a specific part of your body, a correlation could be made for an underlying mass or disorder through manual examination and testing. Today, diagnostic medicine with machines—including the X-ray and ultrasound—might penetrate "beneath the flesh to unearth its pathological secrets" but as iconic technologies of scientific medicine, they ironically seem to shift the authoritative reliance on the medical gaze (Lau 2020; Lavine 2011, 591). **Layers of skin, layers of tendrils, layers of visibility.** If we cannot see the symptoms in images, then they cannot exist. As my friend Kelly explains, "It's almost like putting glasses on the medical gaze, so to speak, has caused a really fundamental disruption in the observation of symptoms" (Kelly O'Donnell, personal communication 2024).

Still, for a patient to view the materiality of their pain as captured in an image is a powerful experience, even as imaging technologies "are marked by continuing struggles over cultural authority and cultural inscription—over who will have the authority to define the role and meaning of these technologies and determine how they will be institutionalized" (Treichler, Cartwright, and Penley 1998, 9).[4] If the MRI scan was a validation of the mass that I long felt existed, but could not identify, then seeing the laparoscopy photos was a shocking revelation of the extent to which the disease ravaged my body. I had, of course, googled endometriosis numerous times, but the images that appeared on the screen were—at least to me—abstract renderings. They weren't an indication of *my pain*, but something similar, a possibility of what *could* exist within my body. Something to identify with, I suppose, or to visually understand my own experiences, to find a hidden language that evokes emotion. Perhaps medical imaging can be how we understand our own selfhood.

At the post-surgery consultation, my surgeon opened my patient folder—this thick pile of papers that encompassed my body's archive—and pulled out a series of laminated prints to show me and Geoff. White paper with four color photographs, each looking approximately the same to the untrained eye: a square featuring a dark vignette surrounding a circle featuring an abstract jumble of flesh-colored background, red or dark brown squiggles or tiny circles, and shadows of the unknown. **Powerful, validating, cathartic, earth shattering. Nobody knows the depths of pain experienced, no matter how much we write or share or explain.** These were images that my surgeon captured during the excision, and as she explained details of the procedure she pointed to some of the photographs. These red and dark brown squiggles? Those were endometrial lesions. The shadows or yellowish tints above the flesh? Adhesions. Here's my left ovary, nearly annihilated by scarring, collapsed from the weight to the back of my uterus.[5] As she drew attention to specific photographs to connect the seemingly disparate medical elements to her expert words, I felt still. I think I laughed in surprise or shock. "Words alone," Deborah Padfield expresses, "or at least the type of language that abounds in the clinic, relying on more generic descriptions such as pain intensity, location or frequency, are seldom able to produce the type of shared experience as images, relying as these do on shared perception" (2021, 154).[6] The highly technical biomedical images are used by trained experts to convey specialized knowledge and years of training, but the moment of sharing here, between clinician and patient, fails to fully capture the co-construction of knowledge or the distinctions between what is being shared and what is being perceived. At this moment of sharing, of coproduction, with these photographs, I see and understand what the surgeon viewed through the laparoscope, and the shared dialogue between us makes real the experience of the disease. Our various expertise exists in a horizontal hierarchy, each dependent on the other for holistic information. Between the three of us, layers of expertise weave together—surgeon, sufferer, supporter—and for a moment

5 This is making me think of bell hooks's *All about Love*.
6 See also Sontag (1977).

there in the consultation room, together we materialize endometriosis.

I imagine the tendrils of endometriosis, all the adhesions and squiggly lines, floating out of the laparoscopy photographs, mixing with the words and questions from me . . . floating upward to the space around us and adhering to the walls. There it grows and spreads, an invasive creature, wrapping itself around all the objects in the room, surrounding the three of us huddled around the photographs. It is deep burgundy, with dark chocolate shadows, but almost glowing, as if it is freed. Here, in all its glory, is the pain of endometriosis manifested, no longer made invisible by medical skepticism or gaslighting, but real, real beyond clinical words, real enough to justify all that Geoff and I had gone through for years of begging to be seen. Here are the tangled tendrils of past and present, the invisibility surrounding the disease utterly, completely, shattered.

2
Etiology

Endometriosis is, quite frankly, a disease of "diagnostic uncertainty," at least until it is confirmed with pathology (Denny 2009). As one gynecologist explained to me, the disease spreads in the body much like cancer does. It primarily affects one in ten people with a female reproductive system, when the tissue that normally lines the uterus—the endometrium—grows outside of it, often on the ovaries, fallopian tubes, and pelvic lining. It can grow on organs too: on bladders, bowels, kidneys, and, in rare cases, on the lungs and brain. Just like in the uterus, every month the displaced endometrial tissue acts as it's engineered to behave—thickening, breaking down, and bleeding with each menstrual cycle. Since the tissue cannot shed out of the body, it becomes trapped and inflamed, causing immense pain and, over time, forms adhesions that glue organs and pelvic tissues together, often within the ligaments of the uterus, cervix, appendix, bladder, and rectouterine pouch—the seemingly empty space behind the uterus (between the vagina and rectum) where I learned my own mass was growing.[7] The disease

7 Most endometrial growths are not malignant or cancerous and occasionally, the endometrial tissues "can even invade distant anatomical structures such as the lungs, nose, or armpits" (Baruch 1999, 92).

usually presents as pelvic pain, heavy and painful periods, bowel and urinary disorders, chronic fatigue, and immense nausea. Because endometriosis primarily affects the female reproductive organs, it falls under the domain of gynecology and reproductive health. Many endometriosis suffers tend to first be diagnosed when facing fertility issues connected to consistent pelvic pain, and it is only then that their suffering is taken seriously. The field's focus of fertility also means that the increasing numbers of endo sufferers who do not—or do not want to—consider their fertility options face an even longer battle to obtain a diagnosis. Indeed, for some it takes repeated temporary treatments before a doctor finally approves a hysterectomy, a solution that a patient might be requesting from the beginning. For others, hysterectomy is presented as the only, and often heartbreaking, solution, even though hysterectomy may not cure the disease.

Historian Cara E. Jones argues that while endometriosis is "representative of the sexualized and reproductive status of women's health in general," the myopic focus on the uterus makes us miss the bigger picture—that is, this is not just a "woman's disease" (Jones 2014). This isn't anything new. Newspaper articles in the 1980s blamed sufferers for delayed childbirth, regularly describing the disease as a "working woman's disease" or the "career woman's disease"—to which feminists responded that they were "typical of the obscurantist sexist, classicist, racist hype that is often initiated by doctors" (Jaffe 1986, 31).[8] As Jones explains, such perspectives cause a rift between endometriosis as a fertility issue versus an inflammatory chronic pain condition, thereby resulting in reproductive health issues being tied to gendered expectations and roles, mainly due to a language problem that constructs all reproductive concerns as *women's* health. It's probably why medical and self-help literature on endometriosis tends to be haunted by a specter of hysteria's wandering womb (Jones 2015, 1084).[9] The rift additionally creates persistent gaps in women's health research such that endometriosis remains undervalued for a condition that affects over 190 million

8 For an overview of this history of "career woman's disease," see Sanmiguel (2000).
9 On the "wandering womb," see King (1998) and Meyer (1997).

women, trans, and nonbinary people worldwide (with rare cases in cis men as well) (Ellis, Munro, and Clarke 2022). Recent studies, moreover, have stressed the non-gynecological aspects of the disease, declaring it as an inflammatory chronic pain condition that can be disabling and affect a person's quality of life. Endometrial pain is not merely a condition of endometrium gone haywire. It is a complex disease, "with heterogenous symptom expression and phenotypes, including superficial endometriosis, invasive deep-infiltrating endometriosis, and ovarian endometriosis" (Wahl et al. 2021, 89). The pain experience is not always rooted in the "bleeding" but can be a result of complications from the disease itself, particularly the adhesion of tissues, when pain can be felt from "jolting movements" such as exercise or riding in a car (Helosvuori and Oikkonen 2023, 5).

Still, endometriosis has been, and still tends to be, situated in a wider set of omissions and constructions relating to women's health. The discourse around the disease heavily centers on privileging a woman's reproductive capacity over her experiences of chronic pain and disability. Here, then, endometriosis falls within the scope of other gendered conditions in which the masculine defines the standard for health, such that "illness common to women are systematically ignored or misattributed as evidence of mental illness, deviant behavior or a lack of self-care" (Hudson 2022, 22). This includes: fibroids, polycystic ovary syndrome, fibromyalgia, migraines, and brain trauma—all conditions "in which painful and disabling symptoms (mostly amongst women) have been systematically and historically dismissed, ignored or delegitimized."[10]

Even as increased studies confirm endo sufferers perceive their disease experiences through the lens of pain rather than fertility, their clinical experiences regularly prioritize the latter. Abby Norman empathically makes this point in her book, *Ask Me About My Uterus,* describing her surgeon's disinclination to perform a hysterectomy in the likelihood that Norman would "change her mind"—even though Norman had never expressed or considered her fertility (2018).[11] Conservative treatment

10 A hysterectomy, especially combined with an oophorectomy (removal of ovaries), can arguably improve one's quality of life, but unlike mastectomies, are not for *saving* life-threatening conditions (though improving one's pain is *saving* one's life!), and for that reason—as well as concerns about reproduction—are often promoted as a last option, usually as an elective surgery (Hudson 2022, 22). See also Abel (2021); Foxhall (2019); Casper and O'Donnell (2020); Barker (2005).

11 Kerri Baruch similarly emphasized this point a decade earlier: "Although endometriosis has been reported to be one of the major causes of infertility in the United States, this theme emerged as a concern for only a minority of the women interviewed" (1999, 94).

options still tend to focus on preserving fertility. While the range of hormonal and surgical treatments can significantly improve one's quality of life, mental health, and productivity, they are stopgap measures that are repeatedly encouraged by doctors and endured by patients before a full hysterotomy is offered as a (permanent) solution.[12]

12 And, of course, it begs the question about fundamental questions about gender identity. See Elson (2004).

I did not want that option.
Not until we exhausted all avenues to conceive.
We only wanted one chance to create what's ours.
But truth be told, I was terrified.
There was the promise, you know?
It would miraculously fix the pain.
Never again would I scream in agony, cry all the tears.
Then a voice whispered in the darkness of my mind: but what if it doesn't?
What if you're hoping for something that will never come?
Something that is not even possible? What if this is it?
This is just your life?
But my love . . . what if you survive?

Here, she oscillates between speaking objectively as a medical historian and sharing her subjective experiences. Her shift from first to second person creates a beautiful ebb and flow that paints a more holistic picture. Nicky Hudson argues that the "uncertain ontology" of endometriosis "and the persistent ignorance surrounding its form and trajectory" are constitutive of an indeterminacy, particularly as the disease etiology has yet to be standardized (2022, 23). This persistence of uncertainty is why, since the 1970s, women health activists have demanded endometriosis be perceived not as a "fertility problem" but as a substantial health burden requiring state funding and support. Recent research supports arguments that endometriosis is not merely a "low value" disease, but a complex one caused by various genetic and environmental factors affecting more and more people yearly such that sociologist Kate Seear has termed it a "modern epidemic" more common than breast and ovarian cancer (2018).

A major issue stems from the fact that diagnosis of endometriosis is delayed. On average, it takes seven to ten years to receive a diagnosis, and that's primarily in the Global North where access to medical care and diagnostic imaging tends to be more stable.[13] Even then, the costs are high: one study, for instance, showed that patients with longer diagnostic delays for endometriosis had higher healthcare utilization and costs (Surrey et al. 2020). Diagnostic delays are complicated by the fact that symptoms vary amongst endo suffers and tend to be vague or overlap with other conditions such as fibroids, urinary tract infections, or irritable bowel syndrome. **Diagnosis can take many years; there is almost a gaslighting that occurs until an encounter during a laparoscopy, for example, confirms the very real pain and inflammation. This profound encounter confirms all the thoughts, painful days and nights, and the radical hope a persistent patient has for recognition of a very real experience.** To report on pain in the face of medical sexism and gender health disparities also means that pain alone isn't taken seriously when it is the *only* consistent symptom, as it tends to be in the early stages of the disease or in endo suffers with superficial endometriosis. But in some cases, the disease doesn't cause any visible symptoms, even as it ravages the pelvic area, or pelvic exams produce normal findings, leading doctors to operate with a "working diagnosis" of eliminating all possible disorders before endometriosis is the only viable diagnosis left. This means waiting, trying multiple treatments, being neglected or dismissed, and, of course, suffering. And this is not including the problem of cultural misconceptions about menstruation, in which debilitating pain, projectile vomiting, and heaving bleeding, to name a few, are consistently declared to be part of the "normal" condition of having a menstruating body.

In the 1940s, new pelvic endoscopic techniques were introduced to differentiate between endometriosis and other conditions such as appendicitis and salpingitis (Hudson 2022, 22). Combined with medical history, physical examination, and targeted ultrasound imaging, it was possible to suspect a

13 "People in the Global South who are marginalized and do not have access to healthcare and diagnostic imaging due to poverty and/or cultural stigma surrounding invasive procedures stand to be the most disenfranchised. There needs to be culturally sensitive care available to these groups so that they can have equitable access to procedures that could drastically improve the quality of their lives" (from Virdi and Bhanot's shared collaboration notes).

diagnosis of endometriosis, but mostly when it caused associated conditions that were visible on imaging tests. Not until the 1970s, when laparoscopic techniques were introduced, was surgery presented as an option. Keyhole laparoscopy, in which small incisions are made in the abdomen to excise endometrium from the pelvis, emerged in the 1980s and quickly became considered the "gold standard" for confirming the disease with pathology, as well as a treatment. Still, laparoscopy is problematic as a first-line diagnostic tool (Parasar, Ozcan, and Terry 2017). It is invasive and expensive, and not always useful for deep lesions. And again, because of the variability of symptoms, not all patients who report extreme pain can have major evidence of lesions for laparoscopic excision. Imaging tests such as CT or MRI can also miss deep, severe endometrial lesions.

Supposedly there are new noninvasive tests for accurately diagnosing endometriosis.[14] *Can you imagine what this would mean for sufferers who no longer need to wait years for confirmation? That they can squeeze through the gender health gap and receive medical care as soon as they need it?*

Pain, however, does not always show up on screen. Nor does it always correlate with the severity of endometriosis (Helosvuori and Oikkonen 2023). The measurements—the verbal ratings scale, visual analog scale, brief pain inventory, or McGill pain questionnaire—are limited, in that they "can fail to capture an experience as multifaceted as pain," reducing a complex interplay of alignments to a biomedical form of knowledge that fails to capture a person's embodied experience of pain and disease (Padfield 2021, 151). Tools for measuring pain cannot always "capture the nuances and complexities of persistent pain," and as such, endo sufferers tend to create their own spectrum of pain sensation to determine how and when to seek out clinical care that corresponds to the progression of the illness and symptoms (Helosvuori and Oikkonen 2023, 14). When we're desperate to be believed, when our pain is being dismissed as something "minor" or "tolerable," we look to these imaging technologies in the hopes that embodied sensations of pain are translated to biomedical data. It's not merely

14 The test, "EndoTect," was developed by Dr. Barbara Guinn at the University of Hull, to identify specific proteins that are increased in the urine of endometriosis patients. Announced in 2023, the test supposedly will have the potential to indicate whether patients have deep or superficial endometriosis. A quick search showed that several other noninvasive diagnostic tests for endometriosis launched over the past few years: a similar test created by Hera Biotech, a San Antonio startup (2024), a blood test for microRNA markers created by US company DotLab (2023), AI system IMAGENDO developed at University of Adelaide in Australia in partnership with University of Surrey in UK (2023), a microRNA signature for diagnosing through a saliva test created by French researchers (2022), and a version of a menstrual cup to identify biomarkers created by students at the University of Rochester (2020). I'm sure I've missed some more. None of these tests are certain nor (yet?) advocated as a new gold standard for diagnosing endometriosis.

about verifying the presence of the disease or to link subjective experiences to pathology, it's to establish a connection between our embodied experience and clinical expertise, one that can form expectations about the lived reality of endometriosis.

Sensing pain, Elina Helosvuori and Venla Oikkonen argue, "is not a passive state happening to a person but involves actively distinguishing between the nuances of pain. Embodied experiences of pain engender knowledge" (Helosvuori and Oikkonen 2023, 6). That is, as endo sufferers know all too well, we not only create descriptive language to specify the location and kind of pain, but often, to stress the urgency of the pain to be clinically acknowledged, we also continuously self-assess (*Doubt? No, minimize*) the severity of embodied pain experience. We make decisions on when the pain is manageable, how much over-the-counter pain remedies are needed, and calculate the length of time the hot compress/heating pad/water bottle needs to be placed on the sore spots. Repeatedly, we make this assessment because the trauma of going to emergency care and narrating the same story only to be gaslit or dismissed, has to be measured against the level of energy to be exhausted from this action. Scans and lab tests can be ordered but, most of the time, they tell nothing significant, or at least, they cannot capture the subjective experiences that hide beneath the skin. The skill of managing pain, of untangling the tendrils to become somewhat—even slightly—bearable characterized most of my days. Calculations of treatment versus pain intensity overwhelmed my mind, hours of searching and reading online to find a new combination, a new calculation that would lessen the severity of the aching, throbbing, burning feeling I lived with daily. I learned cilantro could help with the endo bloat; I begged Geoff to go to the store immediately to get me a bunch. **The present and future all involve waiting. Waiting to be believed, waiting for a referral, waiting for a test, waiting for a procedure, waiting, waiting, waiting.**

There was that night I convinced myself that it wasn't too bad, that I could manage it with a soak in a tub of Epsom salts as Geoff suggested. **It was important to include Geoff in this**

composition because he is part of her journey and at times might be the only one beside her in the darkest times of need and vulnerability. He set up the tub and kissed me good night as he headed to bed; I spent an hour, maybe, watching my shows on the iPad and feeling the muscle pain slowly lessen. Then as I got up from the tub and wrapped myself in a towel, the searing agony hit me suddenly in a wave that I'd never experienced before. I collapsed on the floor, sobbing and waiting for it to pass, and later—I don't know how long—I realized I had passed out. The door was closed. Geoff, utterly exhausted, had fallen asleep. Our dog, Lizzie, presumably had joined him. No one was near to hear my cries. Too tired to get up, body too contorted to untangle itself, I decided to stay on the rug until the next wave of pain hit—because it always comes in waves, this I knew for certain. I pulled down the towel from the rack to create a make-shift pillow and—*oh here it is, here is the wave. Oh, this is the worst. I can't do this. I can't do this. I can't I can't I can't*—tried to ease the pain the best I could. I made sure I drank water. But with each successive wave—*I can't I can't I can't*—I ended up throwing up or emptying my bowels, dizziness enveloping my mind; at one point, my vision went blurry. What could I do? *I can't I can't I can't*—I felt like I did everything I possibly could. It had felt good being in the tub, so maybe another bath? I turned on the water and added more Epsom salts. I soaked for a while longer. Then when I got up again, I immediately collapsed on the floor again and the cycle repeated. Then it was daybreak, according to my iPad, for how else would I know, having spent the entire night in the windowless bathroom? I couldn't take it anymore. I wrapped myself with a towel and went into the bedroom to wake Geoff and tell him to call an ambulance. Then, with the last of my strength gone, I collapsed on the bed, only to be woken up when the paramedics arrived. Geoff put one of his T-shirts on me as I was placed on the gurney and taken away. I was acutely aware of how vulnerable and naked I was, covered with just this thin fabric and a blanket, but I didn't care. I had no energy left. It hurt to breathe. *I can't. I want this to be over.*

Please help me.

3
Expertise

We insisted on a note indicating that I am a historian of medicine be included in my patient file. If all the healthcare providers were not going to take me seriously as a patient with embodied expertise and specialized—even if it's subjective—knowledge of endometriosis, then perhaps they would consider me as an intellectual with a doctorate. It's bittersweet to share that this strategy worked. The language they used around me and Geoff was more specific, they were more forthcoming about my condition, and considered me as an equal (*or at least as close to one*) for assessing the many scans and tests that arrived their way.

I keep thinking about the thousands—millions—of disenfranchised people whose embodied experience of the disease was denied or neglected, because their expertise wasn't presumed valuable enough (*authoritative enough?*) to enter the realm of decision-making. They end up floating in a liminal space, where they are both experts and not experts of their own body. Emma Whelan expands on Kristen Barker's term "epistemological purgatory" (2002, 281), describing it as a space where "lived experience of illness is contradicted by a lack of objective confirmation" (2007, 957).[15] And when we layer this perspective upon feminist disability theory, we cannot help but feel lost. The omission is troubling, Jones tells us, especially given the gendered nature of endometriosis (Jones 2016). A pain-centric model of disability provides us a model for understanding the depths of the disease—lived experiences of pain and critiques of the medical infrastructure shape how we can (*how we should*) accept the realities of endo existence (Jones 2016, 58).

Pain has no voice, Elaine Scarry reminds us, but when we give it space to communicate, it can tell a story. The language endo sufferers use to describe their pain encompasses a level of expertise that connects the feeling with the location (*a stabbing in my lower abdomen. sharp and precise. always right here. it is consistent*). We see this too in illness narratives, long beloved

15 Nicky Hudson picks up on this too: "pelvic pain becomes a liminal subjective experience which is willfully ignored in the development of formal definitions" (2022, 24).

sources by historians of medicine for understanding the experiences of the sick in the past. Even seemingly mundane encounters of catching a cold have been documented by people struggling to understand their suffering and their varied attempts of finding medical, moral, and/or spiritual solutions to lessen their burdens (L. W. Smith 2008, 462; Abel 2006; Huisman 2006; Porter 1985).

Merging with medical imaging and clinical encounters, the experience of pain does not become *real* to the world unless the pain can be *seen*. After all, isn't this what it means to live with an "invisible" disease, in that it does not exist until it becomes "visible" to others? As Emily Abel notes, "absence of objective data also increases the difficulty of convincing doctors that problems are 'real'" (2021, 19). Clinicians, of course, work to establish the significance of a patient's pain through the medical gaze, but as many endo sufferers have testified, without associated confirmation through imaging, it is difficult for them to do so (Helosvuori and Oikkonen 2023, 9). This creates an additional challenge in which different forms of expertise clash, making it difficult even to create formal guidelines for assessment. The UK, for instance, did not publish clinical guidelines for managing endometriosis until 2017 (Hudson 2022, 25). As Jeannette Pols succinctly puts it, "the idea of patient knowledge blurs the boundaries with different forms of knowledge, without adding up to the same knowledge" (2014, 84).[16] Pain *is* a form of knowledge scarred on the body and tangled with memory.

Pols argues that patient knowledge—or, patient expertise—requires doing additional work beyond proving that the embodied experience exists. It requires doing work of "*translating* medical parameters into practical courses of action" (Pols 2014, 88). To be seated in a clinical room and converse with a clinician/surgeon/physician about the results of medical imaging means to co-share different perspectives, and hence, different knowledge. When Geoff and I were shown the results of my scans, we affirmed what the surgeon explained with the reality of our experiences: *Oh yes, that bleeding*

16 She continues: "Medical knowledge is used in daily life practices, and hence changes into something else. Oxygen saturation turns into judgmental gazes, prescriptions that sound obvious in the doctor's office bump into old routines. Distinctions between medical and other matters are ultimately irrelevant to patients. To them. Medical practice is always a daily life practice" (Pols 2014, 84).

explains why I keep needing a hot water bottle compress on this specific area of my abdomen, which Geoff keeps regularly refilling for me. The correlation of the medical imaging with my embodied experience gives credibility to the surgeon's assessment of the severity of the endometriosis, which begs an important question that I want to borrow from Pols: "If patient knowledge is co-shaped in medical practices and influenced by medical knowledge and technologies, can we not assume that medical knowledge is *the same* as patient knowledge?" (2014, 77).[17] Why is it one or the other when both are coproduced for a better understanding of the truth of disease experience, especially one as elusive as endometriosis?

17 Of course, there's the epistemic risk factor here as well about whose expertise matters more, if at all. See Kukla (2019).

I open my blue cabinet to take out the early twentieth-century gynecology textbook that I once purchased from a bookstore in Kennett Square that was having a closing-out sale. I don't know anything about its author—Howard A. Kelly—and I'm sure I'll research it another time, but for now, I merely want to see where endometriosis fits in this text from 1908. It's a heavy one, slightly over 660 pages. I set it on my dining table and flip through the glossy pages, letting words and illustrations wash over me until I get to the index. On page 623, there is a listing for "endometriosis," with 22 sub-lists, from "abortion, caused by," to "uterine hemorrhage from." Defining "acute endometriosis" and "chronic endometriosis," the textbook tells us that "this is a rare condition" (1908, 160). There are no special symptoms connected with it; diagnosis is made only through examination of the curetted tissue and histology. I go through the list and flip to the pages, seeking a discussion of endometriosis pain. There's only a discussion in relation to menstruation.

I take out another book, this one from 1946. There's an entire chapter on endometriosis and the second sentence gives me pause: "Once considered a pathological curiosity, endometriosis is today a major gynecological problem. . . . [O]ne may expect to find endometriosis in 1 out of every 4 patients who are operated upon for some pelvic condition" (Holmes 1946, 317). I take out yet another book. "Removal of both ovaries cures the condition, but castration should not be done in women under 40. . . . As many endometriotic nodules as possible should be removed surgically or destroyed by cauterization, because every one of these tiny areas can grow and spread" (Greenhill 1946, 504). Going on eighty years, and hardly anything has changed. Ella Shohat writes of this: "The erasure of women's agency in medical discourse is deeply ingrained in class and racial discourses, grounding the racialized female body differently, and even in opposite ways" (1998, 250). The same language (*except now it's "one in ten" for the most part, with castration—I mean, hysterectomy—increasingly advisable as a cure*) tends to appear in recent literature, and the perspectives of endo sufferers tend to be minimized. I guess the more things (*don't*) change, the more they (*obviously*) stay the same?

Putting aside dusty medical textbooks and looking into books published by endo sufferers, we have a multitude of experiences on endometriosis written through the lens of pain. Kate Seear emphasizes that these early books can be classified as self-help books and were not simply about awareness or increasing access to information about endometriosis: "They aim to also motivate them to take action, propagating the idea that women can manage the disease and their symptoms, or even prevent it from recurring or proliferating. The central message of these self-help books is that endometriosis can be overcome" (2018, 86). Pain, disability, chronic illness, these are the predominant themes in this literature, a need to lessen the suffering of others who are likely being—or will be—misdiagnosed, gaslit, and neglected in their search for a diagnosis.

Recent literature, including works by Abby Norman (2018), Maya Dusenbery (2018), Elinor Cleghorn (2021), Rachel E. Gross (2022), and Gabrielle Jackson (2019), strives to go beyond self-help. Collectively they demand a new call for action, providing deeply researched evidence on the numerous ways women's health and gendered dimensions of pain have been systematically mistreated within the medical establishment, insisting on new funding and new research for the twenty-first century. Here, they carry on the legacy of nearly a century of women's health activists who have demanded the same (Kline 2010; Dudley-Shotwell 2020; Nelson 2015; Smith 1995). The expertise they provide is a different sort, one that materially brings the clinician-patient encounter in the consulting room in sharp relief to community and care, using narration, art, and shared experience to collapse the distinction between physiological and psychological pain (Padfield 2021, 171). They give us a simple promise: that we are not alone.

4
Exposition

I've chosen watercolor as the medium for this composition because of its fluid and changeable nature, much like the nature of endometriosis. The subjective experiences of chronic pain force those who suffer to live in the gray through various stages of their medical journey. This gray area can be considered a liminal space, a blur between what is black and white, between knowing and not knowing. I have used layers and wet-on-wet techniques in this composition to heighten the aesthetic of a blur and revel in the overwhelm. The color palette and tendrils that appear between its layers speak to the compounding impact of living with chronic pain, while visualizing various moments in the paper where Jai invites the reader into her imagination, painting a picture of the tendrils by describing their color, shape, and relentless spread. Lastly, the act of me creating this composition by reading Jai's experiences through a lens of my own subjective experiences with invisible pain allows the birth of something new and perhaps unimagined. We must be radical in our pursuit of understanding with regard to endometriosis. This pursuit extends beyond objective medical research and instead thrives on vulnerability, collaboration, and community.

The unfortunate truth about pain, as Whelan documents, is that "when I experience pain, its reality is insistent and self-evident to me. But only to me. To others, my pain can be nothing more than my *account* of my pain. Not only can my account of my pain never capture fully my experience of it; my account can neither be verified nor disconfirmed by others" (2007, 463). When we attempt to define, measure, theorize, scan it, it exists only as a representation, not an actuality, a brief reprieve from the liminal space in which it lives. "Pain is ineffable and elusive," Whelan says, and I agree, but it can be captured and assessed through layered expertise (*surgeon, sufferer, supporter*), to be recreated as an intersubjective description of lived experience. When we can make the invisible visible, we give credence to a person's reality (Kapsalis 1997). We assure them that what they are going through is real, not imagined, that their body—*body's archive*—is a manifestation of their expertise.

When I see the tangled tendrils within my skin, my body, I hold on to the aesthetics of radical hope **that lie in indicators like joy, rage, pain, and refusal.** I refuse to be cast aside **and these experiences in real life and digital spaces, in majority and minority cultures, in homes and outside spaces,** in the "objective" clinic and the "subjective" bedroom where pain seeks to be defined, **in homes and outside spaces,** together these are all part of the multitude of experiences, **layered and intersectional, they read as a mess of connections that do not need to be sorted to be understood.** Perhaps we need the tangled connections, to let our community tendrils grow.

A

Abbott, J. A., J. Hawe, R. D. Clayton, and R. Garry (2003) "The Effects and Effectiveness of Laparoscopic Excision of Endometriosis: A Prospective Study with 2–5 Year Follow-Up." *Human Reproduction* 18, no. 9: 1922–27.

Abel, Emily K. (2006) *Suffering in the Land of Sunshine: A Los Angeles Illness Narrative*. Critical Issues in Health and Medicine. New Brunswick, NJ: Rutgers University Press.

Abel, Emily K. (2021) *Sick and Tired: An Intimate History of Fatigue*. Studies in Social Medicine. Chapel Hill: The University of North Carolina Press.

B

Barker, Kristin Kay (2002) "Self-Help Literature and the Making of an Illness Identity: The Case of Fibromyalgia Syndrome (FMS)." *Social Problems* 49, no. 3: 279–300.

Barker, Kristin Kay (2005) *The Fibromyalgia Story: Medical Authority and Women's Worlds of Pain*. Philadelphia: Temple University Press.

Baruch, Kerri (1999) "Endiometriosis: Bleeding Body and Soul." *Agenda: Empowering Women for Gender Equity* 41, Education and Transformation: 92–95.

Bhanot, Nimisha (2015) *Badass Desi Pinups*. Artist's website: https://www.nimishabhanot.com/badassdesipinups.

Biernoff, Suzannah (2021) "Picturing Pain." In *Encountering Pain: Hearing, Seeing, Speaking*, edited by Deborah Padfield and Joanna M. Zakrzewska. London: UCL Press.

C

Carel, Havi (2008) *Illness: The Cry of the Flesh*. Stocksfield: Acumen.

Casper, Stephen T., and Kelly O'Donnell (2020) "The Punch-Drunk Boxer and the Battered Wife: Gender and Brain Injury Research." *Social Science & Medicine* 245: 112688.

Cleghorn, Elinor (2021) *Unwell Women: A Journey of Medicine and Myth in a Man-Made World*. London: Weidenfeld & Nicolson.

D

Daston, Lorraine, and Peter Galison (2007) *Objectivity*. New York: Zone Books.

Denny, Elaine (2009) "'I Never Know from One Day to Another How I Will Feel': Pain and Uncertainty in Women with Endometriosis." *Qualitative Health Research* 19, no. 7: 985–95.

Dudley-Shotwell, Hannah (2020) *Revolutionizing Women's Healthcare: The Feminist Self-Help Movement in America*. New Brunswick, NJ: Rutgers University Press.

Dusenbery, Maya (2018) *Doing Harm: The Truth about How Bad Medicine and Lazy Science Leave Women Dismissed, Misdiagnosed, and Sick*. New York: HarperCollins.

E

Ellis, Katherine, Deborah Munro, and Jennifer Clarke (2022) "Endometriosis Is Undervalued: A Call to Action." *Frontiers in Global Women's Health* 3: 902371.

Elson, Jean (2004) *Am I Still a Woman? Hysterectomy and Gender Identity*. Philadelphia: Temple University Press.

F

Foucault, Michel (1975) *The Birth of the Clinic: An Archaeology of Medical Perception*. New York: Vintage Books.

Foxhall, Katherine (2019) *Migraine: A History*. Baltimore: Johns Hopkins University Press.

G

Greenhill, J. P., ed. (1946) *The 1946 Year Book of Obstetrics and Gynecology*. Chicago: The Year Book Publishers.

Gross, Rachel E. (2022) *Vagina Obscura an Anatomical Voyage*. New York: W. W. Norton & Company.

H

Helosvuori, Elina, and Venla Oikkonen (2023) "Sensing Pain: Embodied Knowledge in Endometriosis." *Health (London)* 28, no. 6: 937–52. https://journals.sagepub.com/doi/10.1177/13634593231214938.

Holmes, Walter R. (1946) "Endometriosis." In *Progress in Gynecology*, edited by Joe V. Meigs and Somers H. Strugis, 317–27. New York: Grune & Strutton.

Howell, Joel D. (1995) *Technology in the Hospital: Transforming Patient Care in the Early Twentieth Century*. Baltimore: Johns Hopkins University Press.

Hudson, Nicky (2022) "The Missed Disease? Endometriosis as an Example of 'Undone Science.'" *Reproductive Biomedicine & Society Online* 14: 20–27.

Huisman, Frank, ed. (2006) *Locating Medical History: The Stories and Their Meanings*. Baltimore: Johns Hopkins University Press.

J

Jackson, Gabrielle (2019) *Pain and Prejudice: A Call to Arms for Women and Their Bodies*. London: Piatkus.

Jaffe, Carrie (1986) "Endometriosis—What Is It?" *Off Our Backs* 16, no. 2: 31.

Jones, Cara E. (2014) "Taking the Woman out of Women's Health." *Nursing Clio* (blog). https://nursingclio.org/2014/03/13/taking-the-woman-out-of-womens-health/.

Jones, Cara E. (2015) "Wandering Wombs and 'Female Troubles': The Hysterical Origins, Symptoms, and Treatments of Endometriosis." *Women's Studies* 44, no. 8: 1083–1113.

Jones, Cara E. (2016) "The Pain of Endo Existence: Toward a Feminist Disability Studies Reading of Endometriosis." *Hypatia* 31, no. 3: 554–71.

Joyce, Kelly (2005) "Appealing Images: Magnetic Resonance Imaging and the Production of Authoritative Knowledge." *Social Studies of Science* 35, no. 3: 437–62.

K

Kapsalis, Terri (1997) *Public Privates: Performing Gynecology from Both Ends of the Speculum*. Durham, NC: Duke University Press.

Kelly, Howard A. (1908) *Medical Gynecology*. New York: Appleton.

King, Helen (1998) *Hippocrates' Woman: Reading the Female Body in Ancient Greece*. London: Routledge.

Kline, Wendy (2010) *Bodies of Knowledge: Sexuality, Reproduction, and Women's Health in the Second Wave*. Chicago: University of Chicago Press.

Kukla, Rebecca (2019) "Infertility, Epistemic Risk, and Disease Definitions." *Synthese* 196, no. 11: 4409–28.

L

Lau, Travis Chi Wing (2020) "The Crip Poetics of Pain." *Amodern* 10. https://amodern.net/article/the-crip-poetics-of-pain/.

Lavine, Matthew (2011) "The Early Clinical X-Ray in the United States: Patient Experiences and Public Perceptions." *Journal of the History of Medicine and Allied Sciences* 67, no. 4: 587–625.

Meyer, Cheryl L. (1997) *The Wandering Uterus: Politics and the Reproductive Rights of Women*. New York: New York University Press.

N

Nelson, Jennifer (2015) *More than Medicine: A History of the Feminist Women's Health Movement*. New York: New York University Press.

Norman, Abby (2018) *Ask Me about My Uterus: A Quest to Make Doctors Believe in Women's Pain.* New York: Nation Books.

P

Padfield, Deborah (2021) "The Photograph as a Mediating Space in Clinical and Creative Encounters." In *Encountering Pain*, edited by Deborah Padfield and Joanna M. Zakrzewska, 147–76. Hearing, Seeing, Speaking. London: UCL Press.

Parasar, Parveen, Pinar Ozcan, and Kathryn L. Terry (2017) "Endometriosis: Epidemiology, Diagnosis and Clinical Management." *Current Obstetrics and Gynecology Reports* 6, no. 1: 34–41.

Pols, Jeannette (2014) "Knowing Patients: Turning Patient Knowledge into Science." *Science, Technology, & Human Values* 39, no. 1: 73–97.

Porter, Roy (1985) "The Patient's View: Doing Medical History from Below." *Theory and Society* 14, no. 2: 175–98.

Prasad, Amit (2005) "Making Images/Making Bodies: Visibilizing and Disciplining through Magnetic Resonance Imaging (MRI)." *Science Technology & Human Values – SCI TECHNOL HUM VAL* 30: 291–316.

S

Sanmiguel, Lisa Michelle (2000) "From 'Career Woman's' Disease to 'an Epidemic Ignored': Endometriosis in United States Culture since 1948." PhD diss. University of Illinois at Urbana-Champaign.

Saorsa, Jac, and Rebecca Phillips (2019) *Like Any Other Woman: The Lived Experience of Gynaecological Cancer*. Cardiff: Cardiff University Press.

Scarry, Elaine (1987) *The Body in Pain: The Making and Unmaking of the World*. New York: Oxford University Press.

Seear, Kate (2018) *The Makings of a Modern Epidemic: Endometriosis, Gender and Politics*. London: Routledge.

Shohat, Ella (1998) "'Lasers for Ladies': Endo Discourse and the Inscriptions of Science." In *The Visible Woman: Imaging Technologies, Gender, and Science*, edited by Paula A. Treichler, Constance Penley, and Lisa Cartwright, 240–70. New York: New York University Press.

Smith, Lisa Wynne (2008) "'An Account of an Unaccountable Distemper': The Experience of Pain in Early Eighteenth-Century England and France." *Eighteenth-Century Studies* 41, no. 4: 459–80.

Smith, Susan L. (1995) *Sick and Tired of Being Sick and Tired: Black Women's Health Activism in America, 1890–1950*. Philadelphia: University of Pennsylvania Press.

Sontag, Susan (1977) *Illness as Metaphor*. New York: Farrar, Straus and Giroux.

Surrey, Eric, Ahmed M. Soliman, Helen

Trenz, Cori Blauer-Peterson, and Ashley Sluis (2020) "Impact of Endometriosis Diagnostic Delays on Healthcare Resource Utilization and Costs." *Advances in Therapy* 37, no. 3: 1087–99.

T

Treichler, Paula A., Lisa Cartwright, and Constance Penley (1998) "Paradoxes of Visibility." In *The Visible Woman: Imaging Technologies, Gender, and Science*, edited by Paula A. Treichler, Constance Penley, and Lisa Cartwright, 1–17. New York: New York University Press.

W

Wahl, Kate J., Paul J. Yong, Philippa Bridge-Cook, Catherine Allaire, and EndoAct Canada (2021) "Endometriosis in Canada: It Is Time for Collaboration to Advance Patient-Oriented, Evidence-Based Policy, Care, and Research." *Journal of Obstetrics and Gynaecology Canada*: 43, no. 1: 88–90.

Whelan, Emma (2007) "'No One Agrees Except for Those of Us Who Have It': Endometriosis Patients as an Epistemological Community." *Sociology of Health & Illness* 29, no. 7: 957–82.

World Health Organization (2023) "Endometriosis: Key Factors." https://www.who.int/news-room/fact-sheets/detail/endometriosis.

Mediating Fatigue: From Promotional Material of Pharmaceuticals in the 1960s to Statistical Maps of Brain Dysfunction in Present-Day Neuroimaging Research

Paula Muhr and Milton Fernando Gonzalez Rodriguez

This chapter examines how different kinds of images have been deployed in disparate medical contexts to render long-term fatigue—an elusive and quintessentially intangible pathological physical and mental condition—visually communicable and epistemically explorable in the mid-twentieth and early twenty-first centuries. Historically, fatigue has been a vaguely defined concept whose semantic borders and theories of etiology have shifted over the centuries (Vigarello 2020). Equated with intense tiredness and exhaustion that most commonly follow overstimulation or overexertion, fatigue was, at different times, attributed to the loss of bodily humors, spiritual failings, depletion of energy, or diminished physical force. Defined in such broad terms, fatigue was not considered inherently pathological during most of its history (Rabinbach 1990; Shorter 1993).[1] This changed in the second half of the nineteenth century. With the advent of laboratory-based investigations that deployed novel techniques of scientific visualization, such as chronophotographs and graphical tracing, fatigue was framed as a physiological deficiency of the working human body, understood through the body-machine analogy

1 For a diverging interpretation that links fatigue to the ancient Greek medical discourse on melancholia, see Schaffner (2016).

(Mosso 1906; Kesselring 2013; Rabinbach 1990). Redefined as a distinctly pathological condition related to "the breakdown of mental and physical system" (Rabinbach 1990, 39), fatigue entered the medical discourse and came to be regarded as a disorder of the nervous system. It was expanded to include heterogeneous symptoms, including apathy, muscular pain, irritation, and weakness, and codified into distinct clinical categories, such as neurasthenia.[2] The late nineteenth century also marked the emergence of medical research into the neuropathology of chronic mental and physical fatigue, which has been ongoing ever since (Kesselring 2013).

Throughout the twentieth century, chronic fatigue vacillated in the medical discourse between an unspecific symptom of ill physical or mental health, and a medical disorder in its own right (Berrios 1990; Shorter 1993). The current nosological designation of chronic fatigue syndrome (CFS) as a distinct disorder was introduced in the late 1980s (Holmes et al. 1988) and later underwent multiple updates of the case definition and diagnostic criteria (Carruthers et al. 2003; Carruthers et al. 2011; Fukuda et al. 1994; Committee on the Diagnostic Criteria for Myalgic Encephalomyelitis/Chronic Fatigue Syndrome 2015).[3] Over the past few decades, CFS has been continually considered a highly controversial disorder that is difficult to reliably diagnose, leading to nowadays predominantly female patients often being dismissed as simulators (Geraghty and Esmail 2016). Similar disbelief about the physical reality of patients' disabling fatigue-based symptoms has also haunted more recent and possibly CFS-related disorders such as long Covid (Byrne 2022).[4] Thus, despite a century and a half of empirical investigation and the currently intensifying biomedical research into its pathophysiological underpinnings (Friedman 2019), chronic fatigue remains an elusive condition that persistently evades medical explainability and thwarts continued attempts to develop effective treatments.

From the mid-1800s to the present day, medical and physiological discourses on fatigue have encompassed a multiplicity of images, including photographs, curves, drawings, graphs,

2 On the conceptualization of neurasthenia, see Beard (1869), Gosling (1987), and Gijswijt-Hofstra and Porter (2001). On the gender and class aspects of neurasthenia, which in the US and many European countries tended to be more often attributed to upper-class men, see Lian and Bondevik (2015).

3 Currently, the most commonly used nosological designation of the disorder is myalgic encephalomyelitis/chronic fatigue syndrome (ME/CFS). The term *myalgic* encephalomyelitis was first used in the mid-1950s to describe the outbreak of an unknown illness among hospital staff in London during an epidemic of poliomyelitis (Anonymous 1956). Holmes et al. (1988) introduced the label CFS as a descriptive designation for a fatigue-related condition initially linked to the Epstein-Barr virus but for which the causal link to the virus became doubtful. Carruthers et al. (2003) shifted to the umbrella term ME/CFS, emphasizing that this multisymptomatic condition can be triggered by a pathogen but also by a stressful event or physical injury. However, whether ME and CFS are two names for the same medical condition or two distinct conditions remains debated (Jason et al. 2016). To circumvent this debate and retain the focus on fatigue, the designation CFS will be used here. For historical analyses that differently relate CFS to the nineteenth-century concept of neurasthenia, see Shorter (1993) and Straus (1991). For a sociocultural analysis of the historical construction of CFS, see Lian and Bondevik (2015).

4 For a medical comparison of CFS and post-Covid-19, see Komaroff and Lipkin (2023).

electromyography signals, and functional magnetic resonance imaging (fMRI). These have been mobilized to make different aspects of this slippery condition perceivable, measurable, explorable, graspable, and communicable. Providing an exhaustive overview or even a broad typology of the varied uses of scientific visualizations of fatigue across different historical contexts and medical specializations is not this chapter's intended goal. Instead, the aim here is twofold. First, by focusing on two disparate case studies, we intend to perform in-depth analyses of select context-specific uses of images in mediating the production and dissemination of biomedical knowledge of fatigue in different historical contexts. Second, through such an unusual juxtaposition of two mutually independent case studies, each written by a separate author, we want to exemplify the heterogeneity of context-specific functions that diverse images have fulfilled in the medical discourse on fatigue. To achieve this twofold aim, we selected two case studies from different historical periods and medical contexts, characterized by different conceptual framings of fatigue and the use of different types of images, whose separate analyses necessitated employing two different methodological approaches.

The first case study, by Milton Fernando Gonzalez Rodriguez, addresses fatigue as an unspecific symptom of ill health and examines how novel medical treatments for this vague symptom were negotiated in the advertisements of invigorating pharmaceuticals in the 1960s in Latin America. The explicitly gendered images of fatigued and/or indefatigable male subjects that appear in this context were aimed at prescribing physicians and, to a lesser degree, potential users. Yet, by tracing multidirectional "exchanges among culture, lived experience, and medicine" (Schaffner 2016, 11), Gonzalez Rodriguez shows that the meaning of these seemingly approachable medical images is far from self-evident, and their semantic readability is not a given. Through a detailed epistemic semiotic analysis of the exemplary advertisements of three performance-enhancing medications, Gonzalez Rodriguez discloses ideological, discursive, and symbolic aspects of this medical imagery.[5]

5 An epistemic semiotic analysis builds on the notion that images document states "of being, but also of knowing (*episteme*)" (Gonzalez Rodriguez 2022, xiii), and hence entails reviewing visual cues in terms of purpose, relatedness, referentiality, and content, as well, as legibility, circulation, and articulation.

He discusses the targeted deployment of images as tools that both challenge and reinforce long-standing cultural assumptions about fatigue through metaphorical promises of therapeutic benefits that are closely linked to the claims of medical advancement in understanding fatigue. This case study thus demonstrates how the visual communication of medical knowledge about the newly developed fatigue-reducing treatments, which strived for informativeness and persuasiveness, was encoded into images through strategies that responded to and influenced context-specific cultural values.

The second case study, by Paula Muhr, focuses on two scientific papers published in the late 2010s in specialized international neurology journals, which report novel findings of the emerging neuroimaging research into the neurophysiological mechanisms of CFS. This case study thus introduces a change in perspective. It addresses fatigue as a distinct, although still contested, multisymptomatic neurological disorder and examines images—in this case, functional brain maps—that are produced in a research context and explicitly target a specialist audience.[6] By approaching brain maps as operative images (Krämer 2009)—visual inscriptions that open new spaces for interacting with the object they visualize—Muhr investigates how researchers create such images as epistemic tools for obtaining new empirical findings on CFS's underlying neuropathology. Specifically, she draws on science and technology studies (STS) (Latour 1999) to analyze the protracted process through which these seemingly straightforward images are produced within specific experimental arrangements. Of interest here are not images as polished outputs of experiments, but the complex and highly context-specific operations of image-making that differ from experiment to experiment yet remain invisible in the resulting images.[7] As we will see, these operations entail an intertwining of physical measurements, algorithmic processing, statistical modeling, theoretical assumptions, and expert human judgment. Among other aspects, Muhr's analysis reveals the implicitly gendered character of brain maps, which, unlike the images discussed by Gonzalez

6 Functional brain maps frequently migrate from specialized journals into mass media, reaching lay audiences. However, since this case study examines how such maps function within a particular research context, their circulation and reception in nonspecialist settings will not be addressed here.

7 Statistical maps of brain activity and connectivity can be visualized in different ways. These include grayscale brain sections superimposed with colorful blobs that designate statistically significant activation patterns, as well as more abstract graphs of connectivity patterns. Thus visualized, brain maps may appear straightforward, yet they are uninterpretable for a lay audience (Muhr 2022). Muhr, therefore, chose not to include stand-alone figures of brain maps in this chapter but only to integrate them into her schematic visualizations of the brain maps' production process.

Rodriguez, is not readily apparent on the surface of brain maps. Overall, Muhr traces how brain maps are currently utilized to expand the medical understanding of CFS and deliver much-needed preliminary visual evidence for the neurophysiological reality of patients' subjective experiences of chronic fatigue.

Jointly, the two mutually complementary case studies comprising this chapter aim to show that scientific images of fatigue cannot be reduced to passive illustrations of preexisting medical notions. Instead, Gonzalez Rodriguez and Muhr argue that different types of images operate across heterogeneous medical contexts as dynamic visual devices that mediate the production and shape the dissemination of historically situated biomedical knowledge of fatigue, thus influencing how this elusive pathological condition is understood and experienced by specific audiences.

Case Study 1: Portraying Fatigue in Pharmaceutical Advertisement

Intake of substances for performance enhancement is a century-old practice.[8] There is an even longer history of using special plant- and animal-based preparations, various types of fluids and secretions, and even human and animal parts in the hope of increasing levels of vigor, vitality, and performance.[9] In the early twentieth century, a pharmacological understanding of roborant medicines derived from plants emerged (Toomey 1929), resulting in a long-lasting interest in substances that could mitigate fatigue, or manage the illness's symptoms and perceived reduced performance. The extensive work on testosterone in the first decades of the twentieth century resulted in the creation of substances with anabolic effect (Kochakian 1946). By the 1960s, roborant medicines were available across the world in the form of pills, drops, or injectable solutions, recommended for daily use.[10]

Building on an epistemic semiotic approach (Gonzalez Rodriguez 2022), the following discussion focuses on the advertisements mobilized by European laboratories to promote Vibolin, Sostenon, and Festavital as invigorating medicines

8 Changes in lifestyles and increased demands on economic production associated with capitalism are believed to have exacerbated the prevalence of fatigue-related symptoms (Thomas 2018).

9 See among others the discussion in Lieutaud (1816), Powell (1849), Inman (1860), Stevens (1909), and Wood (1928).

10 Across Latin America, innovations in medicine evoked a sense of "unbridled optimism borne by new technologies" (Cueto and Palmer 2014, 149) in the second half of the twentieth century.

across Spanish-speaking Latin America, particularly in Mexico and Chile. Whereas Vibolin and Sostenon are preparations based on anabolic steroids, Festavital is a multivitamin compound enriched with other ingredients (e.g., pancreatic enzymes). By situating the images of promotional material within the multitudes of efforts made to reach patients,[11] we see how biomedical knowledge was coded and mediated through technical images and specific visual styles, and which narratives about fatigue as an illness or a symptom of illness were privileged and mobilized.[12]

By the 1960s, fatigue, affecting millions worldwide, was often directly linked to deficient intake of vitamins and minerals.[13] Amidst advancements in chemistry, biology, and pharmacy, fortified stimulants, such as anabolic steroids, became a new way to combat fatigue, despite limited information about their adverse effects. Vibolin and Sostenon, originally developed by the well-established Dutch pharmaceutical company Organon Laboratories, came to the market between 1961 and 1964. Although these medicines would probably not be approved for their intended purpose today, the drugs gained popularity in the 1960s.[14] With a promise to invigorate users suffering from fatigue, Vibolin captured the imagination and attention of physicians and patients seeking potentially more effective vitality-enhancing drugs. In Mexico and Chile, Vibolin was widely marketed as a roborant medicine, containing not only vitamins and minerals, but also ethylestrenol, an anabolic steroid.[15] Soon after its approval for medical use in 1961, ethylestrenol[16] became available in the form of pills. Like other androgen-anabolic steroids, it accelerates protein synthesis and cell growth, including that of muscles, while having a short-term impact on the maintenance of virilizing traits (Tauchen, Jurášek, and Rimpelová 2021). Even if it is a rather weak muscle growth enhancer, ethylestrenol has also been used in veterinary settings and is routinely screened in animals in cases of suspected illegal steroid use. As for clinical settings, according to the World Health Organization, ethylestrenol remains available in some

11 See Dumit (2012) and Sismondo and Greene (2015).
12 As Armus and Gómez remind us, "The sociocultural history of disease and healing emphasizes the complexity of both illnesses and health as concepts, and not only as problems in themselves but also as tools for discussing other topics" (2021, 60).
13 As in earlier decades, vitamins once again became central to general discussions about various ailments, symptoms, and conditions (see Apple 1996). For a historical perspective on minerals, refer to McDowell (2017).
14 For the history of testosterone, see Morgentaler and Traish (2020), Jordan-Young and Karkazis (2019), and Morales (2013).
15 For a discussion on the history of steroid hormones in the Latin American context, see Laveaga (2005; 2015).
16 Also known as ethyloestrenol or ethylnandrol

countries for the treatment of fibrinolytic activity and debilitating diseases,[17] and is listed as a controlled substance in protocols against doping in sports.[18] Other brand names for ethylestrenol-based drugs have included Dexabolin, Ethylnandrol, Fertabolin, and Neodurabolin.

Organon also launched a campaign to inform doctors across the region about other recently developed drugs. As the text in the advertisement asserts, FIG. 3 this new medication called Sostenon was composed of different testosterone esters, which were gradually released thus leading to a rapid, sustained, and uniform effect.[19] It was particularly marketed as an enhancer of physical vigor, sexual drive, and potency. This claim suggests a sophisticated understanding of the formula's pharmacokinetics and drug delivery, appealing to consumers' desire for reliable and consistent results. The use of specific percentages (80–100 percent of maximum androgenic activity) adds a sense of precision and credibility to the claim, potentially enhancing its persuasiveness.[20] The text suggests that Sostenon contributes to normalizing overall physical vigor, tapping into common concerns among individuals experiencing age-related declines in testosterone levels or hormonal imbalances. In this sense, Organon markets this pharmaceutical innovation as a solution to fatigue as a cluster of ailments or symptoms of an illness experienced by aging men. The advertisement reinforces the logic of stereotypical expectations in terms of performance, vitality, and sexual health. It also links the notions of virility and potency to the encapsulated set of ideas about testosterone (Nieschlag and Nieschlag 2017). One notable claim made in the text states that Sostenon achieves its effects without causing exaggerated or undesirable excitement of the libido—an assertion that addresses potential concerns of hypersexuality or increased aggression as side effects of testosterone therapy. By emphasizing the medication's ability to achieve desired outcomes while minimizing undesirable effects, the advertisement seeks to reassure physicians and patients about its safety and tolerability.

Anabolic therapies had become one of the strategies of pharmaceutical companies to create a market of patients for

17 Mainly such as aplastic anemia and neoplasia.

18 For more details on its prohibited use in sport-related contexts and nonmedical settings, see the International Convention against Doping in Sport (2005), as well as an overview of prohibited substances and methods (Mazzoni, Barroso, and Rabin 2011).

19 Sostenon (Sustanon) is a combination of three testosterone esters (testosterone propionate, testosterone phenylpropionate, and testosterone isocaproate), all of which are androgens/anabolic steroids.

20 In contrast, this kind of explicit information is absent in the advertisements for Festavital and Vibolin.

fatigue-related medicines. Advertisements targeting physicians invited them to recognize the profound impact of fatigue as a pervasive phenomenon affecting individuals across all age groups, genders, and socioeconomic backgrounds.

21 For comparison, see Lysen (2015) on the discursive notion of scientificity prevalent around the 1960s, put in practice to convey an idea of modernity and progress.

Fatigue Management in Images and Words

Advertisements suggest that fatigue is a condition that can be effectively managed with pharmaceutical interventions. The contrast between a slow, old car and a modern, advanced vehicle alludes to the common understanding of fatigue as a state of physical or mental exhaustion characterized by a lack of energy and motivation. A state that could be managed. With the logo, "Cuando las vitaminas solas no bastan" (When vitamins alone are not enough), Organon underlines the fact that micronutrients are not enough to treat tiredness, as it is expected to impair cognitive function and potentially diminish overall performance. The visual centerpiece of the advertisement FIG. 1 is a depiction of an ultrarapid race car speeding across the page.[21] The before-and-after drawings imply that an effective fortifying stimulant is the key to unlocking one's full potential. The image can also be read in terms of the direction the car is going to; the new car races across the page, into the future, whereas the old car jolts along back into the past. The accompanying text is carefully worded to resonate with self-enhancement aspirations. Bold headlines proclaimed the transformative power of Vibolin, promising to banish fatigue, sharpen focus, and unleash boundless energy. The before-and-after drawings operate as promises to potential consumers. Imagined scenarios that serve as a testament to the efficacy of the anabolic formula.

The advertisement begins by identifying the target patient as the one who "does not get better," suffers from various conditions such as "organic poverty," "constitutional weakness," and "lack of defenses." By framing fatigue and lack of energy as a chronic health issue, the advertisement establishes a relatable problem that many individuals may experience. The drug is presented as the solution to these problems, claiming to powerfully promote the "vital tendency" toward "assimilation," "repair," and "health"—all underlined terms in the text. This language emphasizes the drug's purported ability to address the root causes of fatigue and to enhance overall well-being.

The advertisement presents Vibolin's key ingredient, ethylestrenol, as a vital component that promotes repair processes within the body and describes it as an essential eutrophic agent. Additionally, the inclusion of still-popular vitamins, minerals, and trace elements suggests a holistic approach to supplementation, providing essential nutrients necessary for optimal energy levels.

Pharmaceutical solutions for the fast-paced hustle and bustle of modern life that left many drained, weary, and burdened by the weight of exhaustion were a relatively untapped market in Latin America. Following the increased presence of vitamin-fortifying formulas, Hoechst from Germany introduced Festavital across the region. Festavital contained a mixture of vitamins and pancreatic enzymes. The advertisement shown in figure **2**, presumably dated from 1964, states that the medicine is "el primer polivitamínico con minerales, factores lipotrópicos y enzimas pancreáticas" (the first multivitamin with minerals, lipotropic factors, and pancreatic enzymes). If the medicine were taken three times a day after each meal in the form of one or two pills, Festavital would purportedly help to prevent "premature wear," and was recommended for the treatment of chronic digestive conditions and vitamin shortage.

Festavital was a solution for those confined in the weariness of every day. The playful advertisement alluded to a transformative journey from tiredness and lethargy into rejuvenation and renewal. The before-and-after Festavital drawings poignantly capture the evolution of a tired older man from a state of physical exhaustion to one of boundless energy and freedom, all through the power of multivitamin supplementation. In the before setting, on the left side of the page, the advertisement depicts a dejected adult male hunched over in an old-fashioned armchair. He clutches a cane in one hand, while

Cuando
las vitaminas
SOLAS
no bastan ....
VIBOLIN eutrófico
da el impulso vital decisivo
En el paciente que no prospera.... el que padece de "pobreza orgánica", "debilidad constitucional", "falta de defensas".... en el que resultan inadecuados los recursos terapéuticos intrínsecamente más idóneos.... VIBOLIN impulsa poderosamente la tendencia vital hacia la asimilación, la reparación y la salud.... VIBOLIN proporciona un agente eutrófico esencial - etilestrenol - y los factores que aseguran su eficacia: vitaminas, minerales y oligo-elementos....
PRESENTACION:
Fcos. de 25 y
100 Tabletas
VIBOLIN 'Organon' es el roborante racional, idóneo para niños, adultos y ancianos de uno u otro sexo.... es compatible con cualquier otra medicación y seguro y confiable a dosis terapéuticas.
Organon
Kloosterstraat 6, Oss Holanda.
2-266/129-NE
Reg. No. 62617 S.S.A.
Literatura exclusiva para médicos
P. Med. 12191/65 S. S. A.
1966

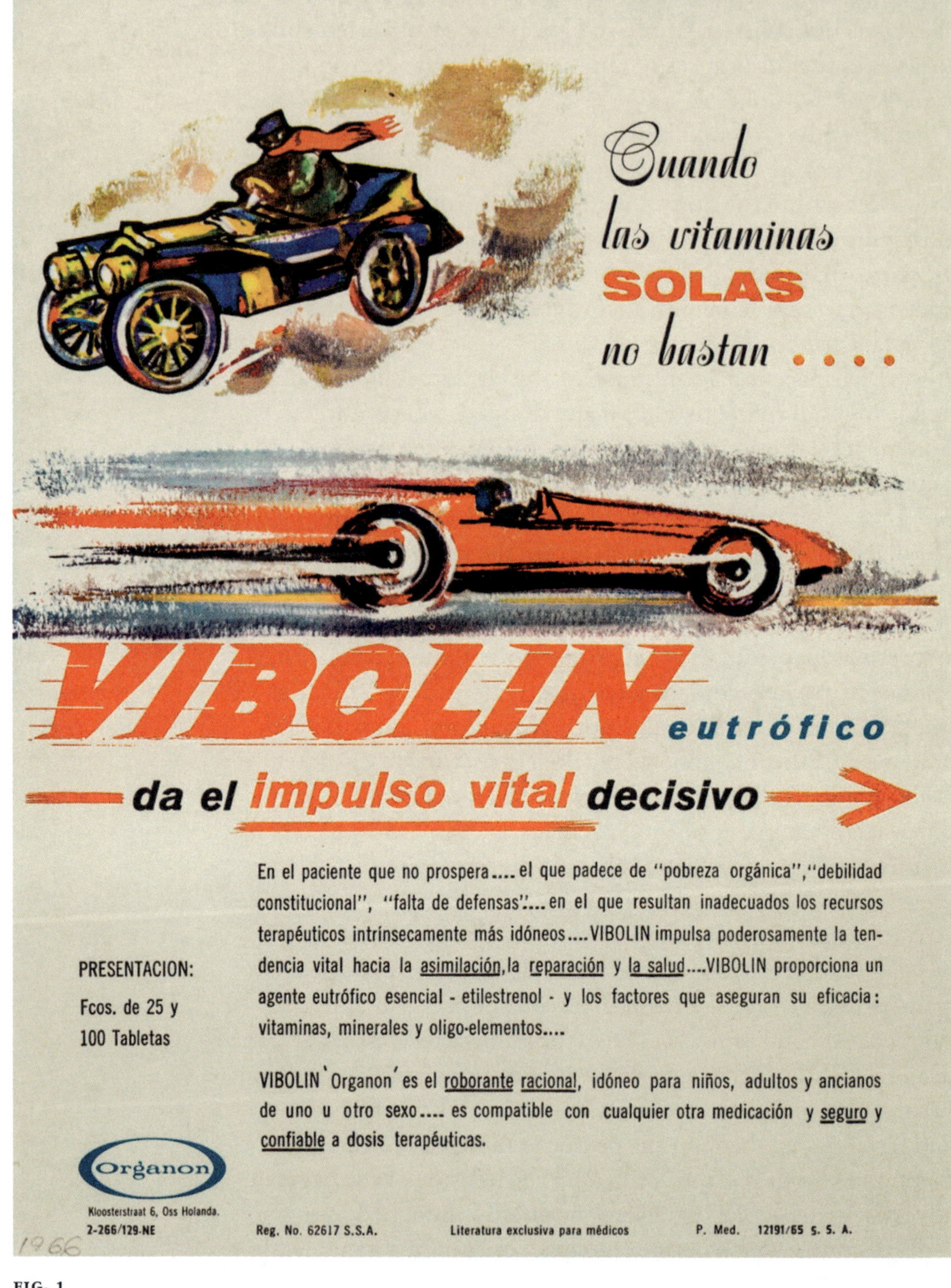

FIG. 1

FIG. 1 Vibolin, Organon, "Aliviar la tos es todo? No para Bredon jarabe, grageas, supositorios: Cuando las vitaminas solas no bastan . . . Vibolin eutrófico da elimpulso vital decisivo," advertisement, 1966. Wellcome Collection. https://wellcomecollection.org/works/tgmaw6my

his legs rest wearily on a footrest. Beside him, hangs a cage containing two birds, which serves as a metaphor for his own perceived sense of captivity by his exhaustion. Because the man is a line drawing, his skin tone is the green background color, emphasizing his sickliness and further reinforcing the sense of resignation and despondency for him and the birds alike. The imagery evokes the essence of stagnation, aging, and lack of vigor in daily life that presumably afflicts many of those male patients seeking medical advice to treat tiredness. On the right side, the advertisement shows a remarkable transformation, made possible by the man's presumed use of Hoechst's Festavital. The effect of the miraculous multivitamin supplementation has allowed him to reclaim his vitality and zest for life. Now sporting a perky mustache and jaunty bowtie, the man zips along on a stand-up scooter, head held high. The two birds, once confined, soar above his head, their wings outstretched in a boundless sense of freedom. The same green of the background is now perceived as verdant and springlike and complements the now rosy glow of his cheeks. The dynamic comparison of the side-by-side visuals reflect the transition from a state of weariness to one of vitality, liberation, and exuberance.

In contrast, the promotional material for Sostenon does not rely on imagined before-and-after scenarios. The image of a cartoon knight wielding a sword and shield serves as a powerful metaphor in the advertisement for synthesized testosterone as a treatment for lack of energy among men. FIG. 3 Instead of a handsome, youthful knight in shining armor, the advertisement wittily depicts the chevalier in question as the target consumer. The stocky, middle-aged warrior, painted in matte hues, lumbers toward the viewer with his sword held high. He is an awkward hero, but nevertheless embodies strength, resilience, and readiness to confront any middle-age-related battle. Drawing on the common symbolism of the knight, the sword iconographically alludes to the vigor needed to conquer challenges and problems, while the shield invokes ideas about the need to protect oneself against external threats and

FIG. 2 Festival, Festal, "Festavital, el primer polivitamínico con minerales, factores lipotrópicos y enimas pancreáticas," advertisement, [1964?]. Wellcome Collection. https://wellcomecollection.org/works/gyzcrv6z

FIG. 3 Sostenon, Organon, "Vigor y virilidad con Sostenon 'Organon,'" advertisement, 1961. Wellcome Collection. https://wellcomecollection.org/works/nzbcx9zc

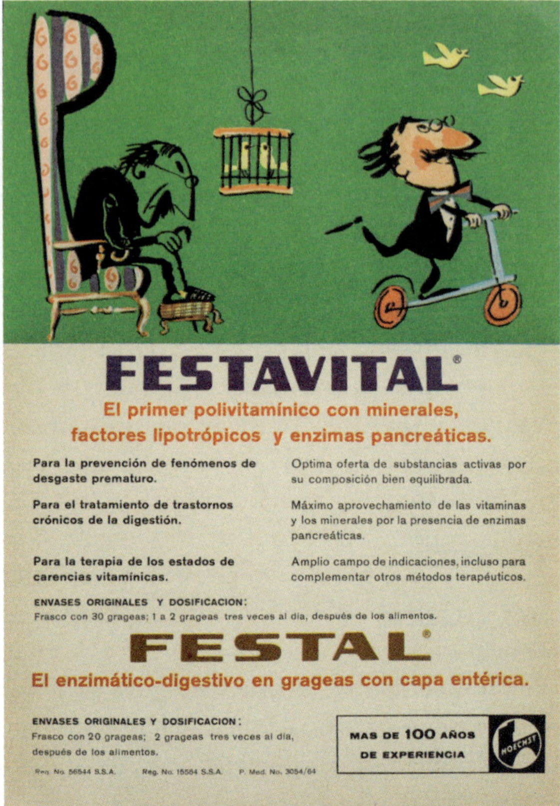

FIG. 2

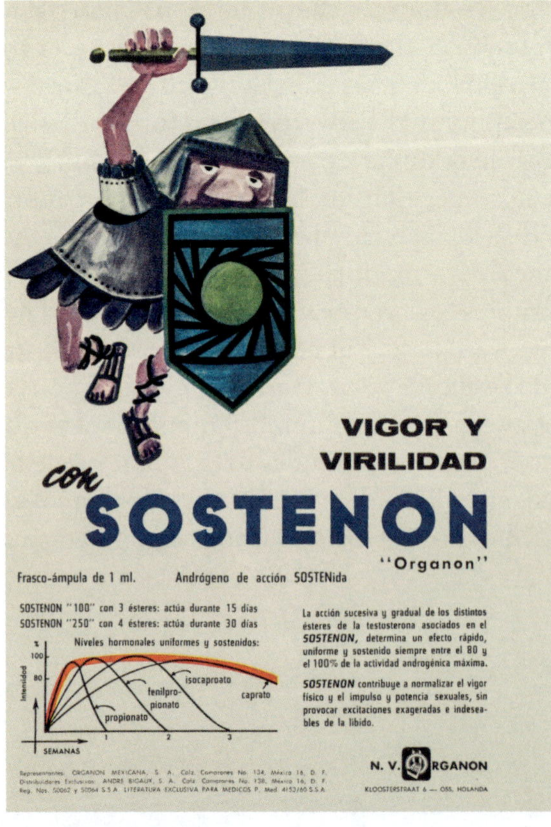

FIG. 3

vulnerabilities. Together, they evoke a sense of vitality and invincibility, reinforcing the message that with synthesized testosterone, individuals can arm themselves against the debilitating effects of impotency and lack of energy and vigor.

22 For a discussion on the pharmaceutical markets in Latin America in the 1960s, see Gereffi (2017).

Mediating and Articulating Efficacy

The introduction of anabolic therapies offered a glimmer of hope in the management of fatigue. In hindsight, the anabolic therapies for tiredness management were not as completely safe as their advertisements claimed. Vibolin's promotional material, for instance, mirrors medical and regulatory standards of the time. Additionally, the cultural and societal context of the 1960s, including prevailing attitudes toward health and medication, would have influenced consumers' perceptions of the advertisement and the product it promotes.[22] Although the main character in the Vibolin advertisement is a man, a notable aspect of the advertisement is its assertion that ethylestrenol is suitable for individuals of all ages and genders, including children, adults, and the elderly. This broad applicability makes the product allegedly accessible to a wide range of consumers, positioning it as a versatile solution for fatigue and diminished general performance across different demographic groups. Another key point emphasized by Organon in the advertisement is the safety and reliability of the fortifying formula. Vibolin is described as compatible with any other medication and safe for therapeutic use at recommended doses. This reassurance regarding safety and compatibility is likely intended to alleviate potential concerns or hesitations that physicians may have about recommending or prescribing this new drug to their patients.

In terms of effectiveness and efficacy, the advertisement employs persuasive language, scientific state-of-the-art terminology, and reassurances regarding safety. In addition to its persuasive appeal, the advertisement subtly seeks to encourage its audience to act. The racing flashy car urges viewers to use available pharmaceutical innovations and embark on their journey to self-enhancement. Time emerges as a trope implicit in the types of vehicles depicted in the images and the velocity at which they can drive. This adds a sense of urgency, compelling target users to act swiftly and emphasizing a stereotypical male-car symbolic relationship. Ultimately, the advertisement for Vibolin is more than just a marketing ploy. It reflects its time, in terms of the state-of-art knowledge about anabolic formulas, and it serves as a testament to an appetite for fatigue management pharmaceutical preparations, an appetite for medicinal efficacy in the management of fatigue.

In like manner, the inclusion of a graphic illustrating Sostenon's absorption and sustained effects adds visual appeal and reinforces the textual claims. The graphic depicts a pharmacokinetic profile showing concentrations of the drug over time, highlighting its modular onset and prolonged duration of action. The claims made align with consumers' desires for effective, safe, and well-tolerated treatments for issues related to physical and sexual health. Additionally, the inclusion of a visual aid enhances the advertisement's credibility, empirical evidence, and clarity, helping consumers visualize how the medication works in the body over time. Scientific jargon and medical terminology lend an air of credibility to the claims made, assuring discerning consumers of Sostenon's rigorous development. References to clinical studies in the form of references to literature in prestigious journals and research findings provide further validation, reinforcing the notion that this drug is not just another passing fad, but a bona fide breakthrough in the field of fatigue management.

Analogously, the leaflet promoting Vibolin emphasizes how effective management of fatigue is essential for enhancing individuals' well-being and functional capacity. The advertisement targeted at physicians is designed to captivate the attention and tap into the desires and expectations of its primary audience, but also those of patients. The fortifying stimulant deploys a combination of scientific terminology and persuasive rhetorical tools. At its core, the advertisement embodied the spirit of an era imbued with a relentless pursuit of self-improvement, optimism, and modernity. An era in which doctors are encouraged to advise patients to use pharmaceutical technologies as much as automobile innovations to achieve self-improvement targets and a sense of fulfillment. Emblazoned with the Organon logo, by then considered a symbol of the quality of European laboratories, Vibolin's advertisement exuded credibility and authority—one of the issues that interest groups, such as the BUKO Pharma-Kampagne, had with this type of advertisement.[23] Western pharmaceutical companies were interested in expanding and solidifying markets of consumers in nations across Africa, Asia, and Latin America (BUKO 1985). Organon's emblem was intended to complement the whimsical cartoon-styled imagery, adding a reference to the pharmaceutical prowess of an innovation developed in the Netherlands.[24] A similar approach was likewise implemented in the promotion of Festavital. Underneath the text and additional information on Festal, enzymatic-digestive pills, the Hoechst logo in the corner of the leaflet boasts "mas [sic] de 100 años de experiencia" (more than one hundred years of experience).

The availability of Festavital, among others, purportedly expanded the horizon of pharmaceutical possibilities for patients of all genders and age groups. Taking vitamins, which had become quite common since the 1950s, was not enough.[25] Hoechst saw the need to develop an enhanced supplement as a solution to those experiencing reduced levels of energy and performance—one that could mitigate all the various physiological, psychological, and environmental factors that contributed to the onset and subsequent severity of fatigue. Additions, such as pancreatic enzymes and lipotropic factors, are presented as a more effective combination to tackle the multifaceted nature of exhaustion, digestive disorders, and "desgaste prematuro" (premature wear and tear of the body). Skeptical of its efficacy, BUKO eventually launched a campaign against the commercialization of Festavital, and by proxy Hoechst, on the grounds that "there is no medical justification for such an irrational mixture" (BUKO 1985, n.p.). The action sought to put pressure on Hoechst to explain why an enhanced supplement was marketed as a medicine that was allegedly

23 BUKO Pharma-Kampagne is an independent organization based in Bielefeld, Germany, that monitors the marketing practices of German pharmaceutical companies.

24 The advertisement concludes by highlighting the manufacturer behind the new drug is a company based in Europe, suggesting a sense of trust and credibility associated with the brand. By emphasizing Organon's endorsement of Vibolin, the advertisement further enhances the product's perceived efficacy and reliability.

25 On the implications and aftermath of the discoveries of vitamins, both in Western contexts and Latin America, see Aguilar Rodríguez (2008), Frankenburg (2009), Rodríguez Osiac (2022).

effective for a series of conditions, without specifying one. BUKO questioned how Festavital was approved in the first place. The main premise of the campaign was to draw attention to the excessive commercialization of vitamin supplements sold by European laboratories in non-Western markets.

Eventually, the multivitamin formula disappeared from pharmacies across the region, as well as Vibolin, although for different reasons. Once anabolic steroids were further researched and it became clear that they were not as safe or effective as advertised, they ceased to be used for (over-the-counter) therapeutic purposes, except for specific cases (i.e., oncology). As for Sostenon (Sustanon), it is still used in modern medicine to treat confirmed testosterone deficiency. An analysis of the advertisement material used to promote Vibolin, Sostenon, and Festavital in Latin America in the 1960s unveils some patterns of how illness is rendered visible. These include the use of imagery that encapsulates how patients experience the conditions they expect pharmaceuticals to mitigate or cure and how advertisers craft a vision of one's future self to the viewer through a combination of claims in both plain terms and medical terminology, and the inclusion of references to the context in which pharmaceutical innovations emerge.

Despite its lack of directly perceptible traits, fatigue has been imaged and thus rendered visible through changing practices of medical visualization. Reviewing the use of visual references in the 1960s, advertisements of medicines prescribed to manage tiredness-related physical symptoms, some patterns emerge. A gendered lens is superimposed on the iconographical representation of fatigue since these are pharmaceutical formulas targeting specific demographic groups. Expectations in terms of performance, vitality, and vigor inform the construction of an idealized, energized body that differs strikingly from an energy-depleted one. Strength is a trait that men apparently ought to exude, and pharmaceutical technologies are a means to attain desired and desirable standards. In the case of advertisement, the goal is to tap into the need of exhausted bodies seeking restoration, implying that fatigue could be pharmaceutically managed.

The male body is used as a reference and target. Lack of vitality is presented as an alteration of an ill-understood condition, yet one that is curable thanks to scientific advances, according to the reviewed promotional material. From this perspective, conclusively, the visibility of fatigue is expressed through an amalgam of symptoms that can be capturable through images and interpretable through cultural references.

Case Study 2: Articulating the Neuropathophysiology of CFS through Functional Brain Maps

Conceptual Framework

Gonzalez Rodriguez's case study showed how fatigue as a vaguely defined sign of ill health was portrayed in pharmaceutical advertisements in the 1960s in Latin America. The following case study shifts the perspective to how CFS, as a specific, albeit contested, multisymptomatic disorder, has been experimentally framed in present-day neuroimaging research with a global scope. Importantly, this case study does not discuss how images mediate existing medical knowledge to the broader public, nor does it approach images "as instruments for [merely] *visualizing* information" (Krämer 2022, 269, emphasis in original). Instead, images are understood here as "tools for *gaining, operating* and *exploring* information" (Krämer 2022, 269, emphasis in original). Accordingly, this analysis examines how researchers deploy a particular cutting-edge neuroimaging technology in specifically designed experimental settings to produce empirical images that operate as active tools for generating new medical insights into the underlying neurophysiology of CFS. It also foregrounds how the context-specific operations involved in producing these images vary across different experiments depending on the research questions posed about CFS.

CFS is a complex, chronic disease characterized by varied symptoms that, besides persistent fatigue, include memory problems, sleep abnormalities, and muscular pain, as well as the defining clinical feature called post-exertional malaise (PEM) that encompasses the exertion-induced worsening of all CFS symptoms (Carruthers et al. 2011). Because of the absence of diagnostic laboratory tests, unknown etiology, and lack of reliable treatments, CFS is often disparagingly equated with hysteria, malingering, or imaginary psychosomatic complaints (Diedrich 2021; Friedman 2019). The view that CFS is entirely psychological or psychosocial causes, thus lacking a biological basis, remains widespread even among medical professionals (Froehlich et al. 2022). However, this view has been contradicted by growing empirical research findings about the CFS patients' multiple physiological anomalies in immune responses, energy metabolism, and nervous system functioning (Rivera et al. 2019; Komaroff 2019). So far, the research findings have remained in the domain of basic science, without applications in clinical practice.

Since 2004, a sustained strand of neurological research has deployed a noninvasive neuroimaging technology called functional magnetic resonance imaging (fMRI) to study the neural basis of CFS patients' elusive symptoms.[26] Using fMRI, researchers indirectly measure neurophysiological correlates of brain activity in living human subjects under controlled experimental conditions.[27] In an fMRI experiment, participants are placed inside a specialized scanner and instructed to perform a particular task (task-based fMRI) or to rest and think of nothing (resting-state fMRI) while the scanner generates imaging data.[28] At the end of the measurement, researchers obtain noisy fMRI data that are illegible even to experts (Muhr 2022). Researchers must submit these data to multiple stages of algorithmic processing and statistical analysis to compute functional brain maps (Huettel, Song, and McCarthy 2009), which they can then interpret, thus making judgments about the experimental subjects' brain activity of interests and correlated cognitive functions.[29]

In medical research, fMRI data are often collected for a group of patients with a particular disorder and a control group that typically consists of healthy subjects. Depending on the type of data analysis performed, the resulting group-level fMRI

26 For the earliest published fMRI-based study of CFS, see de Lange et al. (2004). For a systematic overview of neuroimaging research into CFS until August 2019, which considers diverse imaging technologies besides fMRI, see Maksoud et al. (2020).

27 For a detailed introduction to fMRI, see Huettel, Song, and McCarthy (2009). For a detailed discussion of how fMRI data relate to the neural activity of interest, see Muhr (2022, 304–28)

28 During the measurement, the scanner exposes the participant's brain to a tailored combination of static and dynamic magnetic fields to induce the generation of magnetic resonance signals. The scanner registers the signals and transforms them into sequences of two-dimensional grayscale imaging data that contain information about the subjects' brain anatomy (structural MRI data) and neural activity (fMRI data). Each fMRI experiment starts with acquiring structural MRI before collecting fMRI data. For an accessible account, see Muhr (2022, 275–399).

29 For a succinct discussion of how researchers interpret the patterns of neural activity or connectivity visualized in fMRI maps by correlating them to cognitive function in the neuroimaging research, see Muhr (2022, 238–43, 283–84).

maps can be divided into activation and connectivity brain maps (Huettel, Song, and McCarthy 2009). Activation maps visualize how spatial patterns of statistically significant local task-dependent neural activity of interest differ between patients and control subjects at the group level. Connectivity maps display the differences in the distribution of functional connections across widespread brain regions and networks between patients and control subjects.

In fMRI-based research on CFS, scientists produce functional brain maps aiming to link a particular experimentally isolated aspect of this complex disorder to anatomically localizable dysfunctions of individual brain areas or to disturbances in functional connectivity across distant brain regions. Hence, in the research context, brain maps function as operative images (Krämer 2009; 2022)—they enable scientists to reach and explore the disorder's otherwise inaccessible underlying neuropathophysiology, thus producing new medical insights into CFS and generating visual evidence of its physiological reality. This case study draws on Krämer's (2022, 266–67) claim that the operative images' referentiality, i.e., their ability to provide access to the object they visualize, is neither immediate nor reducible to mimetic similarity. Therefore, of interest here is how the referentiality of fMRI brain maps, understood as a precondition of their knowledge-generating potential, is established through the articulation (Latour 1999) of CFS's neuropathophysiological underpinnings.

As defined by Latour (1999, 142), articulation comprises all experimental interventions that jointly enable the emergence of new insights into a phenomenon of interest through the process of scientific mediation. Importantly, Latour emphasizes the distinctly processual character of articulation. Instead of being a one-off event accomplished in a single step, it involves a chain of successive, interrelated interventions that progressively transform a "mute, unknown, undefined" phenomenon into a well-articulated and hence potentially knowable entity (Latour 1999, 143). Along this chain, the phenomenon of interest is brought into relation to other entities, instruments, models, measurements, inscriptions, and interpretations to draw out its differences. Latour (1999, 69–79) thus designates articulation as the movement along the chain of transformations. He also insists that when scientific images facilitate the articulation of phenomena of interest, the images' referentiality is established through the chains of traceable transformations that underpin the images' production and link each image to a cascade of other images, measurements, protocols, tags, and heterogeneous inscriptions that precede it. Latour thus interchangeably uses the terms *chain of transformations* and *referential chain.*

However, whereas Latour focuses on tracing the sequencing of intermediary steps that form a chain, this analysis highlights the decisions that researchers make at each step to enable the movement along the chain of transformations, thus enacting the articulation of the phenomenon of interest. To emphasize this recalibrated focus, the term *chain of operations* is used here instead of a referential chain. Moreover, as used here, articulation designates the process of linking CFS to its underlying neural basis through the mediation of fMRI with the aim of generating empirical evidence for the physiological reality of patient's experiences of CFS. This case study addresses how such articulation is performed in scientific practice. Accordingly, the analysis does not concentrate on the visual features of brain maps as the empirical output of an fMRI study because, as argued here, such images should not be approached as straightforward representations of CFS's neuropathology. Instead, the focus of analysis is on the chains of operations that underpin the production of brain maps as epistemic tools within concrete experimental setups and on how these operations change across experiments depending on the research questions posed.

Methodologically, the analysis is based on a close reading of two pioneering fMRI studies, one that approached CFS from the clinical perspective of its fluctuating symptom manifestations, whereas the other asked a more technically framed question about potential CFS-related disturbances in neural signal conduction via a specific brain region. Specifically, a team of researchers based in the US published the first fMRI study that explored aberrant patterns of brain activity underlying PEM, a cardinal feature of CFS (Cook et al. 2017). Conversely, a group of Australian researchers authored the first fMRI study that combined resting-state and task-based functional connectivity analyses to examine CFS patients' impaired brainstem connectivity (Barnden et al. 2019).

To trace how the articulation of different aspects of CFS's neuropathology was enacted in these studies depending on the specific research questions their authors aimed to answer, the operations the researchers performed in the four successive stages of each fMRI experiment will be analyzed. While the operations are sequentially described in the methods section of each fMRI study, this analysis will unpack the assumptions underlying each operation. The four successive stages are: first, selecting study participants; second, defining the experimental procedure; third, collecting data; and fourth, processing and analyzing data. The case study's conclusion will discuss the differences in how the articulations of CFS's neuropathology were performed in the two fMRI studies.

Overall, the goal here is not to make overarching claims about the fMRI maps' ability to offer reliable access to CFS's neuropathology nor to identify general conditions under which such reliable access could be achieved. Rather, the aim is to disclose the immense work involved in scientific image-making in fMRI-based research on CFS. While this work remains invisible beyond specialists' circles, it underpins the images' ability to deliver visual evidence for the physical reality of patients' subjective experiences of chronic fatigue, thus effectively countering their dismissal as simulation.

Articulating the Neurophysiology of PEM

As a defining clinical feature of CFS, post-exertional malaise (PEM) denotes patients' "pathological low-threshold fatigability" (Carruthers et al. 2011, 331). It manifests as a delayed exacerbation of patients' diverse symptoms—including pain,

30 For studies that recruit more than two groups, see Washington et al. (2020).

cognitive difficulties, and fatigue—following even mild physical or cognitive exertion. PEM has been investigated by multiple physiological studies (Carruthers et al. 2011, 331–32). However, Cook et al. (2017) were the first to deploy fMRI in an attempt to articulate how PEM, induced under controlled laboratory conditions, affects CFS patients' brain function.

In an fMRI study's initial stage, which precedes data acquisition, researchers select suitable participants by defining inclusion and exclusion criteria. As will be shown, participant selection already partakes in articulating CFS's neuropathology by transforming patients into study participants who exhibit characteristics aligned with the selection criteria. In Cook et al.'s study, which comprised a group of CFS patients and a control group,[30] the focus was on selecting a relatively homogeneous patient sample. This proved challenging as the current research on CFS struggles with diagnosis misclassification due to the parallel use of disparate diagnostic criteria that define cases differently (Nacul et al. 2019). To mitigate potential misclassification, Cook et al. decided not to rely solely on the Fukuda et al. (1994) criteria, as these, although dominant in research, have been increasingly criticized for being "overly inclusive" (Committee on the Diagnostic Criteria for Myalgic Encephalomyelitis/Chronic Fatigue Syndrome 2015, 48) while ignoring PEM as a central CFS feature. Instead, Cook et al. (2017, 88) recruited patients who simultaneously met the Fukuda et al. (1994) and the more stringent Carruthers et al. (2003) criteria. Moreover, to avoid confounding factors that could introduce unwanted neurophysiological variability into fMRI data, Cook et al. excluded from their sample CFS patients diagnosed with psychiatric comorbidities or substance abuse and those receiving immunomodulatory medication.

The joint aim of these operations was to increase the diagnostic specificity of the patient sample by disregarding more ambiguous cases, which abound in clinical practice. It can be assumed that this focus on selecting patients with stringently delineated core CFS symptoms was seen as a precondition for isolating and quantifying the PEM-related exacerbation of these symptoms. However, because of such strict selection criteria, Cook et al. recruited only fifteen patients. Thus, the price for this diagnostic specificity was decreased statistical power of their imaging findings due to the small sample size, which, in turn, potentially limited the statistical validity and reliability of their findings.[31]

The researchers also recruited fifteen healthy control subjects who matched the patients' age and gender. The control subjects were further selected to closely match the patients' weight, height, and varying levels of physical activity (Cook et al. 2017, 88). Such unusually comprehensive matching of bodily features between the groups was epistemically significant. It aimed to minimize the differential non-disease-specific effects that the physical exercise during the experimental procedure could have on patients and control subjects. It also had an added benefit for the subsequent statistical analysis of fMRI data as it reduced the impact that weight and fitness level differences "may have on neurological morphology and function" (Maksoud et al. 2020, 11).

Notably, the study's sample consisted of exclusively female patients. CFS is more frequently diagnosed in women (60–65 percent) than in men (Valdez et al. 2019). Female patients are, therefore, overrepresented in neuroimaging studies, some of which have purely female samples (Maksoud et al. 2020, 11).[32] Although the implicit inscription of gender into fMRI findings through patient sampling is not visible in the brain maps, it has semantic effects. As Cook et al. (2017, 97) emphasized, it remains unclear if the obtained neuroimaging results can be generalized to male patients since the potential role of gender differences in the neuropathology of CFS is unexplored. More problematically, such findings tacitly reinforce the current biased perception of CFS as a predominantly female disorder, which is implicitly stigmatizing (Lian and Bondevik 2015, 932).

In the next stage, Cook et al. defined the conditions of their experimental procedure. Since they aimed to articulate how PEM induced under controlled laboratory conditions

31 On the limited reliability of small-sized fMRI studies, see Button et al. (2013).

32 The current medical gendering of CFS as predominantly female contradicts earlier male-gendered framings of fatigue, as discussed by Gonzalez Rodriguez.

affected CFS patients' brain function, they implemented a pre-test–post-test design, spreading their experimental procedure across three days. Day one entailed the initial acquisition of neuroimaging and non-imaging data. A week later, on day two, participants returned to the laboratory for additional measurements and to perform the PEM-inducing exercise. Finally, 24 hours later, on day three, the researchers collected the second round of fMRI and non-imaging data.

Besides temporally structuring their experimental procedure, Cook et al. specified the PEM-provoking exercise and defined the experimental tasks. They chose a submaximal protocol, a well-established approach for controlled PEM induction in physiological research.[33] It involved a 25-minute steady-state aerobic exercise on a stationary bicycle at an intensity equivalent to 70 percent of each participant's age-predicted maximum heart rate (Cook et al. 2017, 89). Importantly, this standard protocol allowed the researchers to model moderate acute physical exertion—meant to induce PEM in CFS patients—while avoiding physiologically overstressing the participants, which would have introduced confounding physiological effects.

A particularly epistemologically significant aspect of the study was how the researchers designed the experimental tasks that their participants performed during fMRI scanning. In task-based fMRI studies, experimental tasks enable researchers to isolate the differential neurophysiological and cognitive effects of various task components during subsequent data analysis. Hence, the choice of tasks is typically grounded in researchers' assumptions about which cognitive processes are implicated in the phenomenon they study and influenced by the continually evolving theories of the neural basis of cognition (Muhr 2022, 283–285). This was also the case in Cook et al.'s study.

To explore how acute exercise affects CFS patients' diverse physical and cognitive symptoms at the level of neural activity, Cook et al. deployed three separate tasks, which participants executed in sequence. The first was a non-fatiguing

33 For differences between maximal and submaximal exercise protocols, see Noonan and Dean (2000). For different exercise protocols used in CFS research, see Washington et al. (2020).

motor task called finger tapping. During this task, participants were asked to "open and close their right hand, bringing their four fingers in contact with their thumb" at a predetermined rate (Cook et al. 2017, 89). The second was a non-fatiguing cognitive task that entailed simple auditory monitoring and number recognition. During this task, participants listened to a series of numbers from one to ten and had to press a button when they heard the number seven. Unlike the previous two tasks, the third was designed to induce mental fatigue during fMRI scanning and was a modified version of the standardized Paced Auditory Serial Addition Task (PASAT). In the standard PASAT, participants listen to a series of numbers from one to nine, silently adding each new number to the previous one, and are instructed to press the button when the sum of two consecutive numbers equals 10. Initially developed to measure the effects of concussion on the speed of information processing, the PASAT is currently deployed in research for multifactorial assessment of "sustained attention, working memory" and cognitive performance under time constraints (Tombaugh 2006, 65). In the modified PASAT used by Cook et al. (2017, 89), the participants were additionally exposed to distracting visual stimuli in the form of rapidly and randomly changing numbers on the screen that they had to watch while adding the numbers they were hearing.

Based on the above description, it can be argued that Cook et al. designed a complex combination of multiple tasks, each targeting and isolating a particular aspect of the participants' neurocognitive performance in a graded manner. This tailored multiplication of the tasks served to articulate the unknown associations between PEM and the changes in the neural activity underpinning experimental tasks of varying difficulty. Therefore, the tasks were strategically stratified from a non-fatiguing motor over a non-fatiguing cognitive to a mentally fatiguing cognitive task. The tacit assumption guiding this stratification was that PEM, an exertion-induced exacerbation of heterogeneous CFS symptoms, is a cognitively multifactorial and highly variable phenomenon whose explorative fMRI-based decomposition requires a sufficiently complex combination of mutually independent tasks. Moreover, the researchers' decision to modify the standard version of the PASAT and make it more difficult by including distracting elements indicates that they were particularly invested in articulating the neurophysiological effects of PEM that impair CFS patients' ability to perform attention-demanding cognitive tasks.

In the next stage, Cook et al. collected each participant's neuroimaging (fMRI and MRI) and supplementary non-imaging data. Such multimodal data acquisition is a standard approach in fMRI studies because non-imaging data are subsequently incorporated into neuroimaging analyses (Muhr 2022). Yet, the comprehensiveness with which Cook et al. implemented this approach deserves attention. What stands out is the level of detail with which they quantified the participants' exercise-induced changes in symptoms while consistently relating these changes to patients' subjective reports of PEM. On day one of testing, besides acquiring clinical data, Cook et al. (2017, 89) characterized the CFS patients' subjective experience of heterogeneous symptoms (including muscle pain, unrefreshing sleep, fatigue, and memory problems) at baseline using three complementary self-report questionnaires. Directly before and 24 hours after the exercise, participants were administered a visual self-report scale that measured the subjective intensity of ten major CFS symptoms derived from the Carruthers et al. (2003) criteria. Furthermore, while the participants performed the exercise, the researchers collected their cardiorespiratory (oxygen consumption and heart rate), perceptual (subjective rating of perceived exertion and leg muscle pain), and lactate data.

The neuroimaging data were collected on two separate occasions. Each participant's pre- and post-exercise neuroimaging procedures started with the generation of high-resolution anatomical MRI scans, followed by a 25-minute acquisition of fMRI data during the performance of the task sequence (Cook et al. 2017, 89). Over 25 minutes, an fMRI volume that consisted of 40 sagittal slices was collected every two seconds, resulting in a voxel resolution of 3.75 × 3.75 × 5 millimeters.

Simultaneously, the participants' task performance was monitored for correct, incorrect, and omitted responses. During breaks within the tasks, which were divided into blocks, participants were repeatedly asked to rate their perceived levels of mental fatigue. It is apparent that this comprehensive multimodal data collection aimed to integrate various physiological (i.e., cardiopulmonary and lactate data), neurophysiological (i.e., brain activity), and behavioral measurements (i.e., cognitive performance) with the patients' self-reported subjective experiences of the exercise-induced changes in their physical and mental states. Importantly, this integration was pivotal to the researchers' efforts to articulate the neurophysiological basis of CFS patients' subjective experience of PEM.

The fourth stage of articulation involved a long chain of interlinked and increasingly complex statistical data analyses. First, the pre- and post-exercise non-imaging data were analyzed using descriptive statistics and then compared between the patient and control groups. These analyses revealed that, despite reporting greater exertion, patients cycled at significantly lower speeds than controls and, unlike healthy controls, experienced a pronounced exacerbation of all symptoms 24 hours after the exercise (Cook et al. 2017, 90–91). Another relevant finding was that the cognitive performance during scanning improved in control subjects pre- to post-exercise, whereas it significantly decreased in patients. In other words, while controls learned to better perform the PASAT through practice, patients did not.

However, the most insightful results were obtained by analyzing the fMRI data. After applying standard preprocessing steps—including motion correction and normalization—that are required to make the individual subjects' fMRI data mutually comparable (Muhr 2022), Cook et al. first performed whole-brain single-subject analyses for each participant. The resulting single-subject maps served as input for subsequent group-level analyses. In group-level analyses, individual subjects' idiosyncratic task-induced neural responses are treated as noise and eliminated, while amplifying the neural responses shared across the subjects within the group (Muhr 2022, 358). Such statistical aggregation of group effects is meant to identify the disease-specific neural mechanisms common to all patients. Here, the group-level analyses were limited to the predefined regions of interest (ROIS) that, based on their previous fMRI studies of CFS, Cook et al. (2017, 90) hypothesized would be differentially activated in patients and control subjects. They chose the specific ROIS that, according to broader neuroimaging research, partake in motor activity, attention, working memory, and executive functions. Notably, this choice of ROIS was aligned with the cognitive functions that the experimental tasks, including the PASAT, were designed to isolate.

Using the predefined ROIS, Cook et al. performed numerous group-level analyses. FIG. 4 For each of the three experimental tasks, they generated separate fMRI maps that showed the distribution of task-induced statistically relevant brain activations—first at baseline, then post-exercise. They further computed fMRI maps for within-group comparisons of the changes in task-induced brain responses from pre- to post-exercise for each group and each task separately. Next, they produced fMRI maps for between-group comparisons of the changes in task-induced brain responses from pre- to post-exercise for each task separately. Finally, they performed post-hoc analyses to explore "the relationships between metabolic and behavioral data during exercise and brain responses to the PASAT post-exercise" (Cook et al. 2017, 93).

In short, to articulate the neural effects of PEM from their fMRI data, Cook et al. deployed a chain of stratified neuroimaging analyses involving multiple targeted multilevel comparisons within and between groups and pre- versus post-exercise for their three experimental tasks. Each group-level analysis resulted in a separate fMRI map that provided only a partial empirical perspective on the neural effects of PEM. Therefore, to interpret their empirical findings, Cook et al. had to compare the different fMRI maps to one another and thus synthesize their partial, yet complementary, perspectives.

The study's neuroimaging findings are too complex to examine in full detail. Overall, the fMRI maps jointly indicated that the differences in task-induced brain responses between patients and healthy controls, and the changes in task-induced brain responses from pre- to post-exercise in both groups, increased with the task difficulty, becoming most pronounced for the cognitively fatiguing PASAT. The between-group maps for the PASAT were taken to show that, relative to healthy controls, patients exhibited significantly heightened brain responses post-exercise in the brain regions "critical for efficient cognitive processing involving processes associated with attention, error detection, and cognitive control" (Cook et al. 2017, 96). Additionally, the within-group maps revealed that, after the exercise, healthy controls had decreased neural activity and greater performance accuracy on the PASAT, whereas patients showed the opposite development—their cognitive performance declined while their neural activity intensified. Most importantly, the brain maps suggested that the patients' self-reported post-exercise fatigue exacerbation "was significantly and positively related to brain responses in the right inferior parietal and superior temporal cortices" (Cook et al. 2017, 93), thus linking patients' subjective experience of PEM to specific neurophysiological changes.

In sum, the multiple complementary fMRI maps that Cook et al. generated through a chain of interrelated operations FIG. 4 provided preliminary, albeit tentative, empirical insights into possible neural underpinnings of PEM, implicating multiple brain regions. These images also offered cumulative visual support for the physiological reality of patients' subjectively experienced exertion-induced worsening of CFS symptoms. As demonstrated in the preceding analysis, the ability of fMRI maps to fulfill such epistemic functions hinged on the interlinked operations that went into their production, allowing the articulation of the PEM's neural effects in these images. Thus, far from providing direct access to PEM's neural effects, the construction of the highly mediated referentiality of these operative images required extensive work and many

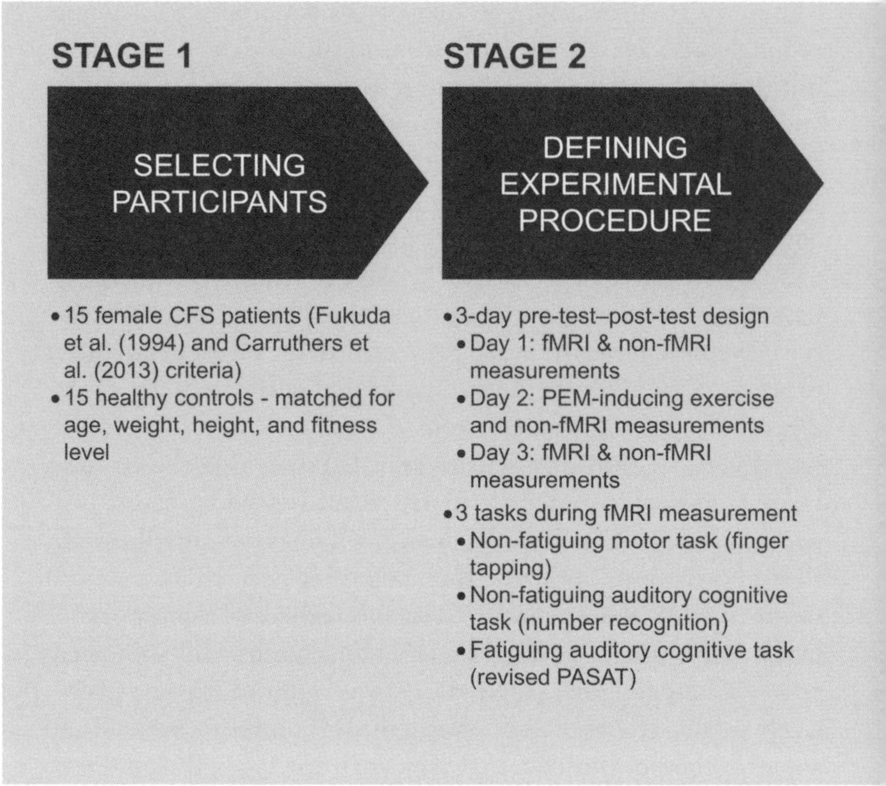

STAGE 1

SELECTING PARTICIPANTS

- 15 female CFS patients (Fukuda et al. (1994) and Carruthers et al. (2013) criteria)
- 15 healthy controls - matched for age, weight, height, and fitness level

STAGE 2

DEFINING EXPERIMENTAL PROCEDURE

- 3-day pre-test–post-test design
  - Day 1: fMRI & non-fMRI measurements
  - Day 2: PEM-inducing exercise and non-fMRI measurements
  - Day 3: fMRI & non-fMRI measurements
- 3 tasks during fMRI measurement
  - Non-fatiguing motor task (finger tapping)
  - Non-fatiguing auditory cognitive task (number recognition)
  - Fatiguing auditory cognitive task (revised PASAT)

FIG. 4

FIG. 4 Chain of operations underpinning the articulation of neural underpinnings of PEM in Cook et al. (2017). Courtesy of Paula Muhr

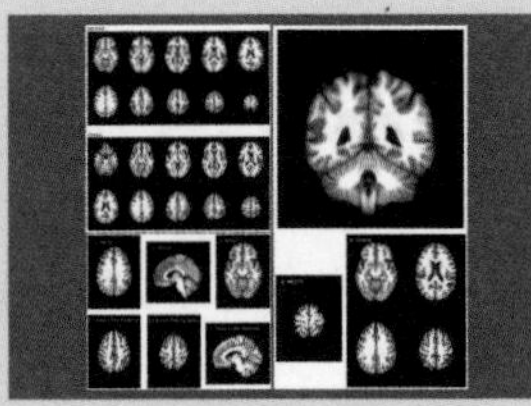

STAGE 3

COLLECTING MULTIMODAL DATA

- Participant characteristics at baseline (3 questionnaires)
- MRI and fMRI pre- & post-exercise
- Task-performance behavioral data during fMRI
- Self-reported symptom assessment: pre- and post-exercise
- Metabolic and behavioral data during exercise

STAGE 4

PROCESSING AND ANALYZING DATA

- Descriptive statistics of non-fMRI data
- fMRI data preprocessing
- Single-subject whole-brain and within-group ROI fMRI activation maps for pre- and post-exercise conditions for each task
- Within-group ROI fMRI activation maps pre- versus post-exercise for each task
- Between-group ROI fMRI activation maps pre- versus post-exercise for each task
- Maps correlating post-exercise PASAT-induced fMRI activations with PEM symptoms

34 The brainstem is the lower part of the brain that connects the brain and the spinal cord.

decisions by researchers, which had to be justified in relation to existing medical knowledge, previous empirical findings, and currently dominant neurological theories. Precisely because the referential quality and the associated epistemic potential of the resulting images are not self-evident, their evaluation necessitates a detailed examination of the chains of operations underlying their production, as performed in this analysis.

Importantly, the chain of operations involved in producing fMRI maps as epistemic tools in CFS research is not standardized. Instead, the choice of operations at each step has to be tailored to a particular research question, meaning that the context-specific adequacy of these operations, which can vary immensely across experiments, needs to be assessed on a case-by-case basis. To exemplify how the fMRI-based articulation changes when researchers pose a different question about CFS's neural underpinnings, we will now analyze Barnden et al.'s 2019 study.

Articulating the Deficient Brainstem Connectivity

Whereas Cook et al. (2017) focused on exploring previously unknown neural effects of CFS's major clinical feature, Barnden et al. (2019, 1) used fMRI to articulate a CFS-related functional brain disturbance that, as they hypothesized, entailed impaired "nerve signal conduction through the brainstem."[34] They derived this hypothesis from previous structural MRI studies that had indicated such a functional disturbance in CFS patients based on neuroanatomical findings. As the following analysis will show, although the articulation comprised the same four stages discussed above, Barnden et al. performed different operations at each stage than Cook et al. to accommodate their specific research question.

To begin with, because their focus was not on CFS's clinical manifestations, Barnden et al. were less concerned with recruiting patients with stringently delineated symptoms. They selected patients based only on the broad Fukuda et al. (1994) diagnostic criteria and did not exclude those with psychiatric comorbidities. Advantageously, these more lenient criteria allowed them to recruit a significantly larger sample of 45 CFS patients, who were predominantly but not exclusively female, thus increasing their findings' statistical power and generalizability across genders.[35] The researchers also enrolled 27 healthy control subjects who matched the patients' age and female-to-male ratio. The large discrepancy in the group sizes, which Barnden et al. did not explain, is puzzling and, as we will see later, presented an obstacle during fMRI analysis.

Next, the researchers defined their fMRI experimental procedure. Since they aimed to articulate the impaired nerve signal conduction through a particular brain region, instead of employing the functional localization approach used by Cook et al., Barnden et al. used the functional integration approach. As discussed earlier, in the localization approach, researchers produce fMRI activation maps to identify the spatial distribution of brain areas activated by a chosen comparison of experimental conditions. Conversely, in the functional integration approach, researchers compute fMRI connectivity maps to infer how spatially distant brain regions "communicate with one another and information is passed from one brain area to the next" (Bijsterbosch, Smith, and Beckmann 2017, 2). The assumption behind statistical functional connectivity analyses, which underpin the production of connectivity maps, is that brain regions whose measured signals correlate over time are functionally connected (Biswal et al. 1995). Typically, such analyses are associated with the resting-state fMRI paradigm that investigates spontaneous fluctuations in brain activity while subjects are not engaged in explicit tasks.[36] More recently, such analyses have been increasingly applied in task-based fMRI studies to examine how the interactions between different brain regions change under different task conditions (Gerchen and Kirsch 2017).

Notably, Barnden et al. used both resting-state and task-based fMRI to articulate the brainstem connectivity deficits in CFS patients compared to healthy controls. Implicit in this decision was the assumption that the connectivity deficits might manifest differently during rest versus an external

35 For the patients' characteristics, see Shan et al. (2018, 280).

36 For an overview of different types of connectivity analyses, which can either be performed on the whole brain or predefined ROIs, see Bijsterbosch, Smith, and Beckmann (2017) and Muhr (2022).

cognitive challenge. In the task-based segment of their study, Barnden et al. employed a variation of the well-known Stroop task, involving color words. Participants were shown word pairs on the monitor and asked to decide if the color of the upper word matched the meaning of the lower word. Barnden et al. selected this task "because it tested the attention and concentration difficulties often reported" by CFS patients (2019, 2). Thus, as in Cook et al.'s study, the task experimentally addressed patients' subjectively experienced disease-related cognitive difficulties.

During the data collection stage, Barnden et al. generated high-resolution structural scans of participants, followed by separate acquisitions of resting-state and task-based fMRI data, each lasting 15 minutes. Compared to Cook et al., they acquired data with considerably higher spatial and temporal resolutions to increase the data's "sensitivity to connectivity changes" (Barnden et al. 2019, 7), a decision that was aligned with their research question.[37] However, the resulting high noise level and signal dropout posed challenges during data processing.

Like Cook et al., Barnden et al. also collected auxiliary non-imaging data. Throughout fMRI acquisition, participants' pulse and respiratory data were measured. Performance metrics, including response times and accuracy, were registered during the Stroop task. However, the study's focus remained primarily on neuroimaging, with less emphasis on physiological and behavioral data. Moreover, clinical symptom characterization was limited to summary scores of participants' physical and mental health issues obtained using a single self-report questionnaire. Although potentially more reductive, this approach aligned with the study's more technically framed research question.

The fourth stage started with substantial preprocessing of the resting-state and task-based datasets. Because fMRI is susceptible to signal distortions in the brainstem during measurement, beyond applying standard preprocessing steps, such as motion correction, Barnden et al. developed a tailored normalization procedure.[38] This operation was required to

37 Altogether, 1,100 resting-state and 1,100 task-based fMRI volumes were acquired. Each fMRI volume, which consisted of 72 sagittal slices, resulting in a voxel size of 2 × 2 × 2 mm, was collected in less than a second (Barnden et al. 2019, 2).

38 For an overview of standard preprocessing steps performed before connectivity analyses, see Bijsterbosch, Smith, and Beckmann (2017, 25–50).

computationally minimize the significant signal dropout in the brainstem, without which data would have been unusable.[39] Additionally, the researchers used the participants' pulse and respiratory measurements to further denoise the fMRI data, reducing the physiological artifacts that might have skewed subsequent connectivity analyses. Barnden et al. judged this preprocessing step necessary because physiological noise in fMRI data is particularly pronounced in the brainstem due to its "proximity to major cerebral arteries" (2019, 6). Hence, whereas preprocessing operations were relatively marginal in Cook et al.'s study, due to the technical challenges of measuring fMRI connectivity in the brainstem, here these operations acquired major epistemic significance.

39 Despite extensive preprocessing, fMRI data from several subjects had to be excluded from the analysis due to "unacceptable signal dropout" (Barnden et al. 2019, 3).

After extensive preprocessing, the researcher defined ten ROIS (regions of interest) for connectivity analyses. Aiming to articulate connectivity deficits within the brainstem, they divided the brainstem into five ROIS, chosen based on earlier structural MRI studies that had implicated them in CFS neuropathology. To explore if potential intra-brainstem connectivity deficits affected connectivity disturbances with other brain regions, Barnden et al. constructed five additional ROIS: one in the cerebellum and four in the bilateral midbrain regions of the hippocampus and the thalamus. These regions were chosen because of their "rich connections" with the brainstem (Barnden et al. 2019, 4). In short, as in Cook et al.'s study, the selection of the ROIS was guided by hypotheses derived from the neuroimaging literature.

To compute the maps, Barnden et al. first submitted their resting-state and task-based fMRI datasets to separate within-group connectivity analyses for patients and healthy controls. However, to perform statistically valid between-group connectivity analyses, they first had to address the disbalance in their group sizes. Since between-group connectivity analyses require equal group sizes for statistical validity, Barnden et al. excluded 18 subjects from the patient group. The final between-group resting-state and task-based connectivity maps were thus computed for equally sized groups and showed the distribution of functional connectivity deficits in CFS patients relative to healthy controls. Additionally, Barnden et al. performed post-hoc analysis to assess the associations between ROI connectivity and the summary symptom severity for each CFS patient in their sample, thus exploring if "impaired brainstem connectivity is an important factor in CFS/ME aetiology" (2019, 5).

As in Cook et al.'s study, the empirical findings were distributed across multiple complementary fMRI maps that had to be interpreted together. The within-group connectivity maps computed separately for patients and controls indicated statistically significant functional connections within the brainstem, as well as between the brainstem and the subcortical nuclei, in each group both during rest and task. The visual comparison of within-group maps revealed that, in both groups, more connections were activated during the Stroop task, when the brainstem "would be actively coordinating cortical arousal and hemodynamic responses," than during rest (Barnden et al. 2019, 5). However, the between-group resting-state map was empty. This negative finding was significant as it suggested the lack of connectivity differences between patients and healthy controls when they were not engaged in explicit cognitive tasks. By contrast, the between-group task-based connectivity map showed reduced functional connections within the brainstem and between the brainstem, the hippocampus, and the thalamus in patients relative to healthy controls. Thus, crucially, their tailor-made chain of operations that combined resting-state and task-based connectivity approaches enabled Barnden et al. to articulate CFS patients' connectivity deficits that became manifest during active cognitive engagement but not during rest. Moreover, the post-hoc analyses suggested a correlation between the impaired brainstem connectivity and the patients' self-reported cumulative symptom severity scores, thus linking these deficits to patients' experience of illness.

Drawing their image-based empirical findings together, Barnden et al. posited that the brainstem connectivity deficits their fMRI maps visualized "can explain autonomic changes and diminish cortical oscillatory coherence which can impair attention, memory, cognitive function, sleep quality and muscle tone, all symptoms of ME/CFS" (2019, 1). Admittedly, this interpretation remained tentative. However, it is noteworthy that the novel medical findings about the potential functional connectivity deficits underpinning CFS, however tentative, were articulated through fMRI maps that also delivered visual support for the physical reality of patients' elusive symptoms. As in Cook et al.'s study, the viability of the tailor-made empirical images to fulfill the attributed epistemic functions depended on the quality of the chains of operations FIG. 5 that underpinned their production and served to establish a referential connection between these images and the fatigue-related phenomena they visualized.

Summing up, let us highlight the differences in how these two studies performed the process of articulation. Whereas Cook et al. aimed to articulate neural correlates of fatigability as CFS's defining clinical feature, Barnden et al. focused on articulating a presumed CFS-related dysfunctional connectivity within and beyond a particular brain region. To address their different research questions using fMRI maps, the researchers lacked standardized image-based solutions. Instead, they had to develop custom-made chains of operations that allowed them to generate new empirical findings about CFS through the mediation of fMRI. As performed by Cook et al., the articulation of CFS's neural basis primarily aimed at reliably linking fMRI and non-fMRI data derived from the detailed characterization of the exertion-induced worsening of clinical features in a homogeneously sampled patient group to the patients' self-reported experiences of PEM. It also entailed a careful dissection of PEM's neurophysiological and cognitive components through stratified experimental tasks. By contrast, the articulation devised by Barnden et al. focused on disentangling how the hypothesized functional connectivity deficits in CFS patients varied between demanding cognitive engagement and rest. Moreover, due to the technological limitations of fMRI, the latter articulation required the inclusion of multiple operations whose goal was to computationally mitigate these limitations.

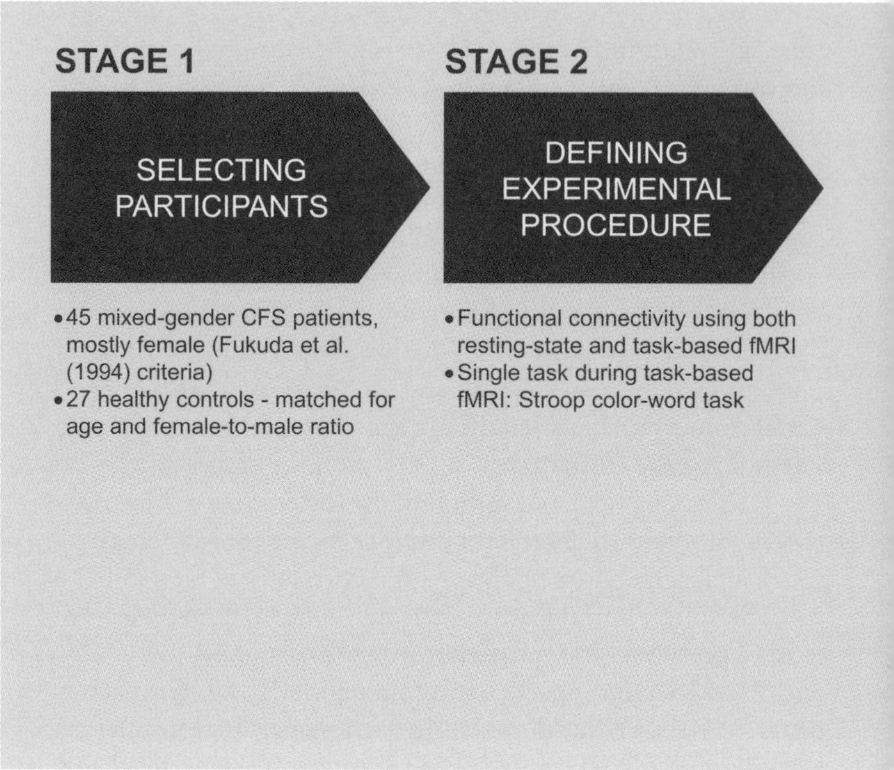

STAGE 1

SELECTING PARTICIPANTS

- 45 mixed-gender CFS patients, mostly female (Fukuda et al. (1994) criteria)
- 27 healthy controls - matched for age and female-to-male ratio

STAGE 2

DEFINING EXPERIMENTAL PROCEDURE

- Functional connectivity using both resting-state and task-based fMRI
- Single task during task-based fMRI: Stroop color-word task

FIG. 5

FIG. 5 Chain of operations underpinning the articulation of connectivity deficits in CFS in Barnden et al. (2019). Courtesy of Paula Muhr

STAGE 3

COLLECTING MULTIMODAL DATA

- MRI, resting-state fMRI, task-based fMRI
- Task-performance behavioral data during task-based fMRI
- Pulse and respiratory data during fMRI measurements
- Summary self-reported scores of symptom severity

STAGE 4

PROCESSING AND ANALYZING DATA

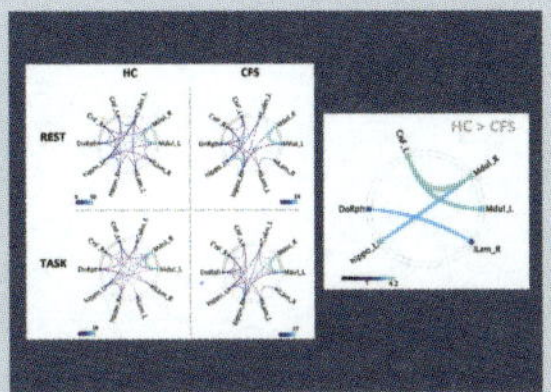

- fMRI data preprocessing:
  - Tailored normalization procedure
  - Data-driven physiological denoising
- Single-subject resting-state & task-based ROI fMRI connectivity maps
- Within-group resting-state & task-based ROI fMRI connectivity maps
- Between-group resting-state and task-based ROI fMRI connectivity maps
- Maps correlating connectivity patterns with CFS symptom severity scores & task performance metrics for each subject

The thus produced fMRI maps made various aspects of CFS's neural underpinning empirically explorable, while also delivering preliminary visual evidence for the physical reality of this still contested illness.

Overall, this case study has traced how the present-day deployment of functional neuroimaging technologies in medical research on CFS has opened new epistemic paths to experimentally articulating the elusive neurophysiological underpinning of chronic fatigue. Yet, it demonstrated that while fMRI mediates access to previously unexplorable aspects of CFS's neuropathophysiology, it also imposes new methodological challenges and limitations that are not readily apparent in the resulting images. Far from being straightforward representations of CFS's neurobiology, fMRI maps, as deployed in research, are highly flexible and versatile knowledge-producing tools whose epistemically pertinent production necessitates an interlinking of a long series of tailored operations that jointly determine what will be made visible in the resulting images and what not. Thus, to understand these images' epistemic import, we need to analyze not how these images look but how they were produced and in which specific contexts.

Conclusion

After a century and a half of medical and physiological research into its pathology and potential treatments, chronic fatigue remains a vaguely understood and elusive condition. To make fatigue tangible and knowable for medical specialists and the wider public, various visualization practices have been deployed in research and clinical practices across historical periods. Rather than providing a general overview of the different kinds of images used and the functions they fulfilled across changing medical contexts, this chapter has aimed to exemplify the diversity of images and their roles by juxtaposing two mutually independent yet complementary case studies. Through his detailed semiotic analysis of the drawings of male subjects in 1960s pharmaceutical advertisements in Latin America, which communicated new medical findings on fatigue treatments and persuaded doctors to prescribe novel medications to patients, Gonzalez Rodriguez has shown how these images both drew on and influenced the cultural experience of fatigue. In her STS-informed analysis, Muhr has examined the complex processes of image-making required to produce fMRI brain maps that present-day scientists use to explore the neuropathophysiological underpinning of chronic fatigue as a distinct nosological category, now predominantly diagnosed in women. Her analysis has revealed how the decisions made during the image-making process inform the resulting brain maps' epistemic efficacy, while remaining invisible on the maps' surface.

Whereas the first case study built on rhetorical visual codes deployed in advertisements intended for mass publications and broad audiences, the latter emphasized the multilayered operational dimensions of images as context-specific tools produced and used in experimental research to generate new empirical findings. The first case study focused on images as a means of negotiating the cultural imaginaries of the ill-understood condition of deflated energy as a target of medical intervention. The second case study zoomed in on the operative conditions under which specific images function as epistemic tools capable of delivering preliminary evidence for the neurophysiological reality of patients' subjective experiences of fatigue. Yet, precisely because of the different visual practices and medical contexts they each examine, the juxtaposition of these two in-depth case studies demonstrates the versatile ways in which images actively mediated the construction of biomedical visions of fatigue across diverse historical contexts.

A

Aguilar Rodriguez, Sandra (2008) "Alimentando a la nación: Género y nutrición en México (1940–1960)." *Revista de Estudios Sociales*, no. 29 (January): 28–41.

Anonymous (1956) "A New Clinical Entity?" *Lancet* 270 (6926): 789–90.

Apple, Rima D. (1996) *Vitamania: Vitamins in American Culture*. New Brunswick, NJ: Rutgers University Press.

Armus, Diego, and Pablo F. Gómez, eds. (2021) *The Gray Zones of Medicine: Healers and History in Latin America*. Pittsburgh, PA: University of Pittsburgh Press. https://doi.org/10.2307/j.ctv1tgx0br.

B

Barnden, Leighton R., Zack Y. Shan, Donald R. Staines, Sonya Marshall-Gradisnik, Kevin Finegan, Timothy Ireland, and Sandeep Bhuta (2019) "Intra Brainstem Connectivity Is Impaired in Chronic Fatigue Syndrome." *NeuroImage Clinical* 24: 102045. https://doi.org/10.1016/j.nicl.2019.102045.

Beard, George (1869) "Neurasthenia, or Nervous Exhaustion." *The Boston Medical and Surgical Journal* 80, no. 13: 217–21. https://doi.org/10.1056/NEJM186904290801301.

Berrios, G. E. (1990) "Feelings of Fatigue and Psychopathology: A Conceptual History." *Comprehensive Psychiatry* 31, no. 2: 140–51. https://doi.org/10.1016/0010-440x(90)90018-n.

Bijsterbosch, Janine, Stephen M. Smith, and Christian F. Beckmann (2017) *Introduction to Resting State fMRI Functional Connectivity*. Oxford Neuroimaging Primers. Oxford: Oxford University Press.

Biswal, B., F. Z. Yetkin, V. M. Haughton, and J. S. Hyde (1995) "Functional Connectivity in the Motor Cortex of Resting Human Brain Using Echo-Planar MRI." *Magnetic Resonance in Medicine* 34, no. 4: 537–41. https://doi.org/10.1002/mrm.1910340409.

BUKO Pharma-Kampagne, ed. (1985) "A Drug Campaign Newsletter." *Mfc Rational Drug Policy Cell* 119(A).

Button, Katherine S., John P. A. Ioannidis, Claire Mokrysz, Brian A. Nosek, Jonathan Flint, Emma S. J. Robinson, and Marcus R. Munafò (2013) "Power Failure: Why Small Sample Size Undermines the Reliability of Neuroscience." *Nature Reviews. Neuroscience* 14 (5): 365–76. https://doi.org/10.1038/nrn3475.

Byrne, Eleanor Alexandra (2022) "Understanding Long Covid: Nosology, Social Attitudes and Stigma." *Brain, Behavior, and Immunity* 99 (January): 17–24. https://doi.org/10.1016/j.bbi.2021.09.012.

C

Carruthers, Bruce M., Anil Kumar Jain, Kenny L. De Meirleir, Daniel L. Peterson, Nancy G. Klimas, A. Martin Lerner, Alison C. Bested, et al. (2003) "Myalgic Encephalomyelitis/Chronic Fatigue Syndrome: Clinical Working Case Definition, Diagnostic and Treatment Protocols." *Journal Of Chronic Fatigue Syndrome* 11, no. 1: 7–115. https://doi.org/10.1300/J092v11n01_02.

Carruthers, Bruce M., M. I. van de Sande, Kenny De Meirleir, N. G. Klimas, G. Broderick, T. Mitchell, D. Staines, et al. (2011) "Myalgic Encephalomyelitis: International Consensus Criteria." *Journal of Internal Medicine* 270 (4): 327–38. https://doi.org/10.1111/j.1365-2796.2011.02428.x.

Committee on the Diagnostic Criteria for Myalgic Encephalomyelitis/Chronic Fatigue Syndrome, Board on the Health of Select Populations, and Institute of Medicine (IOM) (2015) *Beyond Myalgic Encephalomyelitis/Chronic Fatigue Syndrome: Redefining an Illness*. The National Academies Collection: Reports Funded by National Institutes of Health. Washington, DC: National Academies Press. http://www.ncbi.nlm.nih.gov/books/NBK274235/.

Cook, Dane B., Alan R. Light, Kathleen C. Light, Gordon Broderick, Morgan R. Shields, Ryan J. Dougherty, Jacob D. Meyer, et al. (2017) "Neural Consequences of Post-Exertion Malaise in Myalgic Encephalomyelitis/Chronic Fatigue Syndrome." *Brain, Behavior, and Immunity* 62 (May): 87–99. https://doi.org/10.1016/j.bbi.2017.02.009.

Cueto, Marcos, and Steven Palmer (2014) *Medicine and Public Health in Latin America: A History*. New Approaches to the Americas. Cambridge: Cambridge University Press. https://doi.org/10.1017/CBO9781139152174.

D

Diedrich, Lisa (2021) "Illness (In)Action: CFS and #TimeForUnrest." *Literature and Medicine* 39, no. 1: 8–14.

Dumit, Joseph (2012) *Drugs for Life: How Pharmaceutical Companies Define Our Health*. Durham, NC: Duke University Press. https://doi.org/10.1215/9780822393481.

F

Frankenburg, Frances R. (2009) *Vitamin Discoveries and Disasters: History, Science, and Controversies*. New York: Bloomsbury Publishing.

Friedman, Kenneth J. (2019) "Advances in ME/CFS: Past, Present, and Future." *Frontiers in Pediatrics* 7: 131. https://doi.org/10.3389/fped.2019.00131.

Froehlich, Laura, Daniel B.R. Hattesohl, Joseph Cotler, Leonard A. Jason, Carmen Scheibenbogen, and Uta Behrends (2022) "Causal Attributions and Perceived Stigma for Myalgic Encephalomyelitis/Chronic Fatigue Syndrome." *Journal of Health Psychology* 27, no. 10: 2291–2304. https://doi.org/10.1177/13591053211027631.

Fukuda, K., S. E. Straus, I. Hickie, M. C. Sharpe, J. G. Dobbins, and A. Komaroff (1994) "The Chronic Fatigue Syndrome: A Comprehensive Approach to Its Definition and Study. International Chronic Fatigue Syndrome Study Group." *Annals of Internal Medicine* 121, no. 12: 953–59. https://doi.org/10.7326/0003-4819-121-12-199412150-00009.

G

Geraghty, Keith J., and Aneez Esmail (2016) "Chronic Fatigue Syndrome: Is the Biopsychosocial Model Responsible for Patient Dissatisfaction and Harm?" *The British Journal of General Practice* 66, no. 649: 437–38. https://doi.org/10.3399/bjgp16X686473.

Gerchen, Martin Fungisai, and Peter Kirsch (2017) "Combining Task-Related Activation and Connectivity Analysis of fMRI Data Reveals Complex Modulation of Brain Networks." *Human Brain Mapping* 38, no. 11: 5726–39. https://doi.org/10.1002/hbm.23762.

Gereffi, Gary (2017) *The Pharmaceutical Industry and Dependency in the Third World.* Princeton, NJ: Princeton University Press.

Gijswijt-Hofstra, Marijke and Roy Porter (2001) *Cultures of Neurasthenia: From Beard to the First World War.* Amsterdam: Rodopi. https://brill.com/display/title/28323.

Gonzalez Rodriguez, Milton Fernando (2022) *Ontologies and Natures: Knowledge about Health in Visual Culture.* Landham: Rowman and Littlefield.

Gosling, Francis George (1987) *Before Freud: Neurasthenia and the American Medical Community, 1870–1910.* Chicago: University of Illinois Press.

H

Holmes, Garry P., Jonathan E. Kaplan, Nelson M. Gantz, Anthony L. Komaroff, Lawrence B. Schonberger, Stephen E. Straus, James F. Jones, et al. (1988) "Chronic Fatigue Syndrome: A Working Case Definition." *Annals of Internal Medicine* 108, no. 3: 387–89. https://doi.org/10.7326/0003-4819-108-3-387.

Huettel, Scott A., Allen W. Song, and Gregory McCarthy (2009) *Functional Magnetic Resonance Imaging*. 2nd ed. Sunderland, MA: Sinauer Associates Inc., US.

I

Inman, Thomas (1860) *Foundation for a New Theory and Practice of Medicine*. Oxford: Oxford University Press.

J

Jason, Leonard A., Madison Sunnquist, Abigail Brown, Meredyth Evans, and Julia L. Newton (2016) "Are Myalgic Encephalomyelitis and Chronic Fatigue Syndrome Different Illnesses? A Preliminary Analysis." *Journal of Health Psychology* 21, no. 1: 3–15. https://doi.org/10.1177/1359105313520335.

Jordan-Young, Rebecca M., and Katrina Karkazis (2019) *Testosterone: An Unauthorized Biography*. Cambridge, MA: Harvard University Press.

K

Kesselring, Jürg (2013) "On the History of Fatigue." *Touch Neurology* (November). https://touchneurology.com/?p=1240.

Kochakian, Charles D. (1946) "The Protein Anabolic Effects of Steroid Hormones." In *Vitamins & Hormones*, edited by Robert S. Harris and Kenneth V. Thimann, 4: 255–310. New York: Academic Press. https://doi.org/10.1016/S0083-6729(08)61085-7.

Komaroff, Anthony L. (2019) "Advances in Understanding the Pathophysiology of Chronic Fatigue Syndrome." *JAMA* 322, no. 6: 499–500. https://doi.org/10.1001/jama.2019.8312.

Komaroff, Anthony L., and W. Ian Lipkin (2023) "ME/CFS and Long COVID Share Similar Symptoms and Biological Abnormalities: Road Map to the Literature." *Frontiers in Medicine* 10: 1187163. https://doi.org/10.3389/fmed.2023.1187163.

Krämer, Sybille (2009) "Operative Bildlichkeit: Von Der 'Grammatologie' Zu Einer 'Diagrammatologie'? Reflexionen Über Erkennendes 'Sehen.'" In *Logik Des Bildlichen: Zur Kritik Der Ikonischen Vernunft*, edited by Martina Heßler and Dieter Mersch, 94–122. Bielefeld: transcript. https://doi.org/10.1515/9783839410516-003.

Krämer, Sybille (2022) "Reflections on 'Operative Iconicity' and 'Artificial Flatness.'" In *Image, Thought, and the Making of Social Worlds*, edited by David Wengrow, 251–72. Heidelberg: Propylaeum. https://doi.org/10.11588/propylaeum.842.

L

Lange, Floris P. de, Joke S. Kalkman, Gijs Bleijenberg, Peter Hagoort, Sieberen P. van der Werf, Jos W. M. van der Meer, and Ivan Toni (2004) "Neural Correlates of the Chronic Fatigue Syndrome: An fMRI Study." *Brain: A Journal of Neurology* 127, no. 9: 1948–57. https://doi.org/10.1093/brain/awh225.

Latour, Bruno (1999) *Pandora's Hope: Essays on the Reality of Science Studies*. Cambridge, MA: Harvard University Press.

Laveaga, Gabriela Soto (2005) "Uncommon Trajectories: Steroid Hormones, Mexican Peasants, and the Search for a Wild Yam." *Studies in History and Philosophy of Science Part C: Studies in History and Philosophy of Biological and Biomedical Sciences*, Drug Trajectories, 36, no. 4: 743–60. https://doi.org/10.1016/j.shpsc.2005.09.007.

Laveaga, Gabriela Soto (2015) "Hormones, Mexican Peasants, and the Search for a Wild Yam." In *The Pharmaceutical Studies Reader*, edited by Sergio Sismondo and Jeremy Greene, 181–94. Chichester: John Wiley & Sons.

Lian, Olaug S., and Hilde Bondevik (2015) "Medical Constructions of Long-Term Exhaustion, Past and Present." *Sociology of Health & Illness* 37, no. 6: 920–35. https://doi.org/10.1111/1467-9566.12249.

Lieutaud, Joseph (1816) *Synopsis of the Universal Practice of Medicine*. Chicago: E. and R. Parker. https://search.library.wisc.edu/catalog/999625998402121.

Lysen, Flora (2015) "Blinking Brains, Corporate Spectacle, and the Atom Man: Visual Aspects of Science at the Stedelijk Museum Amsterdam (1962)." *Stedelijk Studies Journal* 2. https://stedelijkstudies.com/journal/blinking-brains-corporate-spectacle-and-the-atom-man/.

M

Maksoud, Rebekah, Stanley du Preez, Natalie Eaton-Fitch, Kiran Thapaliya, Leighton Barnden, Hélène Cabanas, Donald Staines, and Sonya Marshall-Gradisnik (2020) "A Systematic Review of Neurological Impairments in Myalgic Encephalomyelitis/Chronic Fatigue Syndrome Using Neuroimaging Techniques." *PloS One* 15, no. 4: e0232475. https://doi.org/10.1371/journal.pone.0232475.

Mazzoni, Irene, Osquel Barroso, and Olivier Rabin (2011) "The List of Prohibited Substances and Methods in Sport: Structure and Review Process by the World Anti-Doping Agency." *Journal of Analytical Toxicology* 35, no. 9: 608–12. https://doi.org/10.1093/anatox/35.9.608.

McDowell, Lee (2017) *Mineral Nutrition History: The Early Years*. Sarasota, FL: First Edition Design Pub.

Morales, Alvaro (2013) "The Long and Tortuous History of the Discovery of Testosterone and Its Clinical Application." *The Journal of Sexual Medicine* 10, no. 4: 1178–83. https://doi.org/10.1111/jsm.12081.

Morgentaler, Abraham, and Abdulmaged Traish (2020) "The History of Testosterone and the Evolution of Its Therapeutic Potential." *Sexual Medicine Reviews* 8, no. 2: 286–96. https://doi.org/10.1016/j.sxmr.2018.03.002.

Mosso, Angelo (1906) *Fatigue*. 2nd ed. London: G. P. Putnam's Sons.

Muhr, Paula (2022) *From Photography to fMRI: Epistemic Functions of Images in Medical Research on Hysteria*. Bielefeld: transcript.

N

Nacul, Luis, Eliana M. Lacerda, Caroline C. Kingdon, Hayley Curran, and Erinna W. Bowman (2019) "How Have Selection Bias and Disease Misclassification Undermined the Validity of Myalgic Encephalomyelitis/Chronic Fatigue Syndrome Studies?" *Journal of Health Psychology* 24, no. 12: 1765–69. https://doi.org/10.1177/1359105317695803.

Nieschlag, Eberhard, and Susan Nieschlag (2017) "The History of Testosterone and the Testes: From Antiquity to Modern Times." In *Testosterone: From Basic to Clinical Aspects*, edited by Alexander Hohl, 1–19. Cham: Springer. https://doi.org/10.1007/978-3-319-46086-4_1.

Noonan, Vanessa, and Elizabeth Dean (2000) "Submaximal Exercise Testing: Clinical Application and Interpretation." *Physical Therapy* 80, no. 8: 782–807.

P

Powell, Hutchinson (1849) "The Modus Operandi of Therapautic Agents." *London Journal of Medicine: A Monthly Record of the Medical Sciences* 1–4: 626.

R

Rabinbach, Anson (1990) *The Human Motor: Energy, Fatigue, and the Origins of Modernity*. New York: Basic Books.

Rivera, Mateo Cortes, Claudio Mastronardi, Claudia T. Silva-Aldana, Mauricio Arcos-Burgos, and Brett A. Lidbury (2019) "Myalgic Encephalomyelitis/Chronic Fatigue Syndrome: A Comprehensive Review." *Diagnostics* 9, no. 3: 91. https://doi.org/10.3390/diagnostics9030091.

Roberts, Harry (1939) *The Troubled Mind: A General Account of the Human Mind, and Its Disorders and Their Remedies*. New York: E. P. Dutton.

Rodriguez Osiac, Lorena (2022) "Una nueva política pública estructural para Chile: Fortificación con Vitamina D." *Andes Pediatrica* 93, no. 6: 791–93. https://doi.org/10.32641/andespediatr.v93i6.4549.

S

Schaffner, Anna Katharina (2016) *Exhaustion: A History*. New York: Columbia University Press.

Shan, Zack Y., Kevin Finegan, Sandeep Bhuta, Timothy Ireland, Donald R. Staines, Sonya M. Marshall-Gradisnik, and Leighton R. Barnden (2018) "Brain Function Characteristics of Chronic Fatigue Syndrome: A Task fMRI Study." *NeuroImage: Clinical* 19: 279–86. https://doi.org/10.1016/j.nicl.2018.04.025.

Shorter, Edward (1993) "Chronic Fatigue in Historical Perspective." In *Ciba Foundation Symposium – Chronic Fatigue Syndrome* 173, edited by Gregory R. Bock and Julie Whelan, 16–22. Chichester: John Wiley & Sons.

Sismondo, Sergio, and Jeremy A. Greene (2015) *The Pharmaceutical Studies Reader*. Chichester: John Wiley & Sons.

Stevens, A. A. (1909) *Modern Materia Medica and Therapeutics*. Philadelphia: Saunders.

Straus, Stephen E. (1991) "History of Chronic Fatigue Syndrome." *Reviews of Infectious Diseases* 13: S2–S7. https://doi.org/10.1093/clinids/13.supplement_1.s2.

T

Tauchen, Jan, Michal Jurášek, Lukáš Huml, and Silvie Rimpelová (2021) "Medicinal Use of Testosterone and Related Steroids Revisited." *Molecules* 26, no. 4: 1032. https://doi.org/10.3390/molecules26041032.

Thomas, Marie (2018) *"Tired All the Time": Persistent Fatigue and Healthcare*. Cham: Springer International Publishing. https://doi.org/10.1007/978-3-319-93913-1.

Tombaugh, Tom N. (2006) "A Comprehensive Review of the Paced Auditory Serial Addition Test (PASAT)." *Archives of Clinical Neuropsychology: The Official Journal of the National Academy of Neuropsychologists* 21, no. 1: 53–76. https://doi.org/10.1016/j.acn.2005.07.006.

Toomey, Thomas Noxon (1929) "The First General Medical Treatise Published in the Western Hemisphere." *Annals of Medical History* 1, no. 2: 215–28.

U

UNESCO (2005) "International Convention Against Doping in Sport." *The Stationery Office Limited*, UNESCO Digital Library, October 19.

V

Valdez, Ashley R., Elizabeth E. Hancock, Seyi Adebayo, David J. Kiernicki, Daniel Proskauer, John R. Attewell, Lucinda Bateman, et al. (2019) "Estimating Prevalence, Demographics, and Costs of ME/CFS Using Large Scale Medical Claims Data and Machine Learning." *Frontiers in Pediatrics* 6: 412. https://doi.org/10.3389/fped.2018.00412.

Vigarello, Georges (2020) *Histoire de la fatigue: Du Moyen Âge à nos jours*. Paris: Seuil.

W

Washington, Stuart D., Rakib U. Rayhan, Richard Garner, Destie Provenzano, Kristina Zajur, Florencia Martinez Addiego, John W. VanMeter, and James N. Baraniuk (2020) "Exercise Alters Brain Activation in Gulf War Illness and Myalgic Encephalomyelitis/Chronic Fatigue Syndrome." *Brain Communications* 2, no. 2. https://doi.org/10.1093/braincomms/fcaa070.

Wood, Thomas Denison (1928) *Teaching How to Get and Use Human Energy*. Bloomington, MN: Public School Publishing Company.

Images of Tuberculosis: Seeing and Understanding an Ancient, Endemic Disease

Stephen A. Geller and
Gideon Manning

Introduction

Prior to the nineteenth century, those who sought to picture disease were not bound to the laboratory or hospital, or even to visual media, as texts alone often created the medical picture of disease.[1] Developments in printing and the later separation of strictly scientific/medical spaces from the public sphere—at isolated physical locations where entry required training and expertise, and concomitant privileged and distinctive knowledge—coincided with a change in the generally accepted ideal conditions for visualizing disease, prioritizing images taken from life and those utilizing the microscope after the advent of compound achromatic lenses in the 1830s.[2] The fundamental argument in favor of both was that they improved accuracy in diagnoses and increased our causal knowledge; in other words, such images and the procedures creating them added "robustness" to the scientific and medical judgments of the time.[3] The nineteenth century's emphasis on visualizing disease, still integral to the scientific culture of contemporary medicine, takes us beyond texts and the physical exam (though still essential) to the development of anatomic pathology, histology, and histopathology and, in time, to modern molecular pathology.

To explore some of the relevant transitions and image production in the nineteenth century, in this chapter we consider images of the endemic disease tuberculosis,

1 The history of pathology before the nineteenth century remains underexplored, although there are now several helpful studies added to those done early in the twentieth century by, for example, Long (1965). Works worth consulting include De Renzi, Bresadola, and Conforti (2018) and Ragland (2022).

2 For discussion of the microscope, and medical instrumentation more generally, see Davis (1981). For the microscope's early impact on ways of seeing, see Snyder (2015). Still worth consulting for an introduction to the history of nineteenth-century biology is Coleman (1977).

3 For an account of "robustness" in philosophy of science, see the essays in Léna Soler et al. (2012).

concentrating on the changes taking place inside the body and the etiology found with microscopy. We examine images rendered approximately a century apart. One, a representation of macroscopic findings produced by René-Théophile-Hyacinthe Laennec (1781–1826), who introduced the stethoscope and mediate auscultation to study the heart and lungs, and another, of the causative micro-organisms themselves, discovered and drawn by Robert Koch (1843–1910), who used innovative preparations and the compound microscope to identify the cause of tuberculosis and establish its communicability. We also consider, by way of contrast, artists' representations of the afflicted patients in their lived experience of the disease in the work of Joseph Severn (1793–1879) and Edvard Munch (1863–1944).

Tuberculosis was visualized both before and after the development of laboratory science, and it continues to affect great numbers of people well into the twenty-first century, especially in the developing world.[4] As a result, tuberculosis itself continues to be a valuable entry point for understanding the changing practices and techniques for picturing disease that animate this volume, allowing us to explore significant episodes in the history of pathology through images.[5]

We begin with a brief retelling of the history of tuberculosis, including the earliest genetic and anthropological evidence including bone involvement in fossils dated to 8000 BCE.[6] This section includes discussion of contemporary pathology and what we know about tuberculosis today.

4 Tuberculosis is a worldwide disease, although the incidence in Western countries is quite low. In 2020, it is estimated that approximately 10 million people developed tuberculosis with 1.5 million deaths, the second greatest number of deaths from an infectious disease in that year of Covid-19. The greatest number of cases occurred in India, China, Indonesia, the Philippines, Pakistan, Nigeria, and Bangladesh (Loscalzo et al. 2022, 1357). For earlier periods, see the details provided in Henschen (1962) and Ackerknecht (1965).

5 The richness of our topic is nicely expressed by Helen Bynum. As she explains, in the nineteenth century, the "effects of the [tuberculosis] lesions had been visualized during life after the advent of stethoscopy (auscultation) and the technique of tapping the body (percussion) to determine whether its solid, hollow, and fluid-filled parts were as they should be. This method of diagnosis continued. So too did examination with a microscope of stained sputum samples to look for [what came to be known as the Koch bacillus], the culture in the [organisms in the] laboratory, and immunological testing with tuberculin. X-rays came to augment all these techniques. Fixed on a photographic plate and later celluloid film, [and now digitally] X-ray pictures provided a permanent visual record in the medical file. Learning to hear the body involved training the ear to differentiate the complex symphony of crackles, clicks, and rattles. Learning to read the skiagram (from the Latin for 'shadow') or X-ray film, meant training the eye to appreciate the inner contours of the body and to make sense of the shadows and spots" (2012, 200).

6 A 9,000-year-old mummy has been found with lesion DNA sufficiently well preserved for confirmation of the presence of the tuberculosis organism by both molecular typing and analysis of the lipids of the cell wall with high performance liquid chromatography. Characteristic macroscopic changes have been seen many times among Egyptian mummies and typical and diagnostic organisms have been confirmed in a psoas muscle of an Inca child from approximately 700 BCE. In the Louvre's Hammurabi stone, from approximately 1750 BCE, there is a description of a chronic lung disease that most likely was tuberculosis. Indeed, the oldest evidence of this disease may be the lesions found in *Homo erectus* fossilized tissue from 2.5 million years ago in East Africa (Kappelman et al. 2008).

Part of our goal in emphasizing our current state of knowledge is to indicate the extent to which specialized knowledge—both scientific and medical—characterizes the pathologists' studies of disease.

In section two, we turn to the nineteenth century and utilize the illustrations of Laennec and Koch. Here, we again specify the technical knowledge and experience necessary to see what they saw, but we also highlight the collaborative and cumulative nature of their work and those on whom they relied as they responded to and helped specify, through their publications, the ideal conditions for visualizing disease. In Laennec's case, we specifically describe how, relying on postmortem study of diseased lungs and a sophisticated didactic image representing progressive stages of the disease, Laennec educated physicians to recognize changes occurring within living patients but from the outside with the use of his invention, the stethoscope. Laennec linked what he heard with his invention to what he had seen postmortem, in effect grounding the art of auscultation in the facts of the morphologioc alterations. In this way, he legitimized the use of the "auditory eye" as a way of seeing inside the body when direct and literal visual inspection of the patient's organs was not possible. Koch, by contrast, focused specifically on understanding the contagious nature of this disease, isolating microorganisms from the body's fluids and then, using his microscope and animal studies, identifying the specific cause of tuberculosis. He relied on sophisticated preparations (staining techniques) as well as techniques for culturing the organism. Both scientists, Laennec and Koch, made choices in how to visualize disease and both relied on more than a static image to do so.

As we explain more fully in section three, the experienced anatomic pathologist thinks and perceives dynamically, envisioning not a singular moment captured in a slide or image but one linked to the past and the future of the part, organ, and patient before them. This differentiates pathologists from the public, even the well-educated public. The pathologist's image of tuberculosis may appear static to the uneducated auditory or literal eye, but to the prepared pathologist it represents a vivid saga that portrays a dynamic battle, including its various beginnings, its many skirmishes, and its paths for denouement.

The message of our contribution, emphasized throughout and highlighted again in our conclusion, is that acoustic impressions, originally conceived of by Laennec, when correlated with macroscopic observations and subsequent microscopic images by Koch, have been vital in expanding the understanding of tuberculosis and the robustness of medical diagnosis. They have served to define what it means to perceive disease. Put simply, these efforts to make clinical judgment more reliable and medical interventions more effective led to a multiplicity of independent and highly technical determinations of the same result: that a patient was suffering from or infected with tuberculosis.

1 A Brief History of Tuberculosis

The history of tuberculosis is too well known to require anything more than brief retelling here.[7] Although the name first appears in 1839 in the work of the German physician Johann Lukas Schönlein (1793–1864), the history of the disease is much older. The Hippocratic corpus, originating in the fifth century BCE, called tuberculosis "phthisis," one of several ancient terms for progressively wasting or consumptive diseases (Nutton 2004, 28). Not necessarily identical with tuberculosis, "consumption," the pre-nineteenth-century English word for tuberculosis, first appeared in the late fourteenth century, and "consumption cough" dates to 1661. The shift in terminology to "tuberculosis" in the nineteenth century highlights a specific anatomic feature of the disease, namely the tubercle, a small tissue mass so named in the sixteenth century.[8] Not to be outdone by later physicians, however, the Hippocratics observed typical tubercular lesions ("phymata") in cattle, sheep, and pigs, although they did not connect them to the same disease. They also believed tuberculosis to be inheritable, which would be consistent with the

7 The literature on the history of tuberculosis is extensive. See, for example, Cummins (1949), Keers (1978), Dubos and Dubos (1952), Herzog (1998), Bynum (2012), Frith (2014), Agarwal et al. (2017). More popular works include Dormandy (2000), Krishnan (2022). For ancient Greece specifically, see the sources reproduced in Meinecke (1927), and for discussion, see Grmek (1989). For the early modern period, see Ragland (2022), which includes details of Franciscus Sylvius de la Boë's precise pathological and anatomical descriptions of tubercles.

appearance of the disease within families who lived in close quarters with one another.[9]

In later antiquity, Aristotle (384–322 BCE), who knew the Hippocratic tradition well and showed extensive interest in medical questions throughout his working life, characterized tuberculosis in animals as contagious within herds, identifying the disease "branchos" and "craurus."[10] He noted in *History of Animals* that both pigs and cattle in herds are susceptible to "cranurus," which can be confirmed in cattle "when the carcase [sic] is opened the lungs are found to be rotten." Pigs also suffer from "swellings about the windpipe" called "branchos," which we now know to be enlarged, infected pulmonary hilar lymph nodes (vol. 1, bk. VIII, sec. 21 and 23). By the first century CE, the Roman author Aretaeus of Cappadocia, who was one of the first physicians to attempt a systematic correlation between disease and anatomic change, defined pthisis explicitly as a condition typified by a cavity or abscess of the lung, with the patient experiencing cough, expectoration, and bloody sputum (hemoptysis) (bk. 1, ch. VIII; cited in Meinecke 1927, 387).[11]

Many other Greek and Roman physicians wrote about tuberculosis, but none more eloquently than Caelius Aurelianus of Sicca, a fifth-century Roman physician and translator whose description rivals that of any later clinician:

8 *Oxford English Dictionary*. https://www.oed.com/?tl=true. Other names for tuberculosis, in addition to "pthisis" and "consumption," include "the White Plague," "the phantom plague," "scrofula," "the Captain of all these Men of Death" (Bunyan 1900), "the King's touch," and "the King's evil." The allusions to royalty were reflections of the prevalent belief that the monarch could cause, and cure, tuberculosis. Each of these names have what philosophers of language since Gottlob Frege would call a different sense (*Sinn*), but this does not preclude them from having the same reference (*Bedeutung*). Thus, when we identify these names with one another—e.g., "pthisis=tuberculosis"—we are making a claim that the two names, each with a different sense, have the same reference. It is precisely in this way that forensic anthropologists working with ancient DNA add to our knowledge of the past, whatever those diseases were once called. Still, for several decades now there has been a widely accepted historiographical claim that the identity conditions of disease and disease concepts changed with the advent of laboratory tests in the nineteenth century (Cunningham 1992). This realization has led many historians to infer that retrospective diagnosis is to be avoided, especially given the different social and cultural contexts that give names their sense. But there is more to history than social and cultural history, and a range of productive questions can be asked about the diseases of the past. While it is clearly true that the means of identifying a patient's disease have changed, just as the robustness of our clinical judgments has increased, whether this entails a different disease is being *referred* to by our different names for them is less clear and the unqualified inference that it does entail this conflates the different senses of disease names with a difference in their reference. In some cases, it is not possible to find a common reference—the information available to the historian is too limited as, for instance, when we are looking at the illness of a single individual—but, in others, it would seem more than possible, especially with respect to endemic diseases (Stolberg 2016). To put the point simply, whether we call it "pthisis" or "scrofula," it is still tuberculosis, just as, to use Frege's famous example, whether we call it "Hesperus" or "Phosphorus," we are still referring to Venus (Frege 1892).

9 We now know that tuberculosis's spread is facilitated by an urban environment with large numbers of people in a confined space. It has been suggested, for example, that the "plague of Justinian," which lasted throughout the sixth and seventh centuries may, at least in part, have been due to the migration of young people from northern and eastern Europe, where they had no contact with tuberculosis, into the urban centers growing around the Mediterranean at that time. This especially vulnerable population sharing a confined space in urban centers would have accelerated and perpetuated the spread of tuberculosis. By contrast, typical plague due to the spread of the organism *Pasteurella pestis* generally abates after a few years and does not usually last for many decades (Dormandy 2000).

10 We use the word "contagious" advisedly. For fuller discussion of the concept in Greek and Roman antiquity, see Nutton (2000).

11 For discussion, see Laios, Androutsos, and Moschos (2017).

> The patients suffer from a latent fever that begins toward evening and vanishes . . . at the break of day. It is accompanied by violent coughing, which expels thin purulent sputum. The patient . . . breathes with difficulty. . . . The skin on the rest of the body is ashen. . . . The eyes have a weary expression, the patient is gaunt . . . but often displays astonished physical or mental activity. In many cases wheezes are heard in the chest. . . . The patients lose their appetite or suffer hunger pangs. They are often very thirsty (cited and translated in Herzog 1998, 5–6).

In its fundamentals, this is precisely what we should expect a contemporary clinician to report after taking a history and examining a patient suffering from chronic tuberculosis: fever appearing worse in the evening, a productive cough with clear or possibly bloody sputum, difficulty breathing, gray pallor, weight loss, hyperactivity, audible wheezing, shifts between hunger and little appetite, and significant thirst.

We know today that tuberculosis is a highly contagious disease caused by the bacterium *Mycobacterium tuberculosis* (MTB). Typically, the lungs and pulmonary hilar lymph nodes are affected but the disease can also involve other parts of the body.[12] In many cases there are no symptoms ("latent tuberculosis"). A small percentage of patients (approximately 10 percent) progress to active disease which, if untreated, leads to death in as many as half the affected patients. Typical complaints of active tuberculosis are chronic cough with the production of bloodstained mucus, fever, high sweats, and weight loss. The pronounced weight loss often seen is the historical basis for the name "consumption." Depending on the site involved, symptoms can vary significantly. For example, bone pain is experienced when tuberculosis involves the bone. Also, back pain and deformity are associated with vertebral body tuberculosis, known as Pott disease after the description by the so-called "best surgeon in England," Percival Pott (1714–1788).[13] Vertebral involvement has been observed in Egyptian mummies in whom the characteristic lesions have

12 We draw freely here on the excellent accounts in Loscalzo et al. (2022, 1357–1382) and Majno and Joris (2004, 556–560).

13 For an account of Pott and his contributions, see Payne (2017).

been seen and, in modern times, demonstrated with histochemical and immunohistochemical methods, as well as molecular studies.[14]

The original focus of tuberculosis organisms in the lung is met with a transient and ineffective acute inflammatory (polymorphonuclear (PMN)) reaction, similar to the body's reaction to any infective agent. When this reaction fails to destroy and isolate the organisms, the area of infection enlarges as more effective chronic inflammatory cells (lymphocytes, monocytes, and macrophages) replace that first futile response, forming a distinct nodule ("tubercle"). The lesions continue to grow, and may begin to show central necrosis, with the influx of more inflammatory cells; it can then be seen with the naked eye on dissection or with imaging techniques, such as X-ray. The inflammatory response leads to cell death, further necrosis, and eventual cavitation, which can be many centimeters in diameter. When the necrosis breaks into small bronchi, the organisms spread throughout both lungs and also to the gastrointestinal system when tubercular material is swallowed. Tubercles can destroy small vessels in the lung with bleeding and hemoptysis. When larger vessels are eroded, hemoptysis can be massive with severe bleeding and death ("Rasmussen aneurysm").[15]

Fibroblasts (cells that elaborate collagen deposition and scarring as attempts to wall off the process) infiltrate at the periphery. The monocytes/macrophages merge as chronicity ensues to form multinucleate giant ("Langhans") cells arranged in a peripheral, palisaded pattern surrounding the antigen-rich tuberculosis. This fibrosing granuloma (an inflammatory nodule, not to be confused with granulation tissue, capillary-rich fibroblasts, typically seen in non-tubercular healing wounds) can limit the spread of the infection although viable organisms can be identified and cultured from granulomas in the laboratory decades after both the original infection and recognizable symptoms. When the necrosis is large enough to see macroscopically it resembles a soft, white cheese and has been termed "caseous" (cheese-like, meaning something resembling pot cheese or cottage cheese). The classic depiction of

14 For references and further detail, see footnote 6.

15 This sequence, though not the precise mechanisms involved, was well known to patients both before and after the nineteenth century and did not require the physician's specialized knowledge. The English poet John Keats, for example, knew death was imminent when he saw significant blood in his sputum. This experience of blood in the sputum has been used in many novels and films, several of which we will mention. Classic pathology findings, both macroscopic and microscopic, can be seen in figures E23–E25 (Grundmann and Geller 1989, 59–60).

tuberculosis, combining macro- and microscopic features, is that of caseating granuloma(s) with chronic inflammatory cells and characteristic multinucleate (Langhans) giant cells.

2
Visualizing Tuberculosis

In 2025, physicians know a great deal about tuberculosis, its signs and symptoms, and how to prevent its spread. How they think about and especially how they visualize the disease, its cause, and pathogenesis, can be traced to two physicians and the reception of their work in the nineteenth century: Laennec and Koch. Laennec saw the effects of the disease's lesions on the lungs post-mortem and then developed techniques for seeing the disease inside the live patient using what we call here the "auditory eye."[16] For his part, Koch saw and demonstrated the causative bacillus of the disease, building on the clinical advances that came before him as well as his own and others' laboratory work with anthrax utilizing the microscope to connect bacteria and disease. We work in the reverse chronological order in this section, and so begin with the more familiar laboratory medicine of today, by starting with Koch and ending with Laennec. In this way, we move from the micro level upward to the gross anatomy and then the clinical encounter. By comparing the two figures, we will see how each depended on collaborators, both scientific and artistic, but in different ways, and how the drive for reaffirming and self-correcting methods in nineteenth-century scientific medicine altered the consensus of how best to see and visualize disease. In other words, the struggle for reliability and effectiveness led to independent and ever more robust derivations of the same result: an identification, through a combination of observation, inference, and experimental manipulation of the presence and progression of tuberculosis in a patient or animal subject.

Koch was one of many to pioneer techniques of photography through the microscope, and photography was in the late nineteenth century taking its cultural place in science and medicine. But, interestingly, in Koch's demonstration of the microscopic appearance of the bacillus utilizing histochemical

16 We take inspiration here from the title of Jacalyn Duffin's classic study of Laennec, *To See with a Better Eye* (1998). Her title is itself inspired by the words of Jean-Nicolas Corvisart that she cites as an epigraph. The better eye to which Duffin refers in Laennec's case is what we call the "auditory eye."

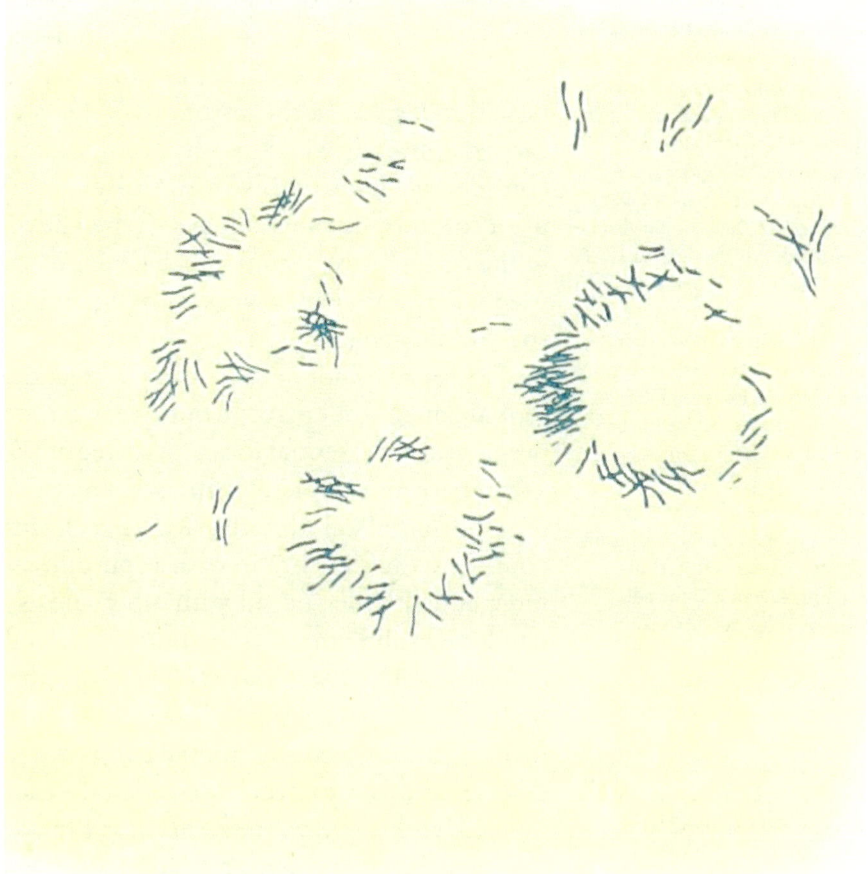

FIG. 1

FIG. 1 Robert Koch's hand-drawn and colored illustration of the blue rod-like structure of *Mycobacterium tuberculosis* seen through the compound microscope. (Koch 1912, Table XXVI, fig. 34.) Wellcome Collection. https://wellcomecollection.org/works/g6yw6n8t

methods, he relied on a color drawing rather than photographs. FIG. 1 Koch drew what he saw under the microscope with his own hand because color photomicrography had not yet been developed and the testimony of his own eyes, and hand, carried epistemic weight with his colleagues. Koch had earned considerable fame for his work studying anthrax in animals prior to studying tuberculosis.[17] When he turned his attention to the latter, he used similar techniques to those he successfully used when studying anthrax, although tuberculosis presented specific challenges.

One does not need to know a great deal about optics to look through a microscope but one must remember that preparation is essential to see anything at all with the device. To prepare his samples, Koch used a methylene blue stain, developed by Paul Ehrlich (1854–1915), with Bismarck brown counter-stain.[18] He began with a sputum sample from a patient independently diagnosed with tuberculosis. Koch then employed solid nutrients including potato slices to grow pure colonies of *Mycobacterium tuberculosis* (the blue rods in figure 1). Animal testing followed when he inoculated that material into susceptible animal subjects to reproduce the disease. In this way, Koch identified the cause of tuberculosis.

Mycobacterium tuberculosis is a small, aerobic (oxygen-dependent), nonmotile bacillus whose outer surface has a high lipid content, contributing to many of its unique characteristics. These led to Koch's early challenges in its isolation using existing staining techniques and the microscope; cells are largely transparent and require careful preparation to be seen. The lipid bilayer with a high mycolic acid content does not stain well with the various staining techniques, including the Gram stain, developed in 1884 by Danish bacteriologist Hans Christian Gram (1853–1938), still widely used to identify most bacteria under the microscope. Koch responded to this challenge by trying many stains before adopting the methylene blue stain of Ehrlich.[19]

Koch first presented the results of his work on tuberculosis in March 1882 at a meeting of the German Physiological

17 In English there is surprisingly little scholarship on Koch outside of discussion of his criteria for disease causation, commonly referred to as "Koch's postulates." An intellectual biography of the more traditional sort is Brock (1988). Gradmann (2009) should also be consulted. For the postulates, see also Carter (2003) and Grimes (2006).

18 The most common stain used today is the Ziehl-Neelson stain, the method of which was also developed by Ehrlich and subsequently refined by Franz Ziehl (1859–1926) and Friedrich Neelsen (1854–1898). With this method the organisms are stained red with carbol fuchsin reagent and the color is resistant to decolorization with acid ("acid-fast"). Other similar stains are used to demonstrate the organism of leprosy, *M. leprae*, the often-seen tuberculosis-like lesions seen in AIDS (*Mycobacterium-avium-intracellulare* complex), and other variants.

19 An excellent summary of Koch's challenges and the rhetorical and scientific choices he made is given in Gradmann (2001, 4–13).

Society in Berlin. Speaking to an audience of experts, including many trained in laboratory science, Koch walked them through his preparations and what the microscope revealed:

> The bacteria visualized by this technique [*Verfahren sichtbar gemachten*] show many distinct characteristics. They are rod-shaped and belong therefore to the group of bacilli. They are very thin and are only one-fourth to one-half as long as the diameter of a red blood cell, but can occasionally reach a length as long as the diameter of a red cell. They possess a form and size which is surprisingly like that of the leprosy bacillus. (Koch 1882, 222; trans. Brock 1999, 110)

Others had looked for the cause of tuberculosis, but none had seen what Koch saw. In his 1882 presentation, he had an explanation for why his results had been missed by previous scientists and physicians. For one, "the bacilli are extremely small structures." For another, they appear "in such small numbers, that they would elude the most attentive observer without the use of a special staining reaction." Thus, in his own telling, it was Koch's preparations that brought the bacilli into view. But even with his preparations, when the bacilli "are present in large numbers, they are generally mixed with finely granular detritus in such a way that they are completely hidden, so that even here their discovery would be extremely difficult" (Koch 1882, 431; trans. Brock 1999, 111). Indeed, before the development of more recent visualization techniques, including immunostains, pathologists were admonished to study slides for at least thirty minutes or more before deciding the organisms were not there.

Many scientists, including Koch's colleague at the Charité Hospital, Rudolf Virchow (1821–1902), remained skeptical.[20] Nevertheless, Ehrlich, who spent two years recovering from tuberculosis, described Koch's presentation as his (Ehrlich's) "single greatest scientific experience" (quoted in Gradmann 2006, 295). In these two responses, there is a parting of scientific generations, and perhaps even a case of

20 Still worth consulting for Virchow's remarkable life and political career is Ackerknecht (1953).

incommensurability involving Germany's greatest cellular biologist and the new advocates of bacteriology.[21] Prior to Koch, consensus had been that tuberculosis was a hereditary disease and Koch's efforts seeking to isolate the pathogenic germs causing tuberculosis provided decisive support for an alternative causal account of disease. Two years after his initial presentation in Berlin, Koch both used illustrations and further elaborated his procedures in an 80-page paper that made explicit what are today called "Koch's postulates" (Koch 1912). These criteria for disease causation feature prominently in nearly every work of contemporary epidemiology.[22]

For our purposes here, the two responses of Virchow and Ehrlich point to something else. Their disagreement revolves around practices of seeing and the need to look beyond a static image and to the concepts involved in scientific disputes. Virchow, whose life bridged the times before and after microscopy became integral to the practice of medicine, was strongly committed to the concept that social conditions led to disease. He believed there was a thus far unidentified causative link between, for example, poverty and disease. The concepts on which Virchow relied to understand Koch's presentation and later research, including Koch's images, prevented Virchow from seeing what Ehrlich saw. This was not mere obstinance on Virchow's part, for he accepted that the bacterium existed and that it was relevant to the story of disease. Nor do we wish to suggest that the common or given elements of what was visible through the microscope were literally different depending on who was looking. The colors, shapes, etc. were the same. However, these common elements do not wholly determine what is seen and certainly not what is understood by what is seen. Virchow's understanding of disease causation informed his judgment and guided how he received Koch's presentation. Thus, in effect, he did not see what Koch and Ehrlich saw.

In the end, Koch accomplished two things with his hand-drawn and colored image of tuberculosis, as well as having his audience examine the preparations themselves. First, strongly suspecting that tuberculosis was caused by bacteria resistant to

21 The transition implied here toward a causal concept of disease, and one that looks specifically to external causes or intrusions into the healthy body, is discussed in Carter (2003).

22 The wide application of Koch's postulates, once modified to accommodate inanimate pathogens, is made in Walker, LeVine, and Jucker (2006, 1–4).

conventional stains available at the time (because of their lipid-rich coating) his laboratory did nothing less than develop reproducible techniques making the organism both visible and open to experimental manipulation. This was a first for a disease that had been killing human beings for thousands of years. The fact that what was seen could be cultured and then used to infect animal subjects militated in favor of the bacillus's existence, adding to the reliability and effectiveness of both science and medicine.[23] In other words, Koch's visualization led to a new way not just of identifying tuberculosis from samples taken from a sick patient but also to widespread hope for a cure.[24] The obstacles to implementing public health initiatives and investment remained political, but the etiological question was resolved.

Secondly, his program initiated myriad microbiologic and chemical studies generally, which in the case of tuberculosis eventually satisfied the early hope for effective medications (e.g., streptomycin, for which Selman Waksman [1888–1973] was awarded a 1952 Nobel prize). Throughout these subsequent studies, images of tuberculosis, as seen through the microscope, continued to play a decisive role, with the X-ray concomitantly allowing clinicians a view of damage to organs in living patients, adding to the robustness of a diagnosis initially limited to the physical exam or a determination postmortem.

Koch's image of the bacillus is far removed from the typical pale and wasted figure of a dying patient with tuberculosis seen in Joseph Severn's portrait of John Keats on his deathbed FIG. 2 or Edvard Munch's portrait of his dying sister being cared for by their mother. FIG. 3 Still, it was from the clinician's knowledge of such patients, and their sputum, that Koch's investigations began. These depictions of the "White Plague"—so named because of the skin color of the terminal patient, which is notably less apparent in those with darker skin tones—are matched by highly descriptive nineteenth-century non-pictorial representations found in writings of Charlotte Brontë, all of whose siblings died of tuberculosis, Edgar Allan Poe, whose poignant writings about his tuberculous wife are

23 The idea that our best argument for scientific realism—that the objects the scientist studies actually exist—is experimental manipulation that both creates new phenomena and investigates other features of nature is persuasively argued in Hacking (1983).

24 Koch's fame coupled with his discovery almost immediately led to expectations that a cure would be forthcoming. Eight years after his discovery of the organism, in 1890 at the International Medical Congress in Berlin Koch would announce he had found a cure: "Tuberkulin." The cure was a combination of glycerin and processed tuberculosis bacteria. Tuberkulin offered no cure, however, killing almost as many as it left unaffected, and only months after his announcement Koch was forced to retract his claims, partially prompted by the failure by Virchow and others to reproduce Koch's findings (Hankin 1891, 248–249). In another lesson about the nonlinear direction of medicine, one eventual consequence of the so-called Tuberkulin scandal was that more exacting tests were enacted before therapeutics were introduced into clinical practice, although Koch himself did not appear to "employ the immunological frame of interpretation" to his cure (Gradmann 2006, 294).

FIG. 2 A sleeping and exhausted John Keats suffering from tuberculosis. Joseph Severn, *John Keats's Death-Bed Portrait*, 1821, pen, ink, and watercolor on paper. Keats-Shelley House, Rome. Property of the Keats-Shelley Memorial Association, all rights reserved

FIG. 3 Munch's sister suffering from tuberculosis and attended to by her mother. Edvard Munch, *The Sick Child*, 1885 or 1886, oil on canvas, 118.5 × 120 cm. The National Museum/ Børre Høstland, Oslo, NG.M.00839

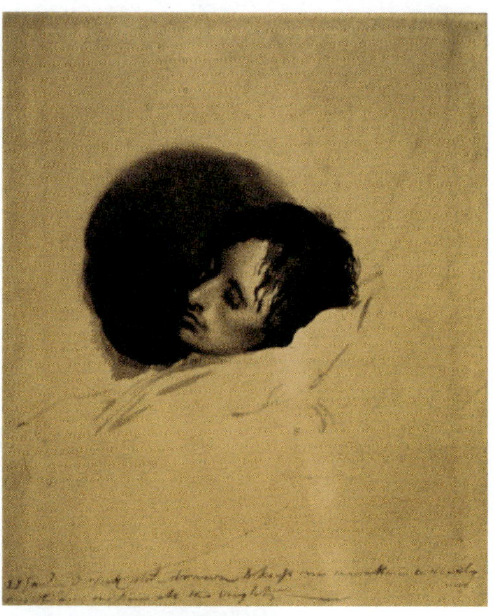

FIG. 2

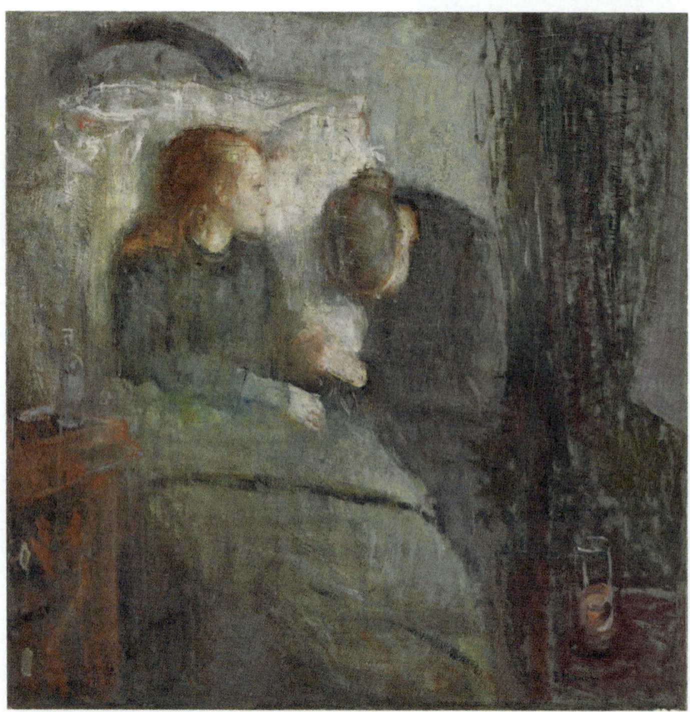

FIG. 3

highly descriptive, Alexander Dumas in his novel *The Lady of the Camellias*, and many others, reflecting the prevalence of tuberculosis.[25]

Non-scientific images of disease like these, whether sketched, painted, or written, depict the patient as seen not just by the physician but by family, friends, and other caregivers. They offer more readily accessible visualizations of tuberculosis than those produced by Koch and later biomedical researchers, for they do not require the educated eye of the physician or pathologist (although the educated eye can see even more in these cases than the rest of us). Instead, all that is required is the competence of having endured the disease oneself or vicariously through others and, of course, an artist's hand or pen. That is, these images fit more closely with the lived experience of the disease from first symptoms until death. However, they do not take us inside the patient's body to visualize the damage wrought to organs or to the microscopic organism causing the disease. These efforts to look inside, to find causes, better serve the interests of the physician seeking ever more reliable and effective means of diagnosis and treatment.

When the physicians of the early nineteenth century turned their attention to this lived experience of the patient, exploiting what was learned during the physical exam as the disease progressed, and then through postmortem study, they were looking inside the body for the cause of disease no less than Koch≈would be doing two generations later. For those working prior to the technical improvements in the microscope in the 1830s, and prior to the advent of bacteriology, one is hard-pressed to find a more important visualization of tuberculosis than René-Théophile-Hyacinthe Laennec's single image of the multiple stages of tuberculosis in the lung from his *Traité l'auscultation médiate et des maladies des poumons et du coeur* (1819). FIG. 4

25 Similarly rich descriptions and performances include Mimi in Puccini's *La Bohème*, Nikolai Dmitrich Levin in Tolstoy's *Anna Karenina*, Hans Castorp and his fellow patients in Thomas Mann's *The Magic Mountain*, and Greta Garbo's portrayal in the 1936 film *Camille*. We do not explore these alternative visualizations, but they are well worthy of further study to understand the multiple ways in which we visualize disease.

26 See for discussion Duffin (1998, 58).
27 For his biography, see Kervran (1960) and Duffin (1998).

Laennec's choice to focus on the actual lung does not mean that he did not rely on a microscope on occasion. He used the microscope to study parasites early in his career and likely also in the study of lesions.[26] But Laennec had a principled reason to resist seeking the cause of tuberculosis at the subvisible level. Primarily a clinician and trained in the French school of pathological anatomy, Laennec adhered to a physiological view of disease interested in functions and he recognized that structurally significant lesions visible at dissection did not necessarily impact an organ's functional role in the body, let alone produce symptoms for the patient. In his words, "Pathological anatomy must not be done with the loupe" (cited and trans. in Duffin 1998, 274). In our words, he reasoned that if a pathological structure visible to the naked eye did not necessarily lead to illness, there was no reason to pursue a microscopic cause of disease. He was wrong, as Koch and later generations of physician-scientists would eventually show, but this only reminds us how significant a change Koch's work and eventual positive reception really were in the late nineteenth century. Even so, Laennec had his reasons, and at the time they were more compelling than any argument claiming tuberculosis had a microscopic cause.

Today, Laennec is best known for the introduction of the stethoscope, but he became a physician of international distinction in the early nineteenth century.[27] He attracted students from across Europe and the Americas; the English physician Thomas Hodgkin came to study with him while still a medical student and was one of the first to introduce the stethoscope to medical practice in England. Laennec was born in Brittany, in the village of Quimper (where he is buried). Laennec's mother died of tuberculosis when he was five years old and he lived with his uncle, a priest, until he was twelve, after which he went to Nantes taking advantage of the newly reformed medical education available in France to study medicine where another uncle, Guillaume-François Laennec, taught. Laennec then went to the University of Paris where he studied with French luminaries such as Guillaume Dupuytren

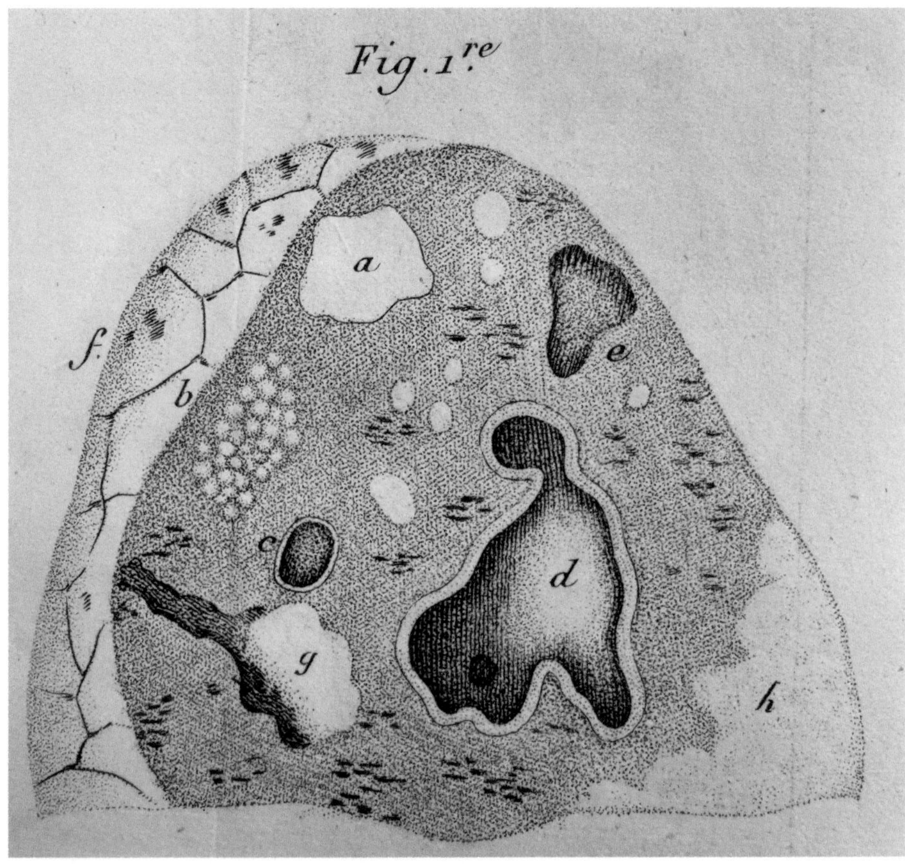

FIG. 4

FIG. 4 Illustration of a lung showing the classic history of tubercles from their early stages at *a* to cavitation at *d* and *e* (Laennec 1819, plate II, fig. 1). Huntington Library, Museum and Botanical Gardens, San Marino, California, RB 475481

(1777–1835) and Jean-Nicolas Corvisart (1755–1821), gaining clinical training at what would later become known as the Charité Hospital. Inspired by the practice of percussion of the chest introduced into France by Corvisart, who translated Leopold Auenbrugger's earlier work into French (Auenbrugger 1808), Laennec termed the use of the stethoscope "mediate auscultation" (literally, indirect listening), in contrast with the then prevalent practice of placing the ear directly on the chest (immediate auscultation). It is likely his nephew, Mériadec Laennec, diagnosed tuberculosis in Laennec using Laennec's own stethoscope; Laennec died at age 45 from the disease.

Laennec's image of the lung visible to the naked eye at dissection in the *Traité* FIG. 4 shows the lung in tuberculosis including cavitation mentioned earlier. The image highlights both Laennec's interest in calling attention to organs as the site of illness, and his reimagining the turbicle as the defining feature of tuberculosis. This was no less a shift in the way diseases were identified than the later shift introduced by Koch relying on germ theory and laboratory science.[28]

About the images in the *Traité*, we know that some of the drawings of pulmonary lesions that were the model for the engravings were done by Laennec's student Adolphe Toulmouche. The evidence is inconclusive about how involved Laennec was in the drafting process and we know nothing of who did the final engravings (Bertoloni Meli 2015, 219).[29] These unknowns, and Laennec's possible reliance on others to draw and produce the images in the *Traité*, do nothing to diminish Laennec's efforts in the clinic and at dissection, seeking to "detect in the live patient unequivocal signs of different disease ... [to provide] a triangulation among general symptoms, sounds detected in the live patient, and lesions found in the cadaver" (Bertoloni Meli 2017, 120). Using his stethoscope, Laennec was able to fix the location of tubercles in the lungs of patients and then, over the course of months and even years, follow their progress from caseation and to their eventual spread. Educating his ear and actively listening, he was able to "relate the perceived organic changes to the state of the patient"

28 It is curious that Koch's later postulates are preempted by Laennec, who articulated five criteria to identify a lesion as the cause of disease. For discussion, see Duffin (1998, 274).

29 Nevertheless, there is strong evidence of Laennec's drawing ability from his notebooks and his earlier engravings of worms of the intestines (Duffin 1998, 17, 55, 221).

(Duffin 1998, 159). It was Laennec's insistence that tuberculosis was a disease to be thought of as a physiological process, leaving organic marks, that allowed for diagnosis in this way. And it was certainly Laennec's auditory eye that determined what was included in the *Traité*'s illustrations.

Laennec's iconic image of the pathological lung in figure 4 is, as Dominico Bertoloni Meli observes, an "idealization" and not the lung of any particular patient; no single specimen would include the range of features present, including a relatively healthy lung represented at *a*, or the several stages of intrusive lesions that could be found postmortem at *b* through g, where the tubercle is present (Bertoloni Meli 2017, 108). The accuracy of Laennec's images has been reaffirmed by the countless demonstrations of pathologists in the past two centuries. Laennec's text also clearly demonstrates the usefulness of the stethoscope, in recognizing the various stages of tuberculosis in the lungs. He devotes more than 30 pages to it, including in sections dedicated to describing "Physical signs of tubercles" and "Symptoms and progress of phthisis" (Laennec 1838, 333, 345).

Part of Laennec's goal is to inform his readers about the pathogenesis of tuberculosis, which he is offering us with figure 4 as a visualization of the progressive nature of this disease. More than this, because of the didactic value of the image he provides, when the stethoscope is used properly, it allows the clinician to understand the changes occurring inside the living patient and thereby to monitor the progress of tuberculosis even in the absence of outward symptoms. By introducing this auditory eye into medicine, Laennec's visualization of disease goes beyond what can be noticed by the untrained observer. Both skill and experience were needed to pick up a stethoscope and use the instrument to picture the state of the lung inside the patient.

Thus, once consensus shifted in his favor, the conditions under which a disease should be seen and diagnosed changed with Laennec just as with Koch two generations later. Evidence of the change appears in many subsequent studies of pathology documenting the lesions of tuberculosis utilizing his blend of pathological anatomy and physiology.[30] These works show what the clinician was looking for, or what the fate of the patient's organs would be, when the physician examined and listened to the living patient. English physicians were not at all surprised by this new trend, having seen it before. Unmentioned by Laennec is Matthew Baillie's *The Morbid Anatomy of Some of the Most Important Parts of the Human Body* (1793), the first book to emphasize the study of pathology by systems and the first English-language text devoted to pathology as a self-standing subject. Baillie also included images to aid in the visualization of disease. A second example, this time owing something to Laennec, comes from Jean Allard Jeançon (1831–1903), a native of France whose professional years were spent mostly in the United States. Jeançon published one of the first atlases of pathology (*Pathological Anatomy, Pathology and Physical Diagnosis: A Series of Clinical Reports Comprising the Principal Diseases of the Human Body: Systematically Arranged in One Hundred Full-Page Illustrations and One Hundred Pages of Text*) in 1882, though the text was largely based on Jean Cruveilhier's *Anatomie pathologique du corps humain* (1829). The color illustrations of the lungs in tuberculosis in Jeançon's book were unsurpassed until the mid-twentieth century, when Frank Netter (1906–1991) depicted the same subjects, with X-ray images and other clinical information, in the Ciba pharmaceutical company's *The Ciba Collection of Medical Illustrations*, originally published in pamphlet form and then as system texts; tuberculosis is covered in "Volume 7: Respiratory System" (1954).

30 For an account of Laennec's reception in Britain, see Nicolson (1993). The speed with which Laennec's diagnostic techniques spread to Britain, is apparent in the guidance offered in both Forbes (1824) and Stokes (1825).

3
Seeing Like a Pathologist

The two images given extended attention in the previous section, from Laennec and Koch, offer differing though complementary views of the same disease. Laennec's provides us with the macroscopic features of early and advanced tuberculosis visible postmortem inside the body that can be easily recognized in almost every case when the affected lung is examined. In contrast, Koch shows us the deadly organism that causes the disease, less than three micrometers (0.000118 inches) long, capable of initiating the complex inflammatory reaction that is the disease. Laennec provided a doorway to establishing the diagnosis by clinical means (physical examination, including percussion and "mediate" auscultation) grounded in morphologic findings postmortem, while the portal Koch opened initiated the understanding of the biology, and subsequent treatment, of the causative organism. Both perspectives, and so both types of visualization, remain essential to the pathologist. In this section we briefly attempt to explain why.

"Pathology" is literally the study of disease (logos + pathos), and in its institutionalized hospital version of today, its investigators are expected to look for the causes of disease affecting the cells, tissues, fluids, and organs of the body. It is the changes to the latter that present as signs and symptoms of the patient detectable to the clinician and to the pathologist in a more complete fashion (Kumar, Abbas, and Aster 2013, 1). This much is clear from the two sides, in addition to diagnosis, of the pathologist's expected expertise: etiology and pathogenesis. In practice, it is only by describing both the origin of a disease and its stages of development that the pathologist justifies a particular diagnosis and treatment.

We believe these expectations make it clear that the pathologist's *modus operandi*—i.e., techniques, rules, procedures, and methods—relies on more than a single time slice of a patient's illness and disease. Though that may be all that we see in the histological image they are provided, they are like the filmmaker who has seen the film before and is therefore able to locate the spliced scene within the fuller reel. In other words, it is dynamic thinking that allows the prepared pathologist to make an informed judgment; it is why they do not see a static image when they look at the images from the previous section.

But how does the pathologist get habituated to their *modus operandi*? Their method is, like any method, a way of doing something. It is a way of diagnosing disease. It is general in the sense that it can be repeated, but also in the sense that it can be applied to every case that comes before the pathologist. How is the profession learned? The learning of pathology is not a training experience in which the same lesson is repeated as many times as necessary but, instead, is based on exposure to as many variables of disease expression as possible and, ultimately, years of experience.[31] Such is the complexity of diagnostic judgment. In other words, the methods and judgment of the qualified pathologist are not a mechanical process, and neither is it wholly propositional knowledge, something that can be articulated in a straightforward way.[32] It falls within the domain of "skillful knowing" that Michale Polanyi (2005) championed in the last century and that Gilbert Ryle (1946) differentiated when he introduced the distinction between "knowing how" to do or make something and "knowing that" some fact or proposition was the case.[33] The pathologist has and acts on both kinds of knowledge, but it is knowledge how to make a diagnosis that characterizes their profession.

Thus, to be clear, we see the pathologist's ideal education in a different light than some of its critics. The influential physician and epidemiologist Alvan Feinstein (1925–2001) lamented that clinicians are "severely restricted by the views of 'disease' provided in still photographs of the camera of pathology" (Feinstein 1967, 105).[34] That may be true of clinicians (and the general public) but, in contrast, the pathologist does not merely interpret a still image. Neither their education nor their *modus operandi*, nor the history of the images on which contemporary pathology builds its foundations, visualize disease solely from straightforwardly static images.

IV
Conclusion

There are many lessons we might draw from the history of tuberculosis and, especially, from the images of Laennec and Koch. In the near term, we expect the combination of science and art, as we know it, will soon be replaced by

31 Stephen Geller owes this observation to personal communication from his teacher and colleague Lotte Strauss, MD (1913–1985), one of the founders of the specialty of pediatric pathology, who learned it from her teacher, the great, early twentieth-century pathologist Paul Klemperer (1887–1964). Klemperer began the study of law at the University of Vienna but transferred to medicine when he heard Sigmund Freud speak. He later became Pathologist-in-Chief at New York's Mount Sinai Hospital and was a principal contributor in establishing the concept of "collagen diseases," including systemic lupus erythematosus (SLE).

32 We wish to thank Alfred Freeborn and Flora Lysen for encouraging us to think further about the habituation of the pathologist and for reminding us of the work of Polyani (1958) and Feinstein (1967), cited later.

33 Ryle's distinction has come in for criticism in recent years, with debate centering on whether "knowing how" is really just a kind of "knowing that." For an effort to move beyond this debate and to emphasize the role of knowing how to do things in science (which would also apply to medicine), see Chang (2017).

34 More recent discussions of clinical judgment that do not share (all) of Feinstein's criticisms include Schön (1988) and Montgomery (2006).

computer-generated graphic images, in some instances reminiscent of the art depicted in the chapter of van der Beugel and Keuck. Diagnosis and prognosis will almost certainly be made with tools of artificial intelligence. But the extent to which visualization of disease will change and the conditions under which it will be ideally conducted, remain to be settled. For the present, however, we see three lessons worth identifying.

First, the visualization of tuberculosis in the nineteenth century presented two shifts in scientific medicine's ideal conditions for diagnosing disease. The ideal conditions altered with Laennec to accommodate an auditory glimpse inside the body, visualizing physiological and anatomic changes in the living patient's internal organs. These conditions included the use of an instrument, a willing patient, relative quiet, and an educated ear. With Koch these conditions changed again, aided by the microscope, to include a laboratory with expertly prepared specimens, which finally allowed the cause of tuberculosis to be seen. In both cases, we find the unstated positivist mantra that "seeing is believing" guiding the diagnostician and scientist. But we also recognize in our history the pragmatist's awareness that what is seen, and that the ideal conditions that allow us to correct and confirm what is seen, are themselves subject to change.

Second, disease is not a single static slide or image of the patient, reducible to what can be visualized in a single moment but, rather, a "screenshot" of a dynamic and evolving process within the patient. The robust concepts of the physician-scientist are needed to understand disease. It is all too easy to miss this vision of the pathologist, which sees beyond the present to the past and the future. Laennec's illustration exemplifies this vision especially well. Only by grasping the stages of disease does the disease get properly identified. FIG. 4

Finally, we recognize the value of collaborative work like that pursed here. The current state of medicine and science is itself a collective enterprise, and no single individual can master the details of either; the amount of information to assimilate is simply too great. No physician operates in isolation today, and the historian's goals cannot be achieved by a single individual working through an archive alone. Historians and scientists, and in this case scientist-physicians, must join forces if they are to come to understand the present by knowing where we have been; only in this way will we be able to understand where we might be going.

A

Ackerknecht, Erwin Heinz (1953) *Rudolf Virchow: Doctor, Statesman, Anthropologist.* Madison: University of Wisconsin Press.

Ackerknecht, Erwin Heinz (1965) *History and Geography of the Most Important Diseases*. New York: Hafner Publishing Company.

Agarwal, Yatish, Rajesh K. Chopra, Dipendra K. Gupta, and Ravinder S. Sethi (2017) "The Tuberculosis Timeline: Of White Plague, a Birthday Present, and Vignettes of Myriad Hues." *Astrocyte* 4, no. 1: 7. https://doi.org/10.4103/2349-0977.217662.

Aretaeus of Cappadocia (1958) *De Causis et Signis Acutorum Morborum (Caus.Ac.); De Causis et Signis Diuturnorum Morborum (Caus. Chr.)*. Edited by C. Hude. Leipzig: In aedibus Academiae Scientiarum.

Aristotle (1995) *Complete Works*. Edited by Jonathan Barnes. Translated by d'A.W. Thompson. Vol. 1. Princeton, NJ: Princeton University Press.

Auenbrugger, L. (1808) *Nouvelle Méthode Pour Reconnaître Les Maladies Internes de La Poitrine Par La Percussion de Cetter Cavité*. Translated by J. N. Corvisart. Paris: Migneret.

B

Bertoloni Meli, Domenico (2015) "The Rise of Pathological Illustrations: Baillie, Bleuland, and Their Collections." *Bulletin of the History of Medicine* 89, no. 2: 209–42. https://doi.org/10.1353/bhm.2015.0034.

Bertoloni Meli, Domenico (2017) *Visualizing Disease: The Art and History of Pathological Illustrations*. Chicago: University of Chicago Press.

Brock, T. D. (1988) *Robert Koch: A Life in Medicine and Bacteriology*. Madison, WI: Science Tech Publishers. https://www.semanticscholar.org/paper/Robert-Koch-A-Life-in-Medicine-and-Bacteriology-Brock/adb4957f150bb94eca5aa124bab6b3d63dcfdfb1.

Brock, Thomas D. (1999) *Milestones in Microbiology: 1546 to 1940*. Washington, DC: American Society for Microbiology. https://www.semanticscholar.org/paper/Milestones-in-microbiology-1546-to-1940-Brock/9da3f4e36c4dd77fb4f1d915f2909e240d2e3ca7.

Bunyan, John (1900) *The Life and Death of Mr. Badman*. New York: R. H. Russell. https://ia801300.us.archive.org/7/items/lifedeathofmrbadm1900buny/lifedeathofmrbadm1900buny.pdf.

Bynum, Helen (2012) *Spitting Blood: The History of Tuberculosis*. Oxford: Oxford University Press.

C

Carter, K. Codell (2003) *The Rise of Causal Concepts of Disease: Case Histories*. London: Routledge.

Chang, H. (2017) "Operational Coherence as the Source of Truth." *Proceedings of the Aristotelian Society* 117: 103–22. https://doi.org/10.17863/CAM.9355.

Coleman, William (1977) *Biology in the Nineteenth Century: Problems of Form, Function, and Transformation*. Cambridge, UK: Cambridge University Press. http://archive.org/details/biologyinninetee0000cole_k5j8.

Cruveilhier, J. (1829) *Anatomie Pathologique Du Corps Humain*. Paris: Baillière.

Cummins, S. Lyle (1949) *Tuberculosis in History*. London: Bailliere, Tindall and Cox.

Cunningham, A. (1992) "Transforming Plague: The Laboratory and the Identity of Infectious Disease." In *In The Laboratory Revolution in Medicine*, edited by A. Cunningham and P. Williams, 209–44. Cambridge, UK: Cambridge University Press.

D

Davis, Audrey B. (1981) *Medicine and Its Technology: An Introduction to the History of Medical Instrumentation*. Westport, CT: Greenwood Press. http://archive.org/details/medicineitstechn0000davi.

De Renzi, Silvia, Marco Bresadola, and Maria Conforti, eds. (2018) *Pathology in Practice: Diseases and Dissections in Early Modern Europe*. The History of Medicine in Context. London: Routledge.

Dormandy, Thomas (2000) *The White Death: A History of Tuberculosis*. New York: New York University Press. http://archive.org/details/whitedeathhistor0000dorm_p3o2.

Dubos, René and Jean Dubos (1952) *The White Plague, Tuberculosis, Man and Society*. Boston: Little, Brown.

Duffin, Jacalyn (1998) *To See with a Better Eye: A Life of R. T. H. Laennec*. Princeton, NJ: Princeton University Press. https://www.jstor.org/stable/j.ctt7zvjqm.

F

Feinstein, Alvan R. (1967) *Clinical Judgment*. Baltimore: Williams & Wilkins.

Forbes, John (1824) *Original Cases with Dissections and Observations Illustrating the Use of the Stethoscope and Percussion in the Diagnosis of Diseases of the Chest*. London: Underwood. http://archive.org/details/originalcaseswit00forb.

Frege, Gottlob (1892) "Über Sinn Und Bedeutung." *Zeitschrift Für Philosophie Und Philosophische Kritik* 100: 25–50.

Frith, J. (2014) "History of Tuberculosis: Part 1: Phthisis, Consumption and the White Plague." *Journal of Military and Veterans' Health* 22: 29–35.

G

Gradmann, Christoph. 2001. "Robert Koch and the Pressures of Scientific Research: Tuberculosis and Tuberculin." *Medical History* 45, no. 1: 1–32. https://doi.org/10.1017/S0025727300000028.

Gradmann, Christoph (2006) "Robert Koch and the White Death: From Tuberculosis to Tuberculin." *Microbes and Infection* 8, no. 1: 294–301. https://doi.org/10.1016/j.micinf.2005.06.004.

Gradmann, Christoph (2009) *Laboratory Disease: Robert Koch's Medical Bacteriology*. Baltimore: Johns Hopkins University Press.

Grimes, D. Jay (2006) "Koch's Postulates: Then and Now." *Microbe Magazine* 1, no. 5: 223–28.

Grmek, Mirko D. (1989) *Diseases in the Ancient Greek World*. Baltimore: Johns Hopkins University Press.

Grundmann, Ekkehard, and Stephen A. Geller, eds. (1989) *Histopathology: Color Atlas of Organs and Systems*. Munich: Urban & Schwarzenberg.

H

Hacking, Ian (1983) *Representing and Intervening: Introductory Topics in the Philosophy of Natural Science*. Cambridge, UK: Cambridge University Press.

Hankin, E. H. (1891) "Professor Virchow on the Consumption Cure." *Nature* 43, no. 1107: 248–49. https://doi.org/10.1038/043248d0.

Henschen, Folke (1962) *The History and Geography of Diseases*. New York: Delacorte Press.

Herzog, H. (1998) "History of Tuberculosis." *Respiration* 65, no. 1: 5–15. https://doi.org/10.1159/000029220.

J

Jeançon, J. A. (1882) *Pathological Anatomy, Pathology and Physical Diagnosis*. Cincinnati: Progress Publishing Company.

K

Kappelman, John, Mehmet Cihat Alçiçek, Nizamettin Kazancı, Michael Schultz, Mehmet Özkul, and Şevket Şen (2008) "First Homo Erectus from Turkey and Implications for Migrations into Temperate Eurasia." *American Journal of Physical Anthropology* 135, no. 1: 110–16. https://doi.org/10.1002/ajpa.20739.

Keers, Robert Young (1978) *Pulmonary Tuberculosis: A Journey down the Centuries*. London: Ballière Tindall.

Kervran, Roger (1960) *Laennec: His Life and Times*. Translated by D. C. Abrahams-Curiel. Oxford: Pergamon Press.

Koch, Robert (1882) "Die Ätiologie der Tuberkulose." *Berliner Klinische Wochenschrift* 15: 221–30.

Koch, Robert (1912) "Die Ätiologie Der Tuberkulose (1884)." In *Gesammelte Werke von Robert Koch*, edited by J. Schwalbe, vol. 1: 454–565. Leipzig: Thieme.

Krishnan, Vidya (2022) *Phantom Plague: How Tuberculosis Shaped History*. New York: Public Affairs.

Kumar, Vinay, Abul K. Abbas, and Jon C. Aster (2013) *Robbins: Basic Pathology*. Philadelphia: Elsevier.

L

Laennec, René Théophile Hyacinthe (1819) *De l'auscultation Médiate: Ou Traité Du Diagnostic Des Maladies Des Poumons et Du Coeur, Fondé Principalement Sur Ce Nouveau Moyen d'exploration*. Paris: Brosson et Chaudé.

Laennec, René Théophile Hyacinth (1838) *A Treatise on the Diseases of the Chest, and on Mediate Auscultation*. Translated by John Forbes. New York: Samuel S. and William Wood.

Laios, Konstantinos, George Androutsos, and Marilita M. Moschos (2017) "Aretaeus of Cappadocia and Pulmonary Tuberculosis." *Balkan Medical Journal* 34, no. 5: 480. https://doi.org/10.4274/balkanmedj.2016.1847.

Long, Esmond Ray (1965) *A History of Pathology*. New York: Dover.

Loscalzo, Joseph, Anthony Fauci, Dennis Kasper, Stephen Hauser, Dan Longo, and J. Larry Jameson, eds. (2022) *Harrison's Principles of Internal Medicine*. 21st edition. New York: McGraw Hill.

M

Majno, Guido, and Isabelle Joris (2004) *Cells, Tissues, and Disease: Principles of General Pathology*. 2nd edition. Oxford: Oxford University Press.

Meinecke, Bruno (1927) "Consumption (Tuberculosis) in Classical Antiquity." *Annals of Medical History* 9, no. 4: 379–402.

Montgomery, Kathryn (2006) *How Doctors Think: Clinical Judgment and the Practice of Medicine*. Oxford: Oxford University Press.

N

Netter, Frank H., ed. (1954) *The Ciba Collection of Medical Illustrations*. Summit, NJ: Ciba Pharmaceutical Products.

Nicolson, M. (1993) "The Introduction of Percussion and Stethoscopy to Early Nineteenth-Century Edinburgh." In *Medicine and the Five Senses*, edited by W. Bynum and T. Porter, 134–53. Cambridge, UK: Cambridge University Press. https://www.semanticscholar.org/paper/The-introduction-of-percussion-and-stethoscopy-to-Nicolson/579803590036f2ed931a64586456c632430550ab.

Nutton, Vivian. 2000. "Did the Greeks Have a Word for It? Contagion and Contagion Theory in Classical Antiquity." In *Contagion: Perspectives from Pre-Modern Societies*, edited by Lawrence Conrad and Dominik Wujastyk, 137–62. Aldershot: Ashgate.

Nutton, Vivian (2004) *Ancient Medicine*. London: Routledge.

O

Oxford English Dictionary (2024) "Tubercule, n. Meanings, Etymology and More." In *Oxford English Dictionary*. https://www.oed.com/dictionary/tubercule_n.

P

Payne, Lynda (2017) *The Best Surgeon in England: Percivall Pott, 1713–1788*. American University Studies. Series IX, History, vol. 205. New York: Peter Lang.

Polanyi, Michael (2005) *Personal Knowledge: Towards a Post-Critical Philosophy*. London: Routledge.

R

Ragland, Evan (2022) *Making Physicians: Tradition, Teaching, and Trials at Leiden University, 1575–1639*. Leiden: Brill.

Ryle, Gilbert (1946) "Knowing How and Knowing That: The Presidential Address." *Proceedings of the Aristotelian Society* 46, no. 1: 1–16. https://doi.org/10.1093/aristotelian/46.1.1.

S

Schön, D. A. (1988) "From Technical Rationality to Reflection in Action." In *Professional Judgment: A Reader in Clinical Decision Making*, edited by J. Dowie and A. S. Elstein, 60–77. Cambridge, UK: Cambridge University Press.

Snyder, Laura J. (2015) *Eye of the Beholder: Johannes Vermeer, Antoni Van Leeuwenhoek, and the Reinvention of Seeing*. 1st edition. New York: W. W. Norton.

Soler, Léna, Emiliano Trizio, Thomas Nickles, and William Wimsatt, eds. (2012) *Characterizing the Robustness of Science: After the Practice Turn in Philosophy of Science*. Dordrecht: Springer. https://doi.org/10.1007/978-94-007-2759-5.

Stokes, William (1825) *An Introduction to the Use of the Stethoscope*. Edinburgh: MacLachlan and Stewart. http://archive.org/details/b21469647.

Stolberg, Michael (2016) "Approaches to the History of Patients: From the Ancient World to Early Modern Europe." In *Homo Patiens: Approaches to the Patient in the Ancient World*, edited by Georgia Petridou and Chiara Thumiger, 497–518. Leiden: Brill. https://doi.org/10.1163/9789004305564_022.

W

Walker, Lary, Harry LeVine, and Mathias Jucker (2006) "Koch's Postulates and Infectious Proteins." *Acta Neuropathologica* 112, no. 1: 1–4. https://doi.org/10.1007/s00401-006-0072-x.

Patterns of Pathology in EEG Research: The "Art and Science" of Analyzing Brainwaves in the Mid-Twentieth Century

Flora Lysen and Marlene Bart

Introduction

"Haven't we tried this before (and failed)?" two researchers recently wondered in an article about the usefulness of electroencephalography (EEG) as a biomarker for neurobehavioral disorders (Ewen and Levin 2022). Ever since the rapid emergence of brainwave research in the 1930s, EEG researchers have been poring over miles of zigzag lines and (big) datasets of brain activity figures to search for "electrophysiological correlates of behavior," including signs that could indicate a person's mental state, mental health, or elements of psychopathology. The hope and promise is that one day, researchers will be able to interpret EEG signals as a meaningful record for diagnostic purposes, as an indicator of diseases in a clinical context, or as a helpful instrument in determining (normal or abnormal) psychological states, mental processes, or perhaps even specific thoughts. Yet, while records of brain activity have become an important and successful clinical tool in the domain of epilepsy and sleep disorder research, they have so far hardly been beneficial in detecting and treating neurobehavioral and neuropathological disorders such as autism spectrum disorder, ADHD, depressive illness, and Alzheimer's disease.[1]

1 Systematic reviews suggest there is (as of yet) little evidence that EEG can serve as a clinically useful biomarker in the domain of psychopathology and mental health or as an aid in treatment (Ewen, Sweeney, and Potter 2019; Widge et al. 2019; Nilsonne and Harrell 2021; Klooster et al. 2024). DL-EEG is predominantly tested for the domain of epilepsy (seizure detection and prediction), brain-computer interfaces (BCIs), and for monitoring of specific cognitive and affective states (Roy et al. 2019).

Despite discouraging results of EEG's utility in the field of pathology, its promise as a classifier of disease persists. Most recently, researchers have pointed to advances in deep learning to propose that meaningful markers can potentially be extracted from big datasets of EEG records (Roy et al. 2019; Wan et al. 2020; Squires et al. 2023). Central to this excitement are references to the unprecedented power of pattern recognition in AI-supported data-driven analysis, which is prospected to "revolutionize diagnosis, detection and treatment" (Squires et al. 2023, 2).[2] While some EEG researchers admit that the field has a history of overselling new technologies of data analysis (Ewen and Levin 2022), there is a persistent hope that new computational power and processing methods may, as two EEG researchers put it "expand what the EEG can 'see' and simultaneously decrease dependence on analyst skill" (Ewen and Beniczky 2017, 7). This last quote is symptomatic; computationally supported EEG is compared to a type of improved vision ("expand what the EEG can 'see'") and is also pitted against the (supposedly) inferior perceptive skills of the human analyst.

2 Most strikingly, unsupervised algorithms in deep learning have been proposed as a way to identify subgroups within disease populations that differ from and extend current diagnostic labels and could shape new diagnostic criteria (Squires et al. 2023).

Discussions of artificial intelligence today frequently revolve around the concepts of finding, recognizing, and discovering patterns. These discussions are heavily focused on recent experiments with deep learning, which build upon machine learning techniques that originated in the 1950s. Despite their ubiquitous appearance in texts, what is meant by patterns is often left undefined and undertheorized. Recently, humanities scholars have started to analyze the concept of pattern as a figure of knowledge with a particularly polysemous character, similar to other mega concepts or hypernyms, such as networks, systems, or structures (Besser 2022). The concept of pattern, especially in the way it is used in discussions on pattern recognition, is characterized by a sedimentation of various (implicit) meanings: it evokes both a conception of correlation (a statistical regularity), as well as a figurative conception of a specific form and spatiotemporal configuration (Schabacher 2023; Besser 2022). Because of its association with a material or perceptible form, the concept of patterns blurs the distinction between order that can be perceptually grasped (visual patterns, auditory patterns) and order that is beyond human perception, such as a statistical pattern. In turn, this association of patterns with perceptibility also strengthens their ontological status: pattern recognition enacts the phenomena of patterns.

Tropes of pattern finding and claims of augmented vision are omnipresent in contemporary discussions about the role of AI and big data in the field of medicine. Imaginaries of computer-aided, pattern recognition-based analysis of medical images revolve around tireless, omnipotent eyes that can cast a view that is "panoramic," integrating images and other clinical data on a new scale that allows for a more comprehensive analysis (Beer 2018, 472), and "deep," detecting subtle patterns and correlations beyond the capacities of human perception and cognition (Engelmann 2020, 626). In popular portrayals, the power of computationally supported image analysis (with deep learning currently at its frontier) is often framed as both prosthetic and super-human; technical systems are presented as amplifying the perceptual capacities of the human, but also as superseding the suboptimal performance of the human image expert (Lysen 2023).

Prompted by these contemporary promises of deep learning's pattern recognition capacities, this chapter examines the history of EEG research to reflect on changing attitudes toward human and mechanically aided analysis of patterns—a historically shifting juxtaposition between the role of automated, machine-supported perception vis-à-vis human interpretive skills. Early histories of brainwave analysis are proposed here as productive case material to shed more light on the epistemological purchase of the concept of seeing and analyzing patterns. At this historical junction in the mid-twentieth century, new ideas about human perception as pattern seeing met with what seemed a preeminent pattern-like object: the brainwave. By the 1950s, it had become established practice to refer to brain activity and EEG records as containing patterns that required interpretation. And in turn, to think of the activities of both human interpreters and computational processes in terms of recognizing patterns. In this chapter, I unpack some of these conceptual zigzag movements, tracing pattern conceptions in the context of EEG analysis from discussion of EEG research in psychopathology and the first international reference *Atlas of EEG* (1941) to EEG researchers adopting the term "pattern recognition" as it was developed in the context of computing.

The research and writing for this chapter were conducted in conversation with and parallel to the work of artist Marlene Bart, who created an augmented reality (AR) piece accessible with a custom-made phone app via the three images embedded in this chapter. These images, referred to as "tableaux" by Marlene, possess an enigmatic iconographic quality. They reference historical material from different time periods in the history of EEG (including, for example, a hidden picture of EEG researcher Erna Gibbs, a diagram of a brainwave measuring system, and a rabbit test subject) as well as fragments from Marlene's experiments with imaging her own body and brain. Layered in these tableaux are visual aesthetics drawn from different domains: 3D scans of body parts, graphic records, rainbow-colored measuring scales, a female chess player in a classic "thinker" pose. Entering the AR piece, visitors can read, hear, and see elements of an intellectual and artistic exploration of pattern concepts that extend far beyond the boundaries of this written chapter. They learn about apophenia (delusions of seeing patterns in random noise), computers playing chess, honeycomb patterns emerging in nature as well as the brainwaves of women included in the 1941 *Atlas of EEG*. In our collaboration, Marlene and I aimed to avoid the hierarchical dynamic where the artist merely illustrates the academic's work, or where the chapter serves as an explanation of the artwork. Instead, the artwork and the text have rubbed off on each other in their creation and are interlinked in their visual and conceptual interests. To provide the reader with some insight into our interactions, this chapter also includes three interludes in the form of vignettes that describe particularly revealing moments in our working process, spanning the period of May 2023 to June 2024.

Searching for EEG Waveforms and Patterns in Psychopathology around 1940

When Hans Berger observed, in the late 1920s, that the brain's alpha waves diminish when a person opens their eyes or engages in mental activity, his discovery spurred enormous efforts to decipher the EEG and correlate neural activity with mental phenomena, including psychopathologies. Furthermore, when researchers found that epilepsy produced a distinct brainwave pattern, many hypothesized that other pathological conditions could similarly be identified through EEG recordings. This enthusiasm for correlation was aligned with a dominant materialist premise—the idea that the physical brain underpins mental processes, human behavior, and thought—which significantly influenced brain research in the twentieth century (Hagner and Borck 2001; Vidal 2009). Consequently, early measurements of the brain's electrical activity were immediately seen as providing a window into the mind and human psychology (Borck 2005). After Hans Berger's first publication in 1929, American researchers in particular rapidly took up EEG research, a development that has been attributed to the US's greater access to, and proficiency with, electronic amplification technology, as well as its substantial funding for neurological research (Millett 2001; Borck 2005). When cerebral curves emerged as electric phenomena, in the 1930s and 1940s, their rise as epistemic things was powerfully imbricated with simultaneous developments in communication and information theory as well as statistical analysis. EEG curves were conceived as very complex signals that could be mathematically quantified and from which—with the help of new approaches in mathematics—a message, i.e., a significant feature, could be extracted from background noise. While neurophysiologists continued to try to understand how anatomical brain structures gave rise to electrical activity, EEG research in the US context was dominated by large comparative measuring operations (Hagner 2004)—as EEG researcher Frederic Gibbs put it, letting "the brainwaves speak for themselves" (Borck 2018, 165).

In the mid-1930s, a number of exploratory research programs aimed to correlate EEG records with a wide range of activity states and classifications: dreaming, paying attention and doing math, menstruating, experiencing a psychosis, and being labeled as a problem child, to name but a few. Personality type research was an active field of study, where EEG records could be conceived as "a pattern of electrical behavior rather than as a series of separate factors, in the same manner as one regards a person's behavior, attitude, or personality as a pattern and not a series of separate factors" (Davis 1941, 101). Another, partially overlapping field was EEG research in abnormal behaviors and psychopathologies, where researchers sought qualitative classifications of different wave forms and rhythms as well as their incidence in various diagnostic groups, such as subjects with depression, sociopathic personality, manic depressive disorder, or paranoia (cf. Gibbs and Gibbs 1964). To do so, this work employed a comparative method by which the range of variation of "normal" and the differences between "normal" and "pathological" were gradually induced from a large collection of EEG records.

What occurred was a back-and-forth movement between EEG and pathological categories established by clinicians. Researchers identified characteristic waves by searching for significant differences in subjects with pathological diagnoses while simultaneously refining pathology classifications based on EEG observations. It appeared that individuals with disorders could display "disordered brainwaves" (Lennox 1942, 594), while those exhibiting unstable behavior were observed to have "unstable records" (Davis 1941, 112). Every aspect of the EEG was a potential candidate to signify abnormality: amplitudes, frequencies, phase relationships between different brain regions, voltage fluctuations, and sudden bursts of activity. Specific signals could be disrupted or exhibit slow activity, be exceptionally fast or asymmetrically localized, and waveforms could be particularly sharp or round.

Many schemata proliferated, but they all depended, to cite one overview article, on measuring the "incidence of the various types of waves and a consideration of the wave forms and patterns" (Pacella and Barrera 1941). On the basis of this comparative research, researchers pointed to potential pathological signs in the record, such as the "spike and wave rhythm," the "square wave," the "fast rhythm," and waves in the shape of a "mitten," a "spindle," or "choppy waves" (Walter 1950, 84). The drive to find indicators of difference in EEG curves was tenacious, even when studies did not deliver the hypothesized results. When two researchers found no "fundamental patterns" that could distinguish 232 patients from mental hospitals from a control series of 500 "normals," they conjectured that some disturbance of the normal pattern could still be considered a "common element" (Davis and Davis 1939, 1019). In this case, "the abnormalities which break into the pattern, rather than the type of pattern itself, constitute the significant difference between the electroencephalograms of these patients and of normal individuals." Even disturbing a pattern could be viewed as a "significant difference," and satisfied this extensive pattern-finding operation (Davis and Davis 1939, 1019).

Research into EEG and psychopathology around 1940 was criticized by researchers who could not replicate findings or found the evidence insufficient (Finley and Campbell 1941; for an overview see Ellingson 1956). An important factor in this failure, as various researchers noted, was the absence of clear pathological classification for mental disorders. Psychopathologies were themselves ill-defined (Walter 1942) and scholars expressed their concerns about the inevitably uncertain results when joined with the technique of EEG. As EEG researcher John Knott put it, with EEG and psychopathology, "two unknowns" were being explained "in terms of each other" (Borck 2018, 201). Many EEG researchers were notably transparent about the nascent and uncertain status of the pattern-finding efforts (Schirmann 2014). Review articles and commentary sections of scholarly papers in the field attest to the way researchers acknowledged and foregrounded the provisional nature of their studies and the speculative dimension of suggested patterns.

Scan the QR code to find additional information about the project and access the augmented reality app on the Patterns of Pathology website: https://www.marlenebart.com/patterns-of-pathology.

Examinations of psychopathology with EEG were characterized by a tentative and explorative attitude and researchers recognized the uncertainties and weaknesses in current research. Nevertheless, there was optimism that with necessary methodological improvements, EEG would eventually become useful as a classification device. Next to the importance of standardization of techniques and clinical case descriptions, two key improvements were frequently highlighted. First, it was pertinent to better establish a uniform way of quantifying "normality" in EEG records in tandem with abnormal EEG patterns. EEG-norm curves were needed to aid more uniform and trustworthy diagnosis. Second, researchers sought to increasingly supplement and replace the expert interpretation of brainwave curves with automated (mechanically aided) computational procedures of analysis. Automated analysis was viewed as a way to realize the potential of EEG for classification. As the next section elaborates, technological optimism about automated interpretation was not uncontested but remained present despite the high costs of developing these techniques and inconclusive results.

Patterns, Collages, Differences

May 2023. Marlene and Flora exchange texts and visual images to inspire practices and processes of writing and making. One image, in particular, catches Marlene's attention: an early twentieth-century illustration of a woman sitting at her desk. Her collaged body forms a diagram, demonstrating how nervous messages travel from the senses to her brain and writing hand. The image epitomizes how women have often been depicted as opaque entities, made transparent through visualization technologies. Marlene "abducts" the image and cuts it into pieces to create animations where the collage talks to multiple versions of herself. These chaotic and absurd female talking heads prompt important questions: What about the position of women in the context of the EEG research? Where are the women? And what would a feminist approach to EEG history look like?

FIG. 1 Marlene Bart, *Patterns of Pathology*, Tableau I, 2024/2025, digital collage and augmented reality. Courtesy of the artist

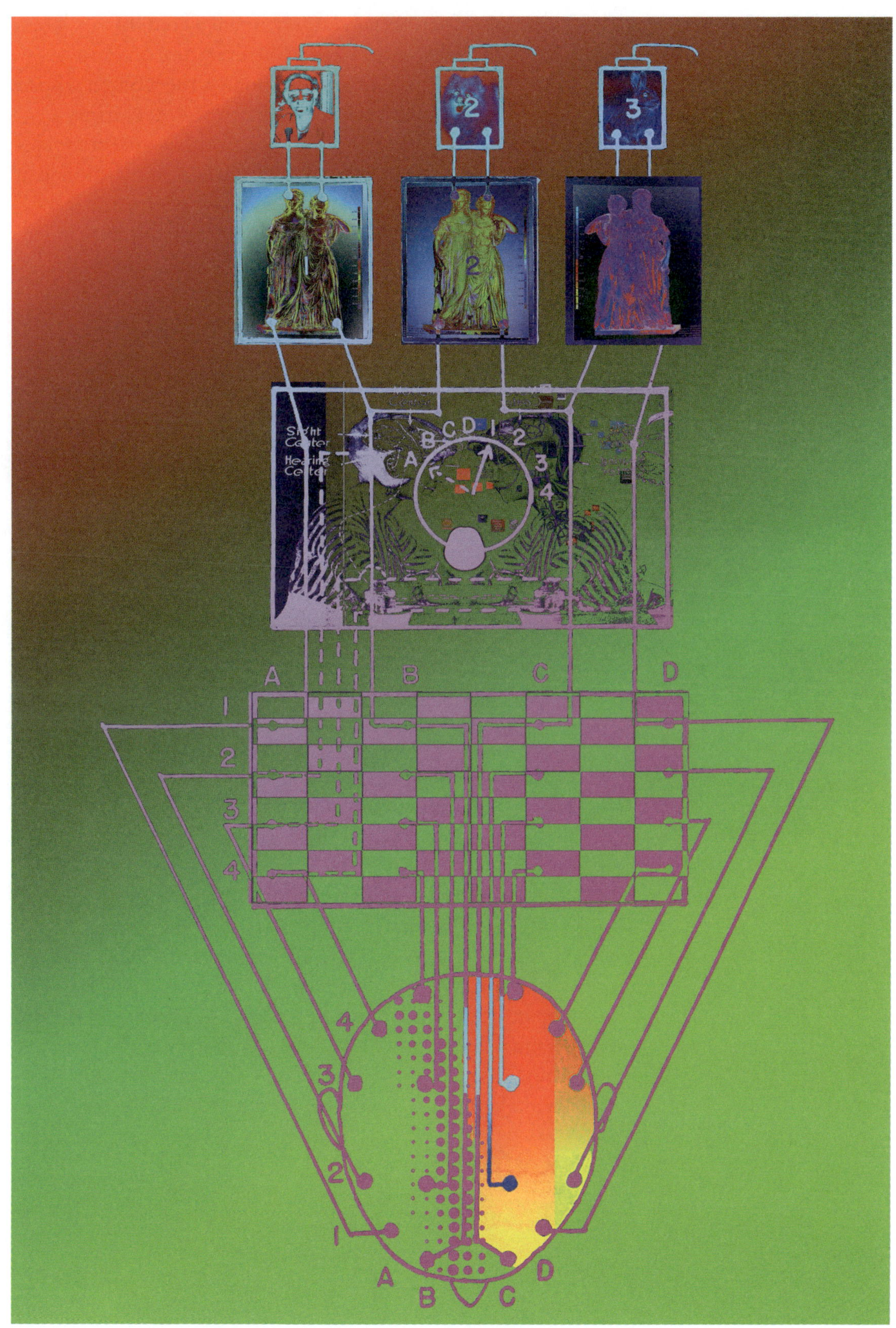
2
3
Sight
Hearing
A
B
C
D
1
2
3
4
A
B
C
D
1
2
3
4
4
3
2
1
A
B
C
D

These questions remain largely unanswered. In mid-twentieth-century scientific literature on innovations in EEG automation technologies, the women whose work underpinned curve computation—measuring, calculating, copying, and punching cards—are often relegated to the footnotes of scientific papers, if mentioned at all. Meanwhile, early EEG research saw a comparatively high number of women assisting and collaborating in lab work, co-authoring scientific papers, and leading EEG laboratories. Yet, their contributions have mostly been overlooked in historical accounts, including Flora's own research. Beyond the question of women's roles, Marlene's work also draws renewed attention to the crucial issue of gender norms embedded in systems of classifying and measuring EEGs. From the first *Atlas of Electroencephalography* (1941), she singles out records of seven women (aged between 30 and 40, the age range between Marlene and Flora) and transforms and merges their data into directives for her augmented reality piece. Female, age 30, no history of mental disease. Female, age 37, epilepsy. Female, age 39, dementia praecox. Female, age 33, no history of seizures. Female, age 36, no history of mental disease. Female, age 33, no history of seizures. Female, age 33, manic depressive disorder. She selectively reproduces these patterns, and not others, melting them together and staging them in a new context, thereby subverting a larger cultural archive or database shaped by a search for gender difference.

Automated Analysis of EEG Versus Human "Brains to Analyze Brains"

The first *Atlas of Electroencephalography*, published in 1941, represents a culminating moment in the large-scale pattern-finding operations of the preceding years. As part of a broader call for standardization in EEG studies, researchers Frederic and Erna Gibbs, based at the Harvard Neurological Unit of Boston City Hospital, published the *Atlas* to offer hundreds of sample electroencephalograms. These exemplary EEG records represented specific normal and abnormal cases and were to be used as a reference document by experts and students. The Gibbs picked these reference curves from thousands of records taken at city and state hospitals and schools, which had been captured with new amplifying and recording systems developed in close collaboration with engineers. The book was meant to help readers train the eye on the most relevant type of material, so as to develop "subjective criteria" (criteria based on experience) that would allow them to rapidly arrive at a diagnosis, even when "complex patterns" were involved (Gibbs and Gibbs 1941, preface). Electroencephalographers Gibbs and Gibbs argued that the trained "seeing eye" of the electroencephalographer would be able to make such visual differentiations "at a glance," akin to the way one can "tell an Eskimo from an Indian" (1941, preface). Such subjective differentiations were often better, the authors contended, than those gathered from a quantitative index.

The "seeing eye" of the electroencephalographer, who had learned to judge complicated patterns at a glance, is a central example in Peter Galison and Lorraine Daston's (2007) well-known study of shifting epistemic virtues in the creation and use of scientific atlas images. The skilled electroencephalographer appears in their analysis of the ideal of the "trained expert" that emerged roughly in the period of the 1930s, when an earlier emphasis on mechanical observation by objective, impartial machines was supplemented by a novel focus on the experienced perception of a trained observer. The human trained expert possessed a perceptive skill that was unconscious and highly proficient in making classifications. This capacity is aptly expressed in the analogy, drawn by the Gibbs researchers, between expert vision and the ability to discriminate between faces and races.[3] This analogy is symptomatic, as Daston and Galison explain, for the period's emphasis on a particular taxonomic capacity of human perception, a way of observing that was always already tied to "the recognition of family resemblance," which the authors describe as "physiognomic sight"

3 The Gibbs' typification of classification as recognizing race is characteristic of wider reverberations of racist ideologies in biometrics. While Daston and Galison do not argue that physiognomic sight directly leads to theories and practices of eugenics, they do link physiognomic sight to a wider preoccupation with "totalistic recognition" also present in Gestalt psychology and racial theories in the 1930s and 1940s (2007, 337–38)

(2007, 314). Physiognomic sight, as Daston and Galison suggest, "puts a face to the data" (2007, 369); any observed phenomenon was viewed has having the potential of a recognizable characteristic. In the context of their study on scientific atlases, they describe physiognomic sight as the perceived ability of both makers and users of these documents to "grasp relationships in ways that were not reducible to mechanical procedure" (Daston and Galison 2007, 314). The example of the *Atlas* aptly shows how the interpretative activities of scientific observers were part of a broader, unfolding debate on human perception and interpretation, in which an emphasis on intuitive classification was significantly tied to the dissemination of ideas from the Gestalt school of psychology in various scholarly domains in the 1930s (a point to which I will return in the last section of this chapter).

Tracing these shifting epistemological ideals in the specific context of EEG research adds new complexity to these observations. While scholars emphasized the perceptive abilities of trained experts, researchers in the field were also keen to develop automated, mechanical procedures for EEG analysis. In light of the previously discussed concerns about the reliability and variability of EEG interpretations, balancing the capacities of automated analysis with the proficiency of the trained expert was considered key. Reflecting on shifting epistemic ideals more generally, Daston and Galison remark that experts did not reject "objective" instruments all together; on the contrary, "they embraced instruments, along with shareable data and images, as the infrastructure on which judgment would rest" (2007, 329). However, the domain of EEG analysis shows an ongoing tension between the status of mechanical instruments as objective observers and as replacements for human interpretation. Forms of analysis were framed not only as a way to speed up calculation, but also as potentially enabling the uncovering of patterns that were invisible to the human eye. In turn, researchers also often emphasized that human expertise was still necessary for successful analysis, though with tentative suggestions that automated analysis might one day be possible.

Soon after Berger published his initial EEG studies, researchers applied the newly emerging mathematical technique of Fourier analysis to brainwave curves. This approach allowed them to decompose complex signals into graphs of specific frequency patterns, which enabled a new form of analysis. Some researchers immediately recognized the potential of these graphical visualizations for pathological classification, thereby enhancing the EEG's utility as a diagnostic tool for analyzing "pathological curves" (Dietsch 1932). However, the manual calculations involved in Fourier analysis were time-consuming, often taking days to complete, and were prone to error. The original records had to be enlarged by approximately 30 times and then traced by hand with a pencil. As Cornelius Borck has noted in his historical studies of EEG, the succeeding development of faster, automatic frequency analyzers (Grass and Gibbs 1938; Walter 1943a; 1943b) was stimulated by the desire to conduct large comparative EEG research to assess psychopathological and personality aspects (Borck 2018, 256). While such machines were praised for potentially offering quicker and more detailed analysis of patterns, researchers repeatedly admitted that human interpretation, often referred to as "eyeballing" or "naked eye" interpretation, remained more reliable for classification purposes. Taking stock of automated analysis methods, in an article published in *Science* in 1947, Frederic Gibbs and his engineer collaborator Albert Grass (1947) noted that none of the manual and mechanical types of frequency analyzers had received general acceptance and that most inventions had been abandoned. And again, a decade later, another review article noted how automated analysis should still be regarded as an instrument supplementing a best-guess approach, since the fundamental neurophysiological coding underlying the EEG was still unknown. "Automatic analysis of the EEG carries a certain magic. The complex patterns generated from moment to moment have always given promise to understanding just beyond measure" (Burch 1959, 827).

On the question whether machine interpretation or human interpretation should predominate in EEG analysis, researchers held differing views and engaged in significant debate. A 1955 EEG paper, for example, clearly advocated for the automated analysis method. Comparing records from patients at a mental hospital, prisoners, and normal subjects, they observed that the use of frequency analysis allows "slight and subtle pattern differences" to be seen "more clearly and more objectively . . . than by means of the usual scanning with the eye" (Kennard, Rabinovitch, and Fister). Conversely, EEG-researcher John Knott complained that "an instrument designed to complement visual analysis should not lead just to further visual analysis" (Burch 1959, 829), since the results would need to be interpreted again, subjectively, by human eyes. For Gibbs and Gibbs, the relation between mechanical and human interpretations was ambiguous. Writing in the second edition of the *Atlas of Electroencephalography* (1950), they argued that some technical assistance was permissible and necessary: electromechanical frequency analyzers and correlators could "reduce a tremendous amount of data into ponderable form" and allow an important "moon's-eye view" (Gibbs and Gibbs 1950, 112). Yet, while such electromechanical analyzers may be more objective, they contended, "accuracy should not be sacrificed to objectivity." It would be "almost impossible" that a future machine would be able to take over the task of interpretation (Gibbs and Gibbs 1950, 112). The analysis of EEG traces should be viewed as an intellectual endeavor, to be executed by a trained expert who knew how to spot patterns in records, in a way that turns the visual analysis of electroencephalograms into "a fairly simple task of recognition" (Gibbs and Gibbs 1950, 112). If an analyzer for complex evaluations and comparisons were to be invented, it would be "cumbersome, exceedingly elaborate, and expensive," the authors contended. And why would anyone want to build such a machine? Electroencephalographers, they noted, "are relatively cheap and portable" (Gibbs and Gibbs 1950, 60).

Of course, problems of efficiency and costs played an important part in researchers' consideration, and considerations of cost-efficiency for computational assistance in the field of medicine deserves its own historical research. However, here I would like to pick up on the theme of efficiency in human-machine interaction only. Researchers increasingly resorted to observations from the domain of perception psychology and operations research to evaluate the capacities of human interpreters. For instance, one team of 1950s EEG researchers wondered if humans could even handle all the new data generated by automatic analyzers, and if perhaps individual differences of electroencephalographers' "data-saturation threshold" should be taken into account (Penuel, Corbin, and Bickford 1955). In the 1950s, studies of the performance of scientific image experts analyzed intra- and interrater reliability, including electroencephalographers (Blum 1954) and mentioned psychological elements as part of broader attempts to optimize image analysis. The *Atlas* authors, too, wondered if the human nervous system was perhaps too taxed by the "powers of integration" necessary for analysis (Gibbs and Gibbs 1950, 68). Although they were optimistic about overcoming these problems, they acknowledged the problem of needing "a brain to analyze a brain" (Gibbs and Gibbs 1950, 68).

Patterns, Mediations, Glitches

February 2024. A video call between Marlene and Flora, with occasional interruptions because of weak Wi-Fi. Some technical breakdowns may actually foster a feeling of genuine connection. They laugh and log back in. While calling, they use a program called "Miro" to mimic an in-person brainstorming session with a virtual whiteboard and sticky notes.

Marlene has prepared a collection of brain research images from different time periods among which are anatomical drawings of the cerebrum, popular science illustrations of neurophysiologists at work, and a screenshot from a 1950s sci-fi horror movie. Some images Flora can identify, but others have become unrecognizably transformed by a sequence of visual edits Marlene performed in Photoshop. Marlene has also

Scan the QR code to find additional information about the project and access the augmented reality app on the Patterns of Pathology website: https://www.marlenebart.com/patterns-of-pathology.

experimented with the Photoshop AI function, which sometimes creates puzzling white voids when provided with prompts about brain activity. In this process of prompting, there is an interesting element of surprise and glitch. There are glimpses of the many automated computations involved in visual data processing, as if peeking into a black-boxed system.

Marlene has also started to connect our mutual study of EEG research to a famous AI origin story: the defeat of chess champion Garry Kasparov in a game against IBM's Deep Blue. For her, the square pattern of the chessboard signifies a masculine vision of cognition, which she plans to playfully sabotage in her AR work. Black-and-white patterns start to appear everywhere in her visual references. The shared whiteboard now also contains storyboards that guide Marlene's collaboration with 3D artist Manuel Farré on the AR work. In this multilayered augmented-reality piece, Marlene starts to play with the aesthetics of high-tech and scientific visualization. Partially underpinning this glossy, contemporary, mediated world are the old records of EEG taken from the 1941 *Atlas of Encephalography*. Marlene has transformed the records taken from the book into numbers in a software program, which feed into the navigation of her AR artwork. In the mid-twentieth century, researchers went to great lengths (using the high tech of their day) to calculate and depict the most accurate wave forms in print. Inevitably, a present-day translation of these very precise 1940s brainwaves adds noise (dust particles, shadows, curves, paper texture) to the records. Marlene realizes this strange sedimentation and welcomes this contaminated data as a way of pointing to inevitable mediations and the instability of the reference pattern in the history of (pathology) classifications.

FIG. 2 Marlene Bart, *Patterns of Pathology*, Tableau II, 2024/2025, digital collage and augmented reality. Courtesy of the artist

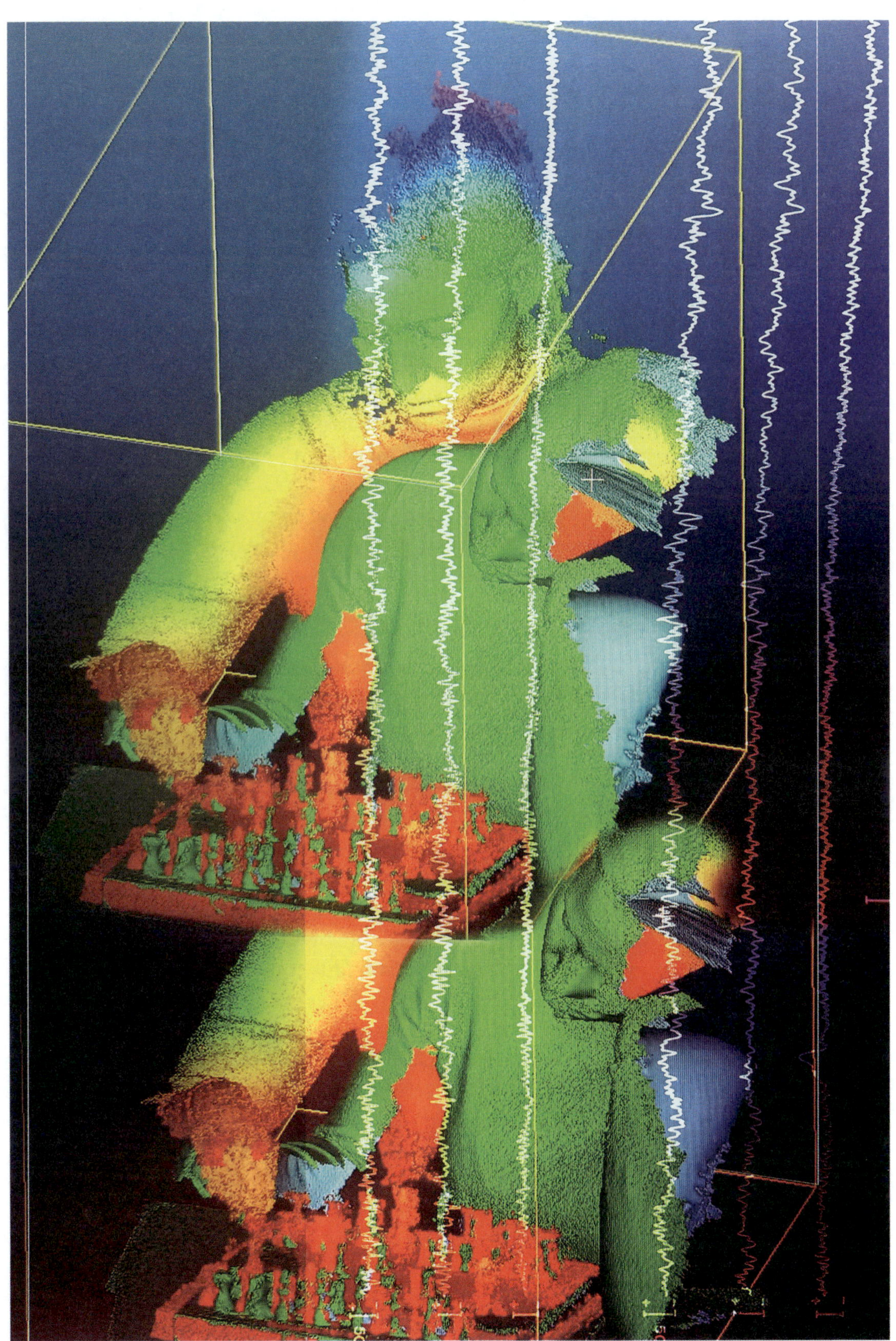

From Gestalten to Patterns to Pattern Recognition

Discussions about human and mechanical interpretations of EEG records were part of a broader debate, propelled by the US-centered context of cybernetics in the 1940s, about the possibility of modeling and mechanizing human perception. In basic terms, this debate centered on whether human perception, as an act of cognition, could be described using the language of information and communication systems and thereby modeled and mechanized through engineering projects. Recently, a number of historical studies have cast renewed attention to these cybernetic discussions (Lee 2020; Geoghegan 2023; Pasquinelli 2023; Üstün 2024), observing how scholars used notions of "Gestalts" to discuss perception, but gradually shifted to a more dominant use of the notion of "patterns" (Üstün 2024). References to Gestalts had spread in the US through the influence of German émigré Gestalt scholars, and were also prevalent in cybernetic discussions through the participation of Gestalt-oriented neurophysiologists and psychologists, including Karl Lashley (who conducted pattern discrimination experiments in rats), Max Wertheimer, Kurt Koffka, Kurt Lewin, Heinrich Klüver, and Kurt Goldstein.[4] Historian Bernard Geoghegan recounts how during a cybernetics-oriented 1949 Macy conference, researchers coming from varying disciplines talked of patterns, from the patterns of firing neurons in the brain, to statistical patterns in data measured by radars, to "patterns of distress" in neurotic patients (Geoghegan 2023, 44).

Notions of patterns were part of a debate between Gestalt-oriented researchers and cybernetics researchers over whether human perception involves processes that can be analytically represented and thus computed, mechanized, and potentially executed by machines (Pasquinelli 2023). In general terms, for Gestalt scholars, perception could be understood as the discernment of visual form and depended on the human capacity to organize sensory experiences into a meaningful whole, an act that was intuitive, instantaneous, and irreducible

4 Gestalt influence also ran along different lines. Cybernetic thinkers and anthropologists Margaret Mead and Gregory Bateson for example, were influenced by Ruth Benedict's Gestalt-inspired 1934 book *Patterns of Culture* (Lee 2020).

to its simple constituents. Conversely, cybernetic theorists drew on Gestalt notions of discerning form, but argued instead that perception could be described as the identification of patterns, a process that could be described in mathematical terms and potentially be automated. Throughout the 1940s and 1950s, cybernetic ideas predominated, the conceptual foundations of Gestalt perception gradually lost significance (Üstün 2024) and were succeeded by an information processing approach by which the finding of patterns was thought to be executable by humans as well as machines.

Patterns had overshadowed Gestalt ideas in various cybernetically influenced domains, including the field of EEG research, though some conceptual tensions between perception as intuition and perception as the discernment of patterns remained. We can see them resurface in discussions about the "seeing eye" of the electroencephalographer versus the perceptual proficiency of mechanical analyzers. The intuitive, at-a-glance classifications that trained electroencephalographers were envisioned to make with the help of the *Atlas of Electroencephalography*, for example, echoed the instantaneous abilities for recognizing different forms foregrounded by Gestalt theorists. This tentative questioning of mechanization in the field of scientific image perception becomes visible, as described in the preceding section, by attending to scientific discussions of electroencephalographers.

Unsurprisingly, cybernetics-oriented researchers involved in EEG work, such as William Grey Walter and, albeit briefly, Norbert Wiener, adhered to a mechanistic and empiricist approach to perception. They viewed the development of mechanisms for computing and automating perception, including the perception of EEG, as a guiding future objective. In the mid-1950s, Wiener collaborated with Mary Brazier and other researchers based in Boston "to find the Rosetta Stone for the script of the brain waves" by means of harmonic analysis of oscillations, a technique dubbed autocorrelation (Wiener 1956, 320; see Brazier and Casby 1952; Wiener and Brazier 1954). While the sizable autocorrelator apparatus was a "spectacle," with automatic rewinding of tape and much "clicking and clatter," it did not lead to considerable new insights and was exceedingly laborious to use (Gevins et al. 1975; Barlow 1997). Two years later, Wiener spoke of the "great hopes" he had for EEG records to finally turn into "really legible form," though he himself had by then abandoned this line of work (1956, 289).

Brainwaves remained stubbornly illegible. Discussions of new measuring techniques in EEG research often concluded by lamenting that without neurophysiological understandings of the mechanisms underpinning nerve activity, analyzers of brainwave curves were groping in the dark. For some researchers, this simply meant that more data needed to be assembled. After hearing Wiener and Brazier talk about the autocorrelation method, biophysicist Walter Rosenblith remarked that "the time has come" that investigators can no longer ask questions by "just looking at an EEG record . . . the success of a method of analysis will have to be here, as elsewhere, measured in terms of the size of the body of data it can encompass and perhaps even predict" (1954, 46).

At the same time that Wiener abandoned his attempts to filter meaningful messages from brainwave signals in the mid-1950s, a shift occurred in ideas about automated image analysis. This shift was propelled by new computational techniques that aimed to model how a human viewer can recognize a form or pattern, regardless of its presentation (for example, recognizing a capital letter "A" even when it differs in size, position, orientation, proportion, and line thickness). Oliver Selfridge, an engineer and former graduate student of Wiener's, devised a technique he dubbed "pattern recognition" and defined it as the "the extraction of the significant features from a background of irrelevant detail" (1955, 91). He explicitly described this engineering endeavor as a simulation, by means of digital computing machines, of the human capacity to recognize patterns—a thing that brains do very well but that machines did not do well yet, he remarked. While some scholars had already started to object to the anthropomorphizing vocabulary of AI researchers, Selfridge deliberately phrased his invention as allowing a machine to "learn" by "experience" to extract the significant elements of a signal, i.e., to "recognize" patterns (1955, 92).

Broadcasting the field of pattern recognition to a wider audience in a *Scientific American* article in 1960, Selfridge and his co-researcher Ulric Neisser set high stakes for mechanizing the human capacity for pattern recognition, positioning it as the very foundation of the field of artificial intelligence. They framed the human capacity for pattern recognition, such as understanding speech and reading print, as the most "basic intellectual skill" that came prior to (and stood at the basis of) more intricate problems of theorem-proving and chess-playing (Selfridge and Neisser 1960). While computers had been successful at simulating these latter two intelligent tasks, they expounded, the more fundamental and everyday work of "cognition, abstraction and perception" involved in pattern recognition proved much harder to generate with a computer program. In ensuing decades, pattern recognition evolved into an amorphous field of research with its own disciplinary identity and a continuously shifting, complex, and partially overlapping relation to work on artificial intelligence (Mendon-Plasek 2020).

Some pattern recognition researchers dismissed the frequent comparisons drawn between machine recognition and human recognition made by others in their field. Associations to artificial intelligence—emphasizing analogies between human cognition and computational systems—gave the pattern recognition field much of its "glamour," two authors noted in an overview of the field, but were far removed from the very practical problems that pattern recognition engineers thought to solve when they tinkered with zip code and print readers, aerial imagery screening machines, and voice recognizers (Kanal and Chandrasekaran 1969, 318). Yet, even stripped of clear correspondences to the human apparatus, they remarked that the "aura of magic and mystery" remained attached to devices of pattern recognition, which were perceived as

Scan the QR code to find additional information about the project and access the augmented reality app on the Patterns of Pathology website: https://www.marlenebart.com/patterns-of-pathology.

executing complex tasks of classification and estimation (Kanal and Chandrasekaran 1969, 318).

Pattern recognition's magic was tested in various research programs in the late 1950s, as a means of counting stars, bacteria, and white blood cells, for detecting bubble chamber patterns and morse code, and also to automate the analysis of EEG tracings (Farley et al. 1962; Uhr 1963). However, a decade later, while researchers reported positive developments for automated pattern recognition in EEG analysis of sleep stages as well as evoked responses by sensory stimuli, as a 1972 review article recounts, its usefulness for clinical diagnosis was still nil (Cox, Nolle, and Arthur 1972). After 40 years of EEG studies, "systematic development of automatic techniques for diagnosis and monitoring of EEG records has not yet begun" (Cox, Nolle, and Arthur 1972, 1141). Reason for this failure was familiar: EEGs lacked standardization.

Electroencephalographers in different departments did not use the same criteria, and more fundamentally there was an "imperfect correlation of clinical observation with disease" (Cox, Nolle, and Arthur 1972, 1142). Because disease entities were graded in extent and also differed per individual it was impossible to design the type of hypothesis for pattern recognition against which the EEG record could be tested. Again, in 1979, half a century after Hans Berger's first publication on EEG, a review article on computerized clinical electroencephalography opened by saying that the total impact of this method had remained limited, "despite rather extensive work. . . . The overriding reason for this state of affairs is that the remarkable skill of the well-trained and experienced electroencephalographer, in his evaluation of the many facets of analysis and interpretation of recordings from the scalp of the electrical activity of the cerebral cortex, has not so far been matched by any single or any combination of computer techniques" (Barlow 1979, 377). Clinical EEG analysis depended on training and experience, and remains, to a considerable degree, "an art rather than a science" (Barlow 1979, 377).

FIG. 3 Marlene Bart, *Patterns of Pathology*, Tableau III, 2024/2025, digital collage and augmented reality. Courtesy of the artist

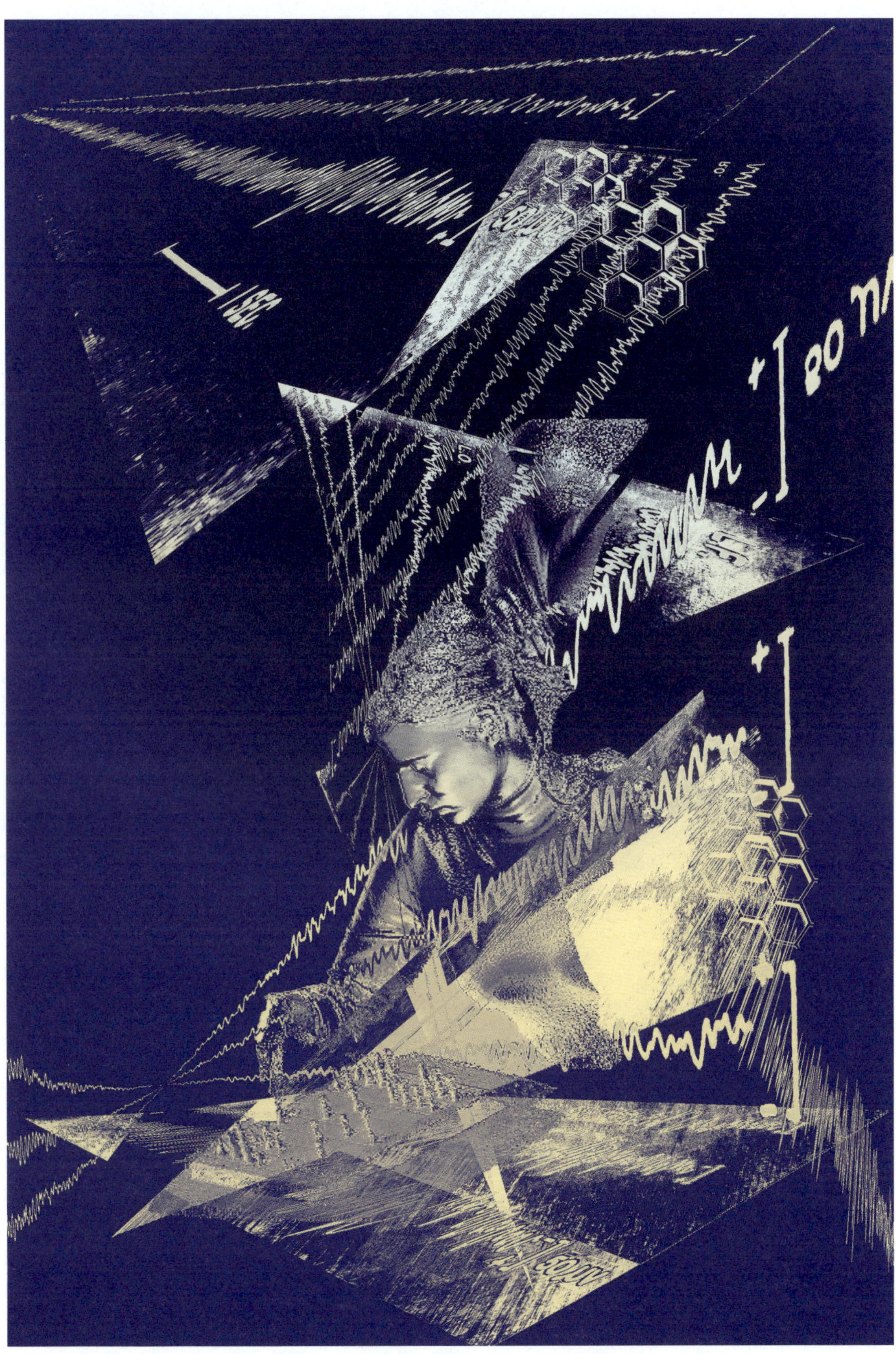

Patterns, Expectations, Intuitions

July 2024. Marlene and Flora visit the Berlin University of Applied Sciences (Hochschule für Technik und Wirtschaft) to explore recent work in deep learning and EEG interpretation. Data scientist Gunnar Klemenz kindly offered to demonstrate how a baseline EEG is measured using an EEG helmet and measurement software. Additionally, he introduces his ongoing research projects with deep-learning classification techniques, including a study into decoding overt and covert (imagined) speech. So far, Gunnar has primarily used himself as a recording subject, training a classification algorithm that should eventually predict which word he imagines. In the future he hopes to increasingly work with data from high-quality EEG databases to conduct his analyses; he wants to expand his scope.

Visiting the lab and participating as subjects provides Marlene and Flora with first-hand experience of the craft of EEG measurement—the meticulous tinkering (and extreme patience) required with hardware, software, and subjects to gather data that underpins deep-learning computations. Their hair keeps getting stuck in the screws of the EEG cap, a device that was freshly 3D-printed by Gunnar earlier that week. After fitting the headcap, testing the setup, and staying very still for 15 minutes, Flora is genuinely excited to hear Gunnar discuss the peaks and plateaus in the EEG record. To her surprise, even a basic experimental setup sparks suspense and anticipation regarding a diagnosis. She hopes to receive, if only rudimentary, some form of classification and judgment.

During a second recording, the erratic behavior of the EEG-measuring apparatus also becomes evident. They aim to capture functional activity in the EEG data by measuring lifting movements of Flora's left and right forearms, one minute for each side. While the left-arm EEG activity showed expected activity in Flora's right hemisphere, the right-arm recording also exhibits significant activity on the right side of her brain. Gunnar cannot immediately explain this activity and searches for a possible recording or processing error. Time is short, however, and they need to transfer the EEG data from the computer to Marlene's USB stick. As Gunnar quickly navigates between different programs, Marlene and Flora are struck by a colorful visualization that was automatically generated as part of the data processing. For Gunnar, this particular picture is not of much use. In his work, he explains, he uses graphic representations of EEG activity per bandwidth over time to quickly grasp the measurements. Ultimately, though, the numbers file with "all the data" is more important to him. Working with this tabular data, he has developed an instinctive sense for the distribution of values across columns and rows—he can usually spot something out of the ordinary. It seems he has developed a type of intuition for the patterns that fit his experiments.

Conclusion: Pattern Recognition beyond Magic, Mystery, and Loss of Human Intuition

Focusing on the field of EEG as an exemplary case, this chapter points to talk of patterns in the period of the 1930 to the 1950s, prior to a more widespread dissemination of the term "pattern recognition" in popular and scientific discourse. The early period of EEG research in the US was characterized by extensive efforts to find patterns, i.e., to correlate EEG records with different psychological and biological conditions. These efforts took the shape of insistent large-scale pattern-finding operations, where researchers persisted in trying to find significant differences, indicated by specific characteristics of the EEG record, as potential classifiers of disease. Researchers in the field demonstrated an exploratory approach, openly acknowledging the provisional nature of their studies. Yet, despite the recognized uncertainties and limitations in current research, there was optimism that EEG would eventually become a valuable classification tool. Since the early years of EEG, computational techniques to calculate typical characteristics of brainwave records were viewed as providing a necessary aid for electroencephalographers, particularly in finding pathological curves. Ensuing mechanical and automated forms of curve calculations were developed and praised in light of their potential to improve analysis in service of classification, but researchers readily acknowledged the promissory and magical appeal of these methods, and admitted that so far, human interpretation remained more reliable for clinical classification purposes. Discussions of clinical diagnosis by means of EEG foregrounded the proficiency of the trained expert electroencephalographer, who could develop a special aptitude to detect patterns in EEG records. This emphasis on human expertise happened in opposition to discussions about the possibility to conduct automated calculations of curves, although practitioners also talked about automated analyzers as assistive tools. A specific emphasis on human capacities for seeing patterns was imbricated with an earlier and ongoing controversy regarding the possibility of mechanizing human perception. The notion of patterns had become ubiquitous in cybernetic discussions, in which it functioned as a partial transformation of notions of Gestalt. A Gestalt-inspired resistance toward the ultimate computational formalization of perceiving form (pattern) was superseded by information theory-influenced ideas of extracting patterns as elementary forms or signals from noisy background. However, we can discern the continuous importance of Gestalt ideas in a persistent emphasis on the immediate, pre-reflexive, and intuitive capacity of human observers.

My analysis of the field of EEG in the period until the mid-1950s has traced one instantiation of a ubiquitous pattern talk prior to the solidification of a notion of pattern recognition in the field of engineering around 1960. After the rise of pattern recognition as technique, the term has come to dominate discussions of perception and judgment in the 1970s, particularly in the field of cognitive science, where cognition was increasingly understood in the mirror of the computational techniques: machine pattern recognition became a model for human pattern recognition (Evans 1968). In a striking turn, however, humans continued to be regarded as more proficient at this (machine-modeled) ability. This emphasis on pattern recognition as a preeminent human capacity obliquely echoes earlier connotations and values about the human intuition and skill for seeing patterns. My historical observations on the field of EEG and automated analysis invite broader reflection on the juxtapositions and amalgamations between human and computer-aided interpretation that continue in present-day discussions, but that take a new form in the most current instantiation of deep learning in medical imaging, including EEG. References to the magic of automated analysis in the 1950s, the glamour of AI, and the "aura of magic and mystery" of pattern recognition in the 1960s show an arguably unsurprising continuity with the contemporary fascination and hype surrounding AI and deep learning.

More importantly, highlighting the conceptual proximity of Gestalts, intuition, and subjective experience to the concept of the pattern recenters the question of what has become of human intuitions in the contemporary development of pattern-recognition-based artificial intelligence. Historicizing the discourse and concepts surrounding patterns allows us to critically assess today's often ambiguous, anthropomorphizing descriptions of AI's supposed beyond-human insights. Tracing decades of human and automated analysis in psychopathology and EEG encourages us to resist the simplistic narrative of a loss of human judgment and intuition in experimental and clinical science amid the black-boxed, techno-solutionist promises of big data analysis in medicine. Instead, the historical zigzag of conceptual developments related to patterns and pattern recognition urges scholars to delve deeper into the infrastructures and conceptions of recognizing patterns. This exploration can reveal how new feelings for algorithms or patterns may emerge in the interplay between humans and computers (as they are used by humans) (Stevens 2017). Such nuance is not intended to downplay the potential harmful effects of the growing contemporary emphasis on—and trust in—mechanical pattern recognition and statistical prediction in medical science. Rather, it seeks to connect these developments to longer histories of conjecture, abduction, and correlation, all encapsulated in that one powerful term: the pattern.

B

Barlow, John S. (1979) "Computerized Clinical Electroencephalography in Perspective." *IEEE Transactions on Biomedical Engineering* BME-26 no. 7: 377–91. https://doi.org/10.1109/TBME.1979.326416.

Barlow, John S. (1997) "The Early History of EEG Data-Processing at the Massachusetts Institute of Technology and the Massachusetts General Hospital." *International Journal of Psychophysiology: Official Journal of the International Organization of Psychophysiology* 26, no. 1–3: 443–54. https://doi.org/10.1016/s0167-8760(97)00781-2.

Beer, David (2018) "Envisioning the Power of Data Analytics." *Information, Communication & Society* 21, no. 3: 465–79. https://doi.org/10.1080/1369118X.2017.1289232.

Besser, Stephan (2022) "Binding Brain, Body and World: Pattern as a Figure of Knowledge in Andy Clark's Work on Predictive Processing." *Poroi* 17 (April). https://doi.org/10.17077/2151-2957.31133.

Blum, Richard H. (1954) "A Note on the Reliability of Electroencephalographic Judgments." *Neurology* 4, no. 2: 143. https://doi.org/10.1212/WNL.4.2.143.

Borck, Cornelius (2005) *Hirnströme: Eine Kulturgeschichte der Elektroenzephalographie*. Göttingen: Wallstein Verlag.

Borck, Cornelius (2018) *Brainwaves: A Cultural History of Electroencephalography*. London: Routledge.

Brazier, Mary A. B., and James U. Casby (1952) "Cross-Correlation and Autocorrelation Studies of Electroencephalographic Potentials." *Electroencephalography and Clinical Neurophysiology* 4, no. 2: 201–11. https://doi.org/10.1016/0013-4694(52)90010-2.

Burch, Neil R. (1959) "Automatic Analysis of the Electroencephalogram: A Review and Classification of Systems." *Electroencephalography and Clinical Neurophysiology* 11 (November): 827–34. https://doi.org/10.1016/0013-4694(59)90133-6.

C

Cox, J. R., F. M. Nolle, and R. M. Arthur (1972) "Digital Analysis of the Electroencephalogram, the Blood Pressure Wave, and the Electrocardiogram." *Proceedings of the IEEE* 60, no. 10: 1137–64. https://doi.org/10.1109/PROC.1972.8877.

D

Daston, Lorraine, and Peter Galison (2007) *Objectivity*. Edited by Peter Galison. Cambridge, MA: Zone Books.

Davis, Pauline A., and Hallowell Davis (1939) "The Electroencephalograms of Psychotic Patients." *The American Journal of Psychiatry* 95: 1007–25. https://doi.org/10.1176/ajp.95.5.1007.

Davis, P. A. (1940) "Evaluation of the Electroencephalograms of Schizophrenic Patients." *American Journal of Psychiatry* 96, no. 4: 851–60. https://doi.org/10.1176/ajp.96.4.851.

Davis, Pauline A. (1941) "Technique and Evaluation of the Electroencephalogram." *Journal of Neurophysiology* 4, no. 1: 92–114. https://doi.org/10.1152/jn.1941.4.1.92.

Dietsch, G. (1932) "Fourier-Analyse von Elektrencephalogrammen des Menschen." *Pflüger's Archiv für die gesamte Physiologie des Menschen und der Tiere* 230, no. 1: 106–12. https://doi.org/10.1007/BF01751972.

E

Ellingson, Robert J. (1956) "Brain Waves and Problems of Psychology." *Psychological Bulletin* 53, no. 1: 1–34. https://doi.org/10.1037/h0042562.

Engelmann, Lukas (2020) "Into the Deep: AI and Total Pathology: Deep Medicine: How Artificial Intelligence Can Make Healthcare Human Again, by Eric Topol, New York: Basic Books, 2010." *Science as Culture* 29, no. 4: 625–29. https://doi.org/10.1080/09505431.2020.1768232.

Evans, Selby H. (1968) "Pattern Identification by Man and Machine: Proceedings of a Planning Conference, Held at Texas Christian Univ., Fort Worth, Texas, 12–13 Dec. 1968." Aberdeen Proving Ground, MD: U.S. Army Human Engineering Laboratories.

Ewen, Joshua B., and Sándor Beniczky (2017) "Validating Biomarkers and Diagnostic Tests in Clinical Neurophysiology: Developing Strong Experimental Designs and Recognizing Confounds." In *Niedermeyer's Electroencephalography: Basic Principles, Clinical Applications, and Related Fields*, edited by Donald L. Schomer, Fernando H. Lopes da Silva, Donald L. Schomer, and Fernando H. Lopes da Silva, 229–46. Oxford: Oxford University Press. https://doi.org/10.1093/med/9780190228484.003.0009.

Ewen, Joshua B., and April R. Levin. 2022. "Neurobehavioral Biomarkers: An EEG Family Reunion." *Journal of Clinical Neurophysiology: Official Publication of the American Electroencephalographic Society* 39, no. 2: 129–34. https://doi.org/10.1097/WNP.0000000000000836.

Ewen, Joshua B., John A. Sweeney, and William Z. Potter (2019) "Conceptual, Regulatory and Strategic Imperatives in the Early Days of EEG-Based Biomarker Validation for Neurodevelopmental Disabilities." *Frontiers in Integrative Neuroscience* 13: 45. https://doi.org/10.3389/fnint.2019.00045.

F

Farley, B. G., L. S. Frishkopf, W. A. Clark, and J. T. Gilmore (1962) "Computer Techniques for the Study of Patterns in the Electroencephalogram." *IRE Transactions on Bio-Medical Electronics* 9, no. 1: 4–12. https://doi.org/10.1109/TBMEL.1962.4322943.

Finley, Knox H., and C. Macfie Campbell (1941) "Electroencephalography in Schizophrenia." *American Journal of Psychiatry* 98, no. 3: 374–81. https://doi.org/10.1176/ajp.98.3.374.

G

Geoghegan, Bernard Dionysius (2023) *Code: From Information Theory to French Theory*. Sign, Storage, Transmission. Durham, NC: Duke University Press. https://www.dukeupress.edu/code.

Gevins, A. S., C. L. Yeager, S. L. Diamond, J. Spire, G. M. Zeitlin, and A. H. Gevins (1975) "Automated Analysis of the Electrical Activity of the Human Brain (EEG): A Progress Report." *Proceedings of the IEEE* 63, no. 10: 1382–99. https://doi.org/10.1109/PROC.1975.9966.

Gibbs, F. A., and E. L. Gibbs (1941) *Atlas of Electroencephalography*. Cambridge, MA: Cummings.

Gibbs, F. A., and E. L. Gibbs (1950a) *Atlas of Electroencephalography,* vol 1: *Methodology and Controls*. Cambridge, MA: Addison-Wesley.

Gibbs, F. A., and E. L. Gibbs (1950b) *Atlas of Electroencephalography*. Boston, MA: Addison-Wesley.

Gibbs, F. A., and E. L. Gibbs (1964) *Atlas of Electroencephalography*, vol. 3: *Neurological and Psychiatric Disorders.* Atlas of Electroencephalography. Boston, MA: Addison-Wesley.

Gibbs, F. A., and A. M. Grass (1947) "Frequency Analysis of Electroencephalograms." *Science* 105 (2718): 132–34. https://doi.org/10.1126/science.105.2718.132.

Grass, A. M., and F. A. Gibbs (1938) "A Fourier Transform of the Electroencephalogram." *Journal of Neurophysiology* 1, no. 6: 521–26. https://doi.org/10.1152/jn.1938.1.6.521.

H

Hagner, Michael (2004) "Das kybernetische Gehirn." In *Geniale Gehirne: Zur Geschichte der Elitegehirnforschung*, by Michael Hagner, 288–96. Wissenschaftsgeschichte. Göttingen: Wallstein.

Hagner, M., and C. Borck (2001) "Mindful Practices: On the Neurosciences in the Twentieth Century." *Science in Context* 14, no. 4: 507–10.

K

Kanal, Laveen, and B. Chandrasekaran (1969) "Recognition, Machine 'Recognition,' and Statistical Approaches." In *Methodologies of Pattern Recognition*, edited by Satosi Watanabe, 317–32. New York: Academic Press. https://doi.org/10.1016/B978-1-4832-3093-1.50021-3.

Kennard, M. A., M. S. Rabinovitch, and W. P. Fister (1955) "The Use of Frequency Analysis in the Interpretation of the EEGs of Patients with Psychological Disorders." *Electroencephalography and Clinical Neurophysiology* 7, no. 1: 29–38. https://doi.org/10.1016/0013-4694(55)90057-2.

Klooster, Debby, Helena Voetterl, Chris Baeken, and Martijn Arns (2024) "Evaluating Robustness of Brain Stimulation Biomarkers for Depression: A Systematic Review of Magnetic Resonance Imaging and Electroencephalography Studies." *Biological Psychiatry* 95, no. 6: 553–63. https://doi.org/10.1016/j.biopsych.2023.09.009.

Knott, J. R. (1941) "Electroencephalography and Physiological Psychology: Evaluation and Statement of Problem." *Psychological Bulletin* 38, no. 10: 944–75. https://doi.org/10.1037/h0059465.

L

Lee, Pamela M. (2020) *Think Tank Aesthetics: Midcentury Modernism, the Cold War, and the Neoliberal Present*. Cambridge, MA: MIT Press.

Lennox, William G. (1942) "Electrophysiology and Epilepsy." *American Journal of Psychiatry* 98, no. 4: 592–95. https://doi.org/10.1176/ajp.98.4.592.

Lysen, Flora (2023) "Errors and Fallibility in Radiology: X-Ray Readings and Expert Radiologists, 1947–1960." *BJHS Themes* 8 (January): 127–41. https://doi.org/10.1017/bjt.2023.5.

M

Mendon-Plasek, Aaron (2020) "Mechanized Significance and Machine Learning: Why It Became Thinkable and Preferable to Teach Machines to Judge the World." In *The Cultural Life of Machine Learning: An Incursion Into Critical AI Studies*, edited by Jonathan Roberge and Michael Castelle, 31–78. Cham: Springer Nature.

Millett, David (2001) *Wiring the Brain: From the Excitable Cortex to the EEG, 1870–1940*. Chicago: University of Chicago Press.

N

Nilsonne, Gustav, and Frank E. Harrell (2021) "EEG-Based Model and Antidepressant Response." *Nature Biotechnology* 39, no. 1: 27. https://doi.org/10.1038/s41587-020-00768-5.

P

Pacella, Bernard L., and S. Eugene Barrera (1941) "Electroencephalography: Its Applications in Neurology and Psychiatry." *Psychiatric Quarterly* 15, no. 3: 407–37. https://doi.org/10.1007/BF01562135.

Pasquinelli, Matteo (2023) *The Eye of the Master: A Social History of Artificial Intelligence*. New York: Verso Books.

Penuel, H., F. Corbin, and Reginald G. Bickford (1955) "Studies of the Electroencephalogram of Normal Children: Comparison of Visual and Automatic Frequency Analyses." *Electroencephalography and Clinical Neurophysiology* 7, no. 1: 15–28. https://doi.org/10.1016/0013-4694(55)90056-0.

R

Rosenblith, W. A. (1954) "Discussion of Correlation Analysis: In 3rd International EEG Congress." *Electroencephalography and Clinical Neurophysiology Supplement* 4: 46.

Roy, Yannick, Hubert Banville, Isabela Albuquerque, Alexandre Gramfort, Tiago H. Falk, and Jocelyn Faubert (2019) "Deep Learning-Based Electroencephalography Analysis: A Systematic Review." *Journal of Neural Engineering* 16, no. 5: 051001. https://doi.org/10.1088/1741-2552/ab260c.

S

Schabacher, Gabriele (2023) "AI and the Work of Patterns: Recognition Technologies, Classification, and Security." In *KI-Kritik / AI Critique*, edited by Andreas Sudmann, Anna Echterhölter, Markus Ramsauer, Fabian Retkowski, Jens Schröter, and Alexander Waibel, 1st edition, 6: 123–54. Bielefeld: transcript. https://doi.org/10.14361/9783839467664-008.

Schirmann, Felix (2014) "'The Wondrous Eyes of a New Technology': A History of the Early Electroencephalography (EEG) of Psychopathy, Delinquency, and Immorality." *Frontiers in Human Neuroscience* 8 (April): 232. https://doi.org/10.3389/fnhum.2014.00232.

Selfridge, Oliver G. (1955) "Pattern Recognition and Modern Computers." In *Proceedings of the March 1–3, 1955, Western Joint Computer Conference*, 91–93. AFIPS '55 (Western). New York, NY: Association for Computing Machinery. https://doi.org/10.1145/1455292.1455310.

Selfridge, Oliver G., and Ulric Neisser (1960) "Pattern Recognition by Machine." *Scientific American* 203, no. 2: 60–68. https://doi.org/10.1038/scientificamerican0860-60.

Squires, Matthew, Xiaohui Tao, Soman Elangovan, Raj Gururajan, Xujuan Zhou, U Rajendra Acharya, and Yuefeng Li (2023) "Deep Learning and Machine Learning in Psychiatry: A Survey of Current Progress in Depression Detection, Diagnosis and Treatment." *Brain Informatics* 10, no. 1: 10. https://doi.org/10.1186/s40708-023-00188-6.

Stevens, Hallam (2017) "A Feeling for the Algorithm: Working Knowledge and Big Data in Biology." *Osiris* 32, no. 1: 151–74. https://doi.org/10.1086/693516.

U

Uhr, Leonard (1963) "'Pattern Recognition' Computers as Models for Form Perception." *Psychological Bulletin* 60, no. 1: 40–73. https://doi.org/10.1037/h0048029.

Üstün, Berkay (2024) "Patterns before Recognition: The Historical Ascendance of an Extractive Empiricism of Forms." *Humanities and Social Sciences Communications* 11 (January): 1–9. https://doi.org/10.1057/s41599-023-02574-1.

V

Vidal, F. (2009) "Brainhood, Anthropological Figure of Modernity." *History of the Human Sciences* 22, no. 1 (February 1): 5–36. https://doi.org/10.1177/0952695108099133.

W

Walter, William Grey (1942) "Electro-Encephalography in Cases of Mental Disorder." *Journal of Mental Science* 88 (370): 110–21, https://doi.org/10.1192/bjp.88.370.110.

Walter, William Grey (1943a) "An Automatic Low Frequency Analyser" *Electronic Engineering* 16 (June): 9–13.

Walter, William Grey (1943b) "An Improved Automatic Low Frequency Analyser" *Electronic Engineering* 16 (November): 236–40.

Walter, Grey William (1950) "Technique – Interpretation." In *Electroencephalography: A Symposium on Its Various Aspects*, edited by Sir Denis Hill, Geoffrey Parr, and William A. Cobb. Paulton and London: MacDonald & Co.

Wan, Zhijiang, Jiajin Huang, Hao Zhang, Haiyan Zhou, Jie Yang, and Ning Zhong (2020) "HybridEEGNet: A Convolutional Neural Network for EEG Feature Learning and Depression Discrimination." *IEEE Access* 8 (February): 30332–42. https://doi.org/10.1109/ACCESS.2020.2971656.

Widge, Alik S., M. Taha Bilge, Rebecca Montana, Weilynn Chang, Carolyn I. Rodriguez, Thilo Deckersbach, Linda L. Carpenter, Ned H. Kalin, and Charles B. Nemeroff (2019) "Electroencephalographic Biomarkers for Treatment Response Prediction in Major Depressive Illness: A Meta-Analysis." *The American Journal of Psychiatry* 176, no. 1: 44–56. https://doi.org/10.1176/appi.ajp.2018.17121358.

Wiener, Norbert (1956) *I Am a Mathematician: The Later Life of a Prodigy; an Autobiographical Account of the Mature Years and Career of Norbert Wiener and a Continuation of the Account of His Childhood in Ex-Prodigy*. New York: Doubleday.

Wiener, Norbert, and Mary A. Brazier (1954) "Discussion of Correlation Analysis: 3rd International EEG Congress." *Electroencephalography and Clinical Neurophysiology* Supplement 4: 41–44.

Imaginary Imaging: Representing the Normal and the Pathological in a Vision of Cell-Based Interceptive Biomedicine

Cornelius Borck and Robert Meunier

1 Introduction: Visualizing a Medicine of the Future and Visual Studies of Science

Images are important for imagination. They help people to create a shared vision of a future toward which they can agree to work. One such vision was recently expressed by the LifeTime Initiative, a multicenter, international research consortium (Rajewsky et al. 2020).[1] The idea is as straightforward as it sounds futuristic: a perfect medicine that does not wait for a disease to develop fully, once it has affected the body, perhaps even destroyed an organ, and made the patient suffer. In "interceptive medicine," visionary medicine would anticipate the course of events and intervene as early as possible to prevent disease manifestation. This perfected medicine would not have to act by drastic means, such as extirpating an affected organ or shutting off a function, but it would guide the system back on course by gently nudging some processes in appropriate directions.

In this chapter, we will analyze in detail one image that forms the core of the LifeTime Initiative's imaginary vision of interceptive medicine as part of a broader "sociotechnical imaginary" (Jasanoff 2015, 4) of precision medicine. FIG. 1 We show how a careful arrangement of visual metaphors and references

1 See the LifeTime Initiative website, https://lifetime-initiative.eu/ (Accessed: June 10, 2024).

helps to naturalize this vision. We support our analysis by contextualizing the image in the history of medical visualization and infographics more generally. We thereby aim to contribute to the visual studies of science by exemplifying how the interrogation of this kind of rhetorical image facilitates a critical assessment of the desirability and feasibility of biomedical projects such as LifeTime and the accompanying changes in the understanding of pathological phenomena.

LifeTime can be seen as part of a larger development in biomedicine built on advances in genetic and epigenetic medicine, multi-omics, and Big Data technologies, which fuel the expectation that prediction and treatment regimens can be individualized (Topol 2014). This larger vision today is commonly referred to as "precision medicine" and seen as replacing standard, disease-specific care by treatment tailored to individual disease trajectories. Advertised by the US National Institutes of Health and announced by President Barack Obama in 2015, precision medicine has been described as naming a promissory agenda (Blasimme and Vayena 2016; Meunier and Herzog 2023), though meanwhile it has been implemented, at least partially, in cancer care as precision oncology (Tsimberidou et al. 2020). Precision medicine creates shared imaginations of a biomedical future, and imaginary images are central in these attempts, precisely because photographs or visual illustrations are not yet available.

Focusing on the image in question, FIG. 1 we further the discussion on functions of visualizations in scientific practice by exploring one of the multiple roles of scientific images in contemporary knowledge society. The Western tradition has always prioritized words over images and linked theory with language (Baigrie 1996). The philosophy of science especially initially neglected and distrusted images, against the proverbial "a picture is worth a thousand words," as mere illustrations of ideas and concepts. History of science and science and technology studies (STS), by contrast, noticed the pivotal role of images and visualization in modern and contemporary scientific practice. Bruno Latour praised visual representations as "immutable mobiles" (Latour 1986, 7), and Karin Knorr-Cetina has suggested to speak of "viscourses" in analogy to discourses (Knorr-Cetina 1999), to name just two voices from the field of visual studies of science that flourished at the turn of the century (Lynch and Woolgar 1990; Kemp 1997; Jones and Galison 1998; Heintz and Huber 2001; Pauwels 2006; Coopmans et al. 2014). Compared to discourse analysis or the toolbox of approaches in STS, the study of visualizations has not (yet) coalesced into a branch of its own with properly established methods. Our chapter builds on and extends this earlier scholarship by investigating a case of visionary science.

The shaping of expectations and their dynamics have become a topic in STS (Konrad et al. 2017). In promissory science (Hedgecoe 2004), visualization relates less to scientific results but is part and parcel of the attempt to promote the project and thereby to make it happen. Describing the image from the LifeTime Initiative as a kind of infographic designed not to visualize data but to convey an idea of what data makes possible, we will argue that this image not only illustrates or explains the project but presents it as realistically achievable. Section II will introduce the image, the LifeTime Initiative, and its scientific background. Section III will zoom in on the different parts and panels of the image in the form of a close reading, focusing on visual metaphors and references to other types of images implicit in the design of the image. Section IV complements this account by zooming out, offering a historicizing reading of the visual rhetoric, and contextualizing it in larger traditions of medical visualization.

We conclude by positioning the image in question in the context of infographics and highlight again the significance of such types of images for the visual studies of science. Close reading and historical contextualization together reveal how the image naturalizes the vision of interceptive medicine, which, by monitoring the normal, aims to make the pathological stand out as its deviation. Our two types of analysis enable a critical assessment of the image and the imaginary to which it belongs. Infographics visualize abstract information and operate by a careful blend of attention to detail and conventions. In our case, the image introduces and stipulates single cell lines as the new locus of the pathological. But when does an individual response turn from being a sign of active resistance into a biomarker of pre-disease? In light of Georges Canguilhem's (1991) analysis of the normal and the pathological, it remains doubtful that an organism's path can be determined as steering toward the pathological before the manifestation of a disease, because life and the living are characterized by varying forms of setting norms rather than passively obeying them or failing to do so. The question of how this argument would apply to single cell trajectories transgresses the horizon of our paper but highlights how a critical assessment of the desirability and feasibility of a project like the one proposed by the LifeTime Initiative can be achieved through the analysis of imaginary images in science.

2
The Image in Question and Its Imaginary

The image on which we focus in this chapter FIG. 1 appeared in a Perspective article in the journal *Nature* titled "LifeTime and Improving European Healthcare through Cell-Based Interceptive Medicine" (Rajewsky et al. 2020). The LifeTime Initiative is a large European research community, involving scientists from almost 100 institutions, and coordinated by Nikolaus Rajewsky (Delbrück Center, Berlin) and Geneviève Almouzni (Institut Curie, Paris). It was set up by researchers in 2018 to articulate a set of shared goals in biomedical research and to acquire large-scale funding. The Initiative garnered support from eighty companies and won a European Commission Coordination and Support Action award. As a result, a Strategic Research Agenda (SRA) document was developed and published on the Initiative's website.[2] The *Nature* article can be seen as a summary of the SRA for the scientific community. The image was created by the professional freelance designer Johannes Richers, who specializes in visual science communication, in collaboration with the artist Karin Kimel.[3]

2 See the LifeTime Initiative website, https://lifetime-initiative.eu/lifetime-strategic-research-agenda-2/ (Accessed: June 14, 2024).

3 Johannes Richers, personal communication. For Richers's work, see https://www.jorichers.com/ (Accessed: June 10, 2024).

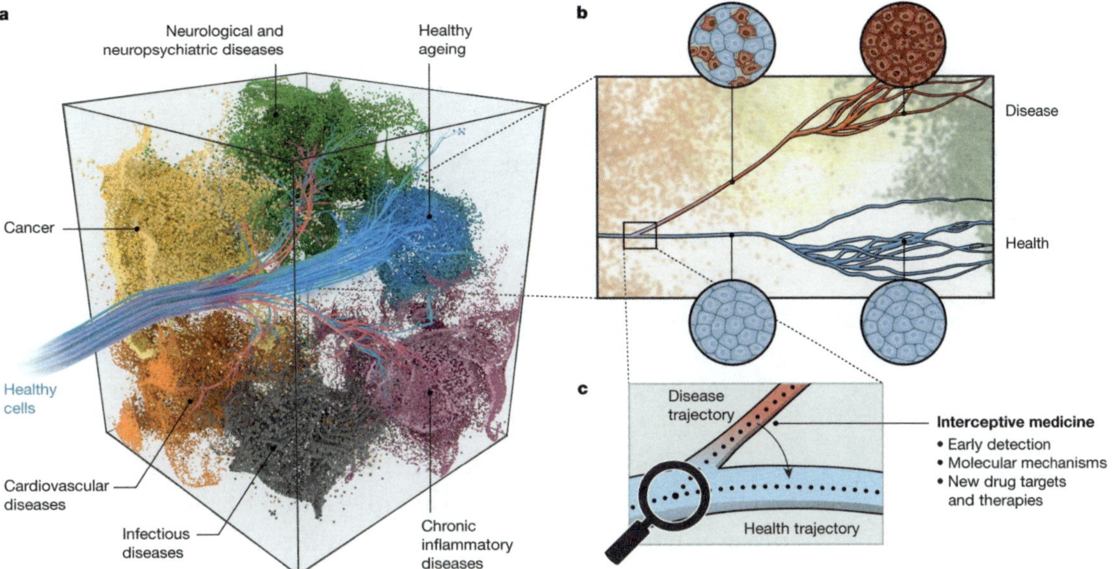

FIG. 1

FIG. 1 The image in question, as it appears in Rajewsky et al. (2020, 379, fig. 1). The image was created by the designer Johannes Richers in collaboration with the artist Karin Kimel.

The LifeTime Initiative was a preparatory action with the aim of establishing a Future and Emerging Technologies Flagship project within the EU Horizon 2020 funding agenda. While this attempt failed, the vision it promoted is further pursued by its proponents, in particular Nikolaus Rajewsky, through activities such as the "LifeTime Conference 2.0" in 2021,[4] the initiation of the "Berlin Cell Hospital,"[5] an Einstein Center for Early Disease Interception,[6] the "Virchow 2.0" proposal for funding by the German Federal Ministry of Education and Research,[7] and a project called "ImmunoPreCept," which has been selected for the German Cluster of Excellence program.[8]

In the context of the recent history of the biomedical sciences, the notion of cell-based interceptive medicine promoted by the LifeTime Initiative and the follow-up enterprises can be seen as part of the precision medicine imaginary (Erikainen and Chan 2019; Meunier and Herzog 2023). Sheila Jasanoff characterizes sociotechnical imaginaries as "collectively held, institutionally stabilized, and publicly performed visions of desirable futures, animated by shared understandings of forms of social life and social order attainable through, and supportive of, advances in science and technology" (Jasanoff 2015, 4). The imaginary of personalized medicine emerged in the context of the Human Genome Project (HGP) in the 1990s and gained currency when nucleic-acid sequencing became faster and cheaper through next-generation sequencing technologies around 2005 (Tabery 2023). Under the assumption that most diseases have at least some genetic components, the possibility to sequence individual genomes suggested an assessment of individual risk, which would in turn enable preventive measures. It was further assumed that the identification of genes associated with disease would lead to the discovery of pathogenic mechanisms and hence new drug targets. In addition, and building on the insight that individuals react differently to drugs, pharmacogenomics was promoted based on the promise to determine which drug will work best for which patient, thus avoiding unnecessary side effects (Hedgecoe 2004).

4 See the LifeTime Initiative website, https://lifetime-initiative.eu/lifetime-conference-2-0/ (Accessed: June 10, 2024).
5 See the Max Delbrück Center website, https://www.mdc-berlin.de/news/news/new-berlin-cell-hospital-announced (Accessed: June 10, 2024).
6 See the Max Delbrück Center website, https://www.mdc-berlin.de/news/news/preparations-new-einstein-center-begin (Accessed: October 29, 2024).
7 See the Max Delbrück Center website, https://www.mdc-berlin.de/de/news/press/virchow-20-von-der-intervention-zur-praevention (Accessed: June 10, 2024).
8 See the Berlin University Alliance website, https://www.berlin-university-alliance.de/excellence-strategy/exzellenzcluster/ImmunoPreCept/index.html (Accessed: June 5, 2025).

The vision of LifeTime, however, significantly differs from this earlier version of genomic medicine as well as from classical biomedicine. First, instead of ascribing a certain disease risk to a person based on their genomic markers, multi-omics cellular biomarkers are envisioned to capture a disease that has already begun. Second, unlike classical screening regimes that can identify diseases shortly before they become symptomatic, the envisioned monitoring seeks to catch diseases closer to their origins. Third, the data-intensive approach is no longer fixated on the genome and inherited risk alleles but acknowledges environmental factors that can push cells on a pathological path, mediated by epigenetic mechanisms. Monitoring cells to detect pathogenesis at the earliest stage is agnostic about the genetic or epigenetic nature of the causes.

How does figure 1 promote this vision? Presumably, even a reader/viewer well-versed in the visual language of contemporary biomedicine will be left perplexed by the image. At first sight, it is reminiscent of many common types of images, from data plots to mechanistic cartoons, to anatomical drawings and high-resolution microscopic images; yet, at the same time, it cannot be directly identified as belonging to any one of these. Additionally, the three panels of the image, A, B, and C, appear to stand in a straightforward relation of magnification, yet they exhibit very different visual styles. The puzzling character of the image results from the fact that it is not a functional image in the sense of the above-mentioned image types that are typically used to present concrete data, models, or other information. The image in question is not related to any specific experiment or data set, nor does it summarize a well-defined area of knowledge in a synoptic manner. Instead, it expresses a scientific vision, and for this purpose it invokes a visual language associated with the fields in which this vision is rooted. The image alludes to various types of images that are associated with biological concepts underpinning the vision and would be used to present the findings once the envisioned research is established. It is through this heterogeneous visual language that figure 1 communicates the idea that underlies the biomedical vision. In terms of its communicative aims, it might be said to be a rhetorical image.

The envisioned research and results would not constitute an entirely new way of doing biomedicine, hence the reference to well-established types of graphs and models. However, the vision suggests a decisive threefold shift: a shift in the focus of research activities that is motivated by a shift in the understanding of disease and entails a shift in the way healthcare would be organized and delivered. At the core of both investigation and intervention is the move from the clinical manifestation of disease, or even the pre-clinical signs captured by classical screening regimes, to the very origin of disease in the body. The question then becomes: How does figure 1 communicate this shift in perspective on disease? To address this question, the following section dissects the structure and elements of the image.

3
Zooming In: Representing Concepts through Visual Metaphors and References

Many images in biomedical research in contemporary life sciences are artificial in the sense that they are not direct inscriptions but render data according to the technical and conventional specifications of a particular visualization style or diagrammatic code. The object of investigation is not the specimen (animal, plant, organ, etc.) as it simply appears to the human eye but a particular aspect that escapes easy recognition—because of minuteness, distance, lack of an appropriate sensory organ, or invisibility for fundamental reasons—but is grasped through data. Scientific images in the life sciences then have to "naturalize" their artificiality by the standardization of visual formats and predefined frames of reference. "A central paradox of biomedical illustration is that a well-crafted image is one that appears not to have been crafted at all," as STS scholar and media theorist Drew Danielle Belsky stipulated the problem. "The expert labor of medical illustrations lies in naturalizing their own artefacts" (Belsky 2022, 219, 223). From microscopes to graphic recording, X-rays, crystallography, immunostaining, optical recording, and color coding, the development of research technologies went hand in hand with the construction, implementation, and standardization of visualization technologies and strategies (Hentschel 2014; Borck 2016; Borck 2017). While figure 1 does not visualize a specific data set, it makes reference to many types of data visualizations and associated data-generating technologies to indicate the scientific basis of the envisioned research. Furthermore, its design relies on visual metaphors familiar from the context of clinical training and the popularization of (patho)physiological knowledge, to express the conceptual frame in which these data-intensive research strategies would play out. Together, these metaphors and references work to facilitate the imaginative performance of the image. They serve as strategic ingredients for making figure 1, despite its promissory nature, scientific and not fantastic. This section first turns to the visual metaphors in the overall design and then to the visual components that constitute references to representations of cellular processes.

Visual Metaphors

Following Rudolf Virchow's (1821–1902) idea that diseases follow a natural path but in the form of a deviation from the healthy track at some specific bifurcation (see below), figure 1 visualizes the theoretical construct of disease trajectories by tracing such bifurcations. Obviously, a point of bifurcation cannot be found as a physical intersection in the body, not even with some future technology's analytic superpowers, because it is the metaphorical representation of the theoretical concept of disease as a deviating path. Furthermore, the image imports a context of corporeal, bodily reality by embedding a repertoire of visual strategies with long-standing traditions for focusing on clinical and therapeutical relevance, as we show in Section IV.

In the image, this corporeal, bodily reality is invoked by the three-dimensional layout of panel A and further stabilized by the zooming-in on panels B and C, alluding to a navigation through the three-dimensional body via different steps of magnification. However, at close inspection, it becomes apparent that each panel exhibits different representational modes rather than an increased magnification, with panel C culminating in the "magnification" of the concept of disease trajectory. Without the textual labels accompanying the graphical elements, panel C would be read as a blood vessel branching off into two smaller ones with small corpuscles moving in them like erythrocytes. This reading comes so "naturally" that it paradoxically stabilizes the alternative meaning that is intended here and only decipherable by the labels "disease trajectory" versus "health trajectory." Zooming in conflates as purposefully as skillfully space with time, cell with organism, anatomy and histology with physiological processes. In the pictorial rhetoric the panels appear as snippets from some organic tissues, but the logic of the representational plane is not one of spatial relations but conceptual distances between "healthy" and "diseased." The tube-like vessels do not connect organs or body parts but run from earlier stages of life on the left to later ones on the right and ultimately—though beyond the frames of the figure—to death.

Panel A visualizes the concept of disease trajectory by blending space and time, as it uses spatial relations for representing different types and degrees of disease. Panel B stabilizes this visual "naturalization" (*sensu* Belsky) by supporting microstructures in the form of quasi-histological vignettes, inserted as magnifications at different cross-sections. Panel C looks like just another cross-section but shows the moment of departure from the healthy path and thereby adds a functional perspective to the static, morphological perspective of panel B. With this combination of panel A visualizing the concept, B the assumed pathological structures, and C the functional perspective, figure 1 uses the zooming-in metaphorically. The scaffolding is employed as an easily recognizable format for graphically explaining the theory behind the project's vision. The dotted lines from panel to panel connect selected areas of interest presumably by "magnification," but these are magnifications only metaphorically, as the mode and content of representation change from panel to panel. The characterization of these modes of representation as "metaphorical" is not meant here as derogative for suggesting the image not to be taken seriously; on the contrary, metaphors are important and necessary cognitive tools for accessing a problem of thinking (Borck 2013) and some questions of theoretical reflection arrive at solutions only in absolute metaphors (Blumenberg 2016). Visualizations can function like metaphors in opening new avenues for scientific research (McAllister 2013). The LifeTime Initiative may be fantastic or far-fetched, but the image functions by way of using the zooming-in as visual metaphor for moving from theory to anatomy to process—thereby substantializing the visionary idea as something altogether corporeal, e.g., bodily and real.

The explicit addition of a magnifying glass at the bottom left of panel **c** demands further comment as it invites us to read it as a visual complement to what Louis Althusser coined the "spontaneous philosophy of the scientists" (Althusser 1990). Usually such a magnifying glass serves to highlight a particular area of interest, to be shown in an insert at higher resolution. Here, however, it appears, at first glance, to be an empty signifier, aimed precisely at the point where the visualization switches from depicting concrete biological structures to highlighting conceptual constructs, namely the branching off of the disease trajectory from the healthy track. This is a form of conceptual focusing, not a higher resolution, and hence the image is empty here. No magnification is shown, because nothing could be visualized about disease at this spot or moment. The magnifying glass focuses literally on the ultimate point where interceptive medicine would have to develop actionability in terms of guiding the monitored entities back on track (as indicated by the arrow right next to the glass). In terms of technical feasibility, this is promissory science, which offers the opportunity for a critical reading in terms of scientific ideology, and yet it encapsulates—again as visual metaphor—the vision's core. The magnifying glass is structurally embedded in the organizing scheme of the figure and its panels; the circular inserts in panel B roughly match the glass in shape and size, thereby providing the imagined histological content. The empty magnifying glass focuses the figure finally on LifeTime's visionary concept and captures it as imaginary imaging.

Visual References

Conceptually at the core of the LifeTime vision lies the idea of cell lineage and cell fate, which connect cells as individual objects with the temporality of disease trajectories. These concepts emerged in the nineteenth century. Virchow had established the notion that each cell in the body originates from another cell, and it is also through this line of work that the idea of cellular trajectories became associated with disease as located in specific tissues:

> Even in pathology we can now go so far as to establish, as a general principle, *that no development of any kind begins de novo, and consequently as to reject the theory of equivocal* [spontaneous] *generation just as much in the history of the development of individual parts as we do in that of entire organisms.* (Virchow 1860, 27; emphasis in original)

With this sentence Virchow makes two important claims. First, he suggests a strictly developmental perspective for analyzing physiological and pathological processes—his famous "cellular pathology." Second, he argues for a complete integration of pathological phenomena (physiological processes gone astray) in this developmental perspective. Cancer, for instance, may present as an entity of itself, a "malignant" tissue growing inside of an organ, but if inspected carefully, cancerous cells show relational ties with physiological cells (Stanger and Wahl 2024). In normal development as much as for pathological processes, it thus became imperative to trace the cells through their divisions and transformations, and figure 1 combines a whole series of strategies for visualizing this. We identify four types of images used to analyze and represent cell lineages that are visually referenced in figure 1: cell lineage or tree diagrams, epigenetic landscape diagrams, T-SNE graphs, and fluorescence microscopy images.

Cell tree diagrams were introduced by August Weismann (1834–1914) in the late nineteenth century to depict the idea that ontogenetic development can be analyzed by tracing each cell division starting from an undifferentiated zygote and the resulting cell generations of increasingly specialized cells in the developing organism (Dröscher 2014). This analysis can in principle be performed for each part or organ separately, as illustrated by figure 2A, the cell lineage of the forelimb of a newt.

Two points can be made regarding Weismann's image. First, it abstracts from the morphological topology of the limb. While the relative position of digits is roughly conserved, anatomical information, e.g., regarding shape and relative size, is omitted. If we imagine the image as framed by a coordinate system, the x and y axes would represent space and time, respectively. But the time axis is relevant mainly to interpret each line of cells individually and does not necessarily represent intervals or indicate synchronicity. The space axis represents spatial differentiation and potentially relative position but no exact distances. The diagram abstracts from the three-dimensional character of the cells, tissues, and organs. Secondly, it is a theoretical image (Dröscher 2014), i.e., it visualizes a theoretical model that is grounded in histological and embryological observations, but it does not report these observations nor their composite. Instead, it represents a certain type of process as a branching process in which the characteristics and potentiality of cells undergo a systematic change. Hence the image in figure 2A contributes to a theoretical argument about development.

Without going into the details of Weismann's theory of the idioplasm and determinants, it is important to note how he connected the idea of a cell lineage to a largely deterministic and internally controlled notion of development. In this

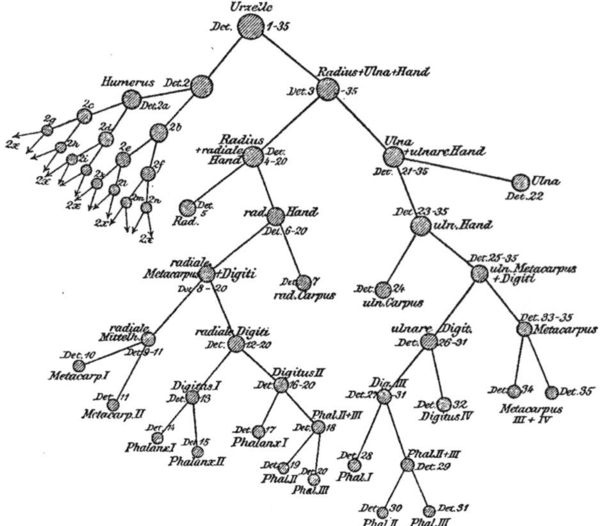

FIG. 2A

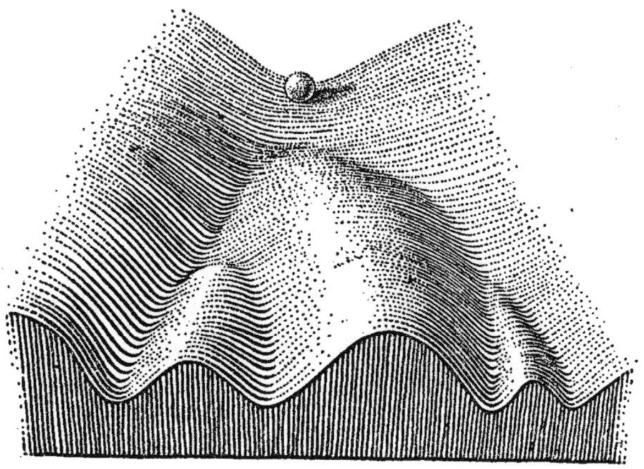

FIG. 2B

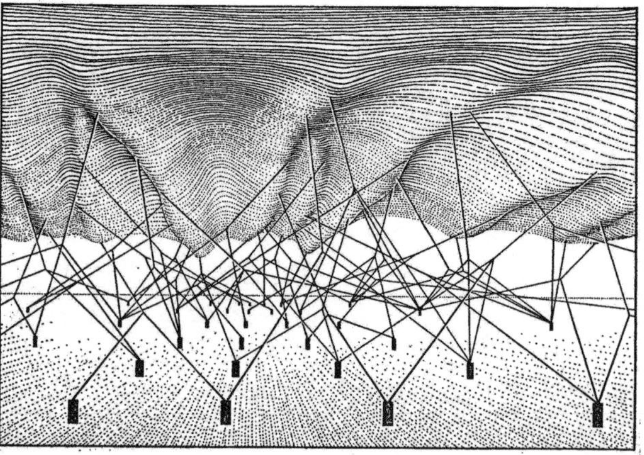

FIG. 2C

FIG. 2A Cell lineage tree diagram from Weismann (1893, 102, fig. 3)
FIG. 2B Epigenetic landscape from Waddington (1957, 29, fig. 4)
FIG. 2C Epigenetic landscape from Waddington (1957, 36, fig. 5)

context, he introduced the notion of cell fate, when he wrote that "the structure which can and will become developed from it always depends on the cell itself, and its fate is determined by the idioplasm it contains, and can only be affected secondarily by external influences" (Weismann 1893, 113–14).

Later embryologists used cell lineage trees more empirically to represent actual observations, albeit in a highly abstract manner. Researchers in this tradition introduced a number of graphical innovations, from a horizontal orientation of the tree to representing cells through letters or numbers, and introduced various peripheral annotations to the diagrams. The idea that ontogeny can be described in its totality by tracing every individual cell is also pursued by the Rajewsky Lab today using a model organism; this work can be seen as delivering a proof of concept for the comprehensive monitoring of cells in humans (Plass et al. 2018). Furthermore, pathological phenomena, especially tumor development, are also described in terms of cell lineages, which speaks to the central Virchowian commitment underlying cellular medicine.

Panel **A** in figure **1** can be read as a horizontal cell lineage tree. To the left of the image there is a bundle of "healthy cells," represented as lines in blue. For the larger part, they are not represented as branching but as existing through time (or possibly as proliferating without significant events). Some of these lineages turn purple, once they branch off to the right; others, deviating to the bottom or top, turn green, yellow, orange, or black, representing different classes of disease. If we follow only the blue lines, they become a cluster of cells that is designated as "healthy aging." This cluster of cells does not represent a specific kind of tissue but rather any kind of tissue as it would develop when healthy aging occurs. This is the core idea of the picture: for any tissue, cells might be affected by various factors, such that they can differentiate into tissues that exhibit disease. As the image suggests, this can happen for tissues constituting various organ systems, such as the cardiovascular system or the nervous system. But it can also happen in several specific ways, i.e., through oncogenesis, infection, or chronic inflammation.

Figure 1A is a visual representation of Virchow's argument that all pathological processes must be understood within a developmental perspective. It shows structural similarities to cell lineage trees and borrows credit from this for the argument that these families of diseases are to be understood as cellular fate, as pathological processes that ultimately must be addressed at the cellular level. Yet, the different colors of the clusters represent these different groups of disease and not specific organs. This highlights an important difference of figure 1A to cell-lineage representations as the one depicted in figure 2A: the spatial relations in the image do not relate to organs or body regions but to abstract families of diseases.

Panel A in figure 1 further differs from a cell lineage tree, because there are no lines or arrows connecting cells. Instead, cell lineages are represented as continuous lines. If we take also panels B and C into consideration, then it seems that these lines are rather like tubes. As mentioned, panel B invokes the idea of blood vessels. As it is common to represent fate as a path, this path could also be a tube. Panel C especially alludes to a branching point in a vessel system where some cells take the "healthy" way, while others do not, and thus embark on a disease trajectory. This can be made sense of when we interpret the image as merging the closely related image types of the cell lineage and the epigenetic landscape.

In the mid-twentieth century, Conrad Hal Waddington (1905–1975) introduced the notion of epigenetics. Unlike in today's use of the term, which emphasizes environmental influence and non-genetic factors in development and heredity, his intention was to describe the complex causal process by which genes act and interact (Baedke 2013). Development was seen as depending to a large degree on cells' ability to differentiate in a robust manner based on epigenetic processes, i.e., not easily affected by perturbations.

The epistemic landscape, FIG.2B like Weismann's tree diagram, was a theoretical, not an empirical image. Waddington used it to communicate a general idea concerning how to think about development. The drawing shows a ball, set to roll down a landscape with ridges and valleys. The ball in movement would be a representation of the composite identity of several cells in a trajectory as it is depicted in the tree diagrams discussed above, and the focus here is not on the emergence of a diversity of cell types but on the robustness of the process leading to a certain cell type. In the logic of the picture, the path of the ball is constrained and thus determined by the shape of the landscape, hence by features external to it. But conceptually, the constraints are located within the cells that are represented by the ball. Waddington complemented the image of the landscape with an image showing the underside of the landscape and how it is shaped by a "complex system of interactions" (1957, 36; see figure **2c**). While the functional role of genes was not known at the time, Waddington takes the pegs in the ground to represent genes and the strings that connect genes and the landscape surface (where some strings are connected to other strings) as representing chemical constituents of cells that depend on genes. Thus, the differentiation trajectory of a series of cell divisions and its resistance to perturbations are determined by internal factors, most notably genes, albeit, importantly, not single genes, but many genes entangled in intricate, holistic interactions. Yet, again, the deterministic nature of cell differentiation is emphasized. The image came to be widely used in biology only a few decades later and in particular in systems biology (Beadke 2013). The diagram was also employed to represent pathological processes, again, especially in the context of cancer.

The tube-like vessels in figure **1** can then be interpreted as Waddingtonian valleys, the dots in panel **c** as the movement of the ball, which, as we saw, in its trajectory represents many cell generations. The branching of the tubes represents situations where the cell diverts from its path and follows another track, due to certain factors that might be genetic or epigenetically (in today's sense) mediated environmental agents. Furthermore, especially the use of the landscape diagram in systems biology and stem cell research, where cells are "reprogrammed" to move up a valley or across a ridge, highlights that cells can not only be traced individually, and their fate be predicted, but that the fate can be technologically controlled by interventions. This association supports the notion of intervention in the vision of interceptive cellular medicine.

While visualizing cell fate in development and disease through cell lineage trees FIG. 2A and the epigenetic landscape diagrams FIG. 2B, C have long histories, the technologies used to observe cells have changed substantially from the late nineteenth to the early twenty-first century. The category of microscopes, for example, has greatly expanded, changing the notion of observation, and the characterization of cells has developed into measuring their molecular constituents.

Molecular analysis was for a long time restricted to homogenized biological samples, which contained a large number of cells. Recently, technologies that resolve analysis to the level of the individual cell have become feasible. These technologies are hailed by many as transformative for biology and biomedicine and figure prominently in the methodological outlook of the LifeTime Initiative (Rajewsky et al. 2020). The most important is single-cell RNA sequencing (scRNA-seq), but also other omics technologies are now applied to the single-cell level. Single cells can be isolated based on microfluidics technologies. Once sorted, different types of molecules can be targeted by appropriate measuring technologies (Chappell et al. 2018). Here, however, we focus on data analysis and visualization techniques. The common algorithm used to analyze single-cell data is t-distributed stochastic neighbor embedding (t-SNE). In most cases, the aim of single-cell analysis is not to characterize or find an individual cell; instead, a large number of cells are measured simultaneously, and the measurements are aggregated to obtain a clustering based on similarities and differences among individual cells. T-SNE is designed to reduce the dimensionality in the data to create clusters in two dimensions (Kobak and Berens 2019).

The procedure results in a specific type of graph, the t-SNE plot. FIG. 3A The dots in the plot each represent an individual cell. The coloring of the dots can be used to transfer

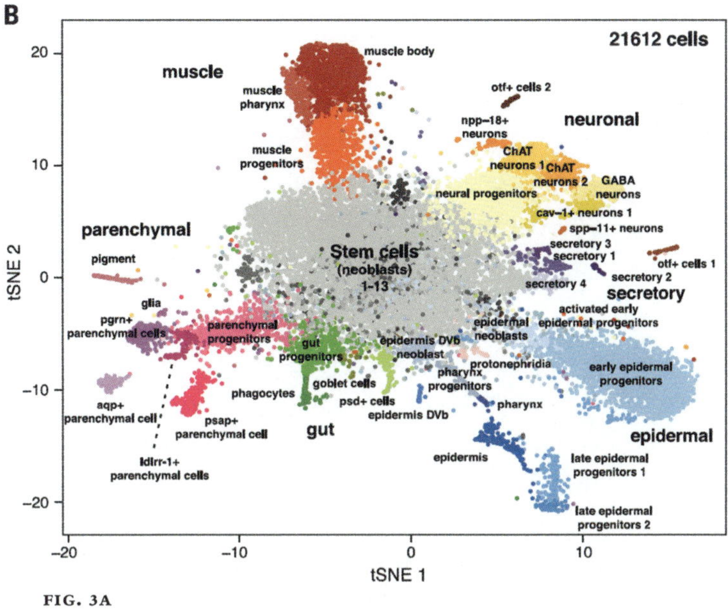

FIG. 3A

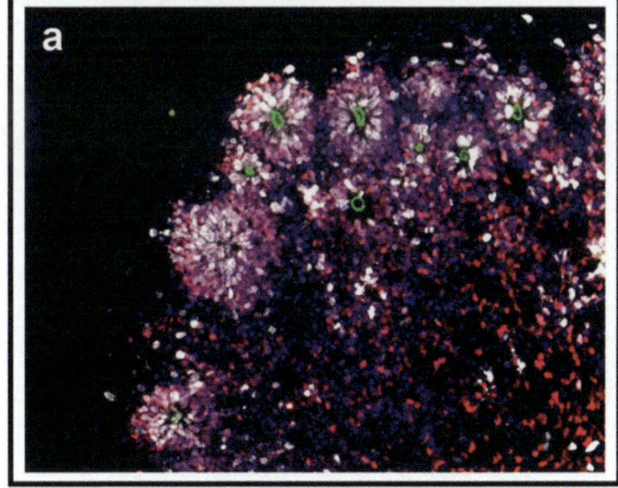

FIG. 3B

FIG. 3A t-SNE plot from Plass et al. (2018, 2, fig. 1b)
FIG. 3B Confocal microscopy image of an organoid from Tang et al. (2022, 4, fig. 4a)

different types of information; most commonly color is used to highlight clusters. Clustering allows researchers to identify groups of cells that are similar in relevant ways, e.g., regarding their RNA transcription profiles. This might indicate functional similarity, for instance, regarding different developmental stages, cellular subtypes within a tissue, or pathological processes. Given that clusters can be interpreted as representing cell types, they can inform the construction of cell lineage trees in a way similar to previous morphological observations of cells. Figure **3A** is derived from a study of the lineage tree of the flatworm species *Schmidtea mediterranea* performed by the Rajewsky Lab (Plass et al. 2018).

While there is a strong tendency to characterize cells and cellular processes on the molecular level, there are still important roles for imaging technologies that capture structural features of cells and tissues. Today, the term microscopy covers a broad range of technologies, from electron microscopy to new types of optical microscopy technologies such as confocal microscopy, allowing for optical sectioning of a tissue sample (Wellmann 2022). These technologies often rely on molecular biology, for instance, regarding the introduction of fluorescent markers. Figure **3B**, for example, is a confocal microscopy image of an organoid (here a brain organoid, see Tang et al. 2022), i.e., a complex three-dimensional cell culture that preserves properties of an organ and is used for modeling development and disease, which is also highlighted as a key technology by the LifeTime Initiative (Rajewsky et al. 2020). Furthermore, the resulting images, albeit reminiscent of photographs, are constructed from data gathered by the optical instrument. In that sense, they are quasi-naturalistic data visualizations, following "(1) historical preferences, (2) the rhetorical power of images, and (3) the cognitive accessibility of data presented in the form of images" (Delehanty 2010, 161). The boundary between data visualization and imaging is thus not sharp.

In the image we analyze here, FIG. 1 cells are not only represented as abstract theoretical constructs, as in the tubes or the dots moving through them. They are also represented as entities subjected to empirical investigation. Indeed, the clusters in panel A represent types of diseased cells (and unspecified healthy tissue) as colored clouds of dots, which can be read in both ways, as the clusters of t-SNE plots or as labeled cells in fluorescence microscopy imaging, as shown in figure 3A and B, respectively. Either way, through these associations, the image suggests how, i.e., by which technologies, the aims of the research enterprise would be pursued. It thereby makes the vision more recognizable for other researchers and embeds it in a set of technologies that are widely seen as not only cutting-edge but as transformative, such as single-cell analysis. Despite allusions to empirical methods, however, the image in question remains, like Weismann's and Waddington's,[FIG. 2] a theoretical image. It does not represent a specific, observed phenomenon but visualizes processes by which diseases, as opposed to healthy aging, emerge from continuous development. The vision it expresses makes speculative assumptions about the origins of disease, i.e., that the origin can be located in individual cells. And in light of the fact that the interventions it suggests are not yet feasible (and that their feasibility can be questioned), it remains promissory.

The theoretical development that it highlights can also be described as indicating a shift in the understanding of pathological phenomena. Building on advances in precision medicine, LifeTime presents a case of data-intensive research. The monitoring required for interceptive biomedicine does not only rely on an incredibly large amount of data, but their analysis in terms of statistically evaluated distributions and internal relations takes on a life of its own. Data-intensive research is not just a question of magnitude but operates with new levels of complexity. Data no longer simply refers to given objects but shows and differentiates relations between them (Meunier 2022; Borck 2022). The "pathological" is no longer a given entity like a tumor specimen in a pathological collection, a calcified artery or necrotizing tuberculum, but constellations of parameters statistically correlated with illness. By visualizing these data volumes as some kind of pathological or organic quasi-tissue, even though the dots do not represent biological particles but their fate in terms of health and illness, figure 1 pathologizes and reifies mere correlations to medical matter. Thus, even though current data-intensive precision medicine is continuous with the molecular biomedical paradigm, the LifeTime image raises the question of whether this transformation of biomedicine ultimately evaporates and dematerializes the conceptualization of the pathological. The image visualizes a futuristic medicine in which diseases as proper, organ-based pathological entities have ceased to exist, both conceptually and because this medicine would intercept with the manifestation.

4
Zooming Out: On the History of Pictorial Rhetoric in Medicine

Section III has zoomed in on the visual references in figure 1 and followed these traces to specific types of scientific imaging by which the figure garners credibility although it is an imaginary image. This section now situates figure 1 in a broader tradition of didactic images in medicine in order to better understand how images facilitate the (re)conceptualization of human bodies and diseases.

We have already mentioned the purposeful scaffolding of the three panels in figure 1, with their intricate change of representational logics (from three-dimensional timespace to morphological structures to dynamic processes). The skillful combination of visual codes and image types clearly points to careful decisions and professional crafting by the designers of the image. Yet, for the historian of scientific visualization, the recognition of creative ingenuity, individual training, and expertise can only amount to half of an answer, as the question of the image's persuasiveness requires a more comprehensive contextualization. The combination of visualization modes exhibited in the image can only claim to be successful if it refers to established visual frames of reference for "naturalizing" something artificial—and even utopian, as in our case (Steiner and Engelmann 2023; Nyhart 2023).

One of the central concepts underlying the image is "disease trajectory." A quick PubMed search of the term shows that, while the concept may have a long history, it only came into broader circulation during the 1990s, increasing to over 1,000 publications per year since the 2010s. Apparently, figure **1** then engages with a concept that is quite specific, yet it represents a trend in the articulation of pathological phenomena. For instance, a recent review on trajectories of lung diseases (Stolz et al. 2022) in the leading medical journal *Lancet* visualized them in far less sophisticated ways compared to the LifeTime image, as it merely arranges different types of lung diseases with their respective causes to segments of a circle in some sort of pie chart. FIG. 4A However, this image combines trajectories also with some underlying histology and thus uses the systematic blending of spatiotemporal relations with "zooming-in" effects for visualizing the different groups, as well as their causes and underlying pathology. Here, we use this image as a visual testimony and pictorial link to what is probably the most significant visual tradition in representing diseases and human pathology: Frank Netter (1906–1991) and his famous illustrated volumes on this subject. FIG. 4B The "Netter approach," which he developed in collaboration with the pharmaceutical company Ciba in the 1950s, relies not on a perfectly "realistic" representation but on a careful combination of overview and detail, highlighting the particular points at issue. The *Lancet* image FIG. 4A clearly engages visual strategies for which Frank Netter had become famous since the end of World War II and thus extends their legacy into the twenty-first century.

Netter was already a successful commercial artist when he entered medical school in the 1920s and reconverted to producing illustrations when his Manhattan-based surgical practice failed in the 1930s because of the Great Depression, quickly attracting commissions from the pharmaceutical industry as he combined graphic skills with background knowledge in medicine and biology. After World War II, his collaboration with the Ciba company developed into the famous *Ciba Collection of Medical Illustrations*, thirteen

FIG. 4A Causes of lung diseases together with their histopathology from Stolz et al. (2022, 931, fig. 6)

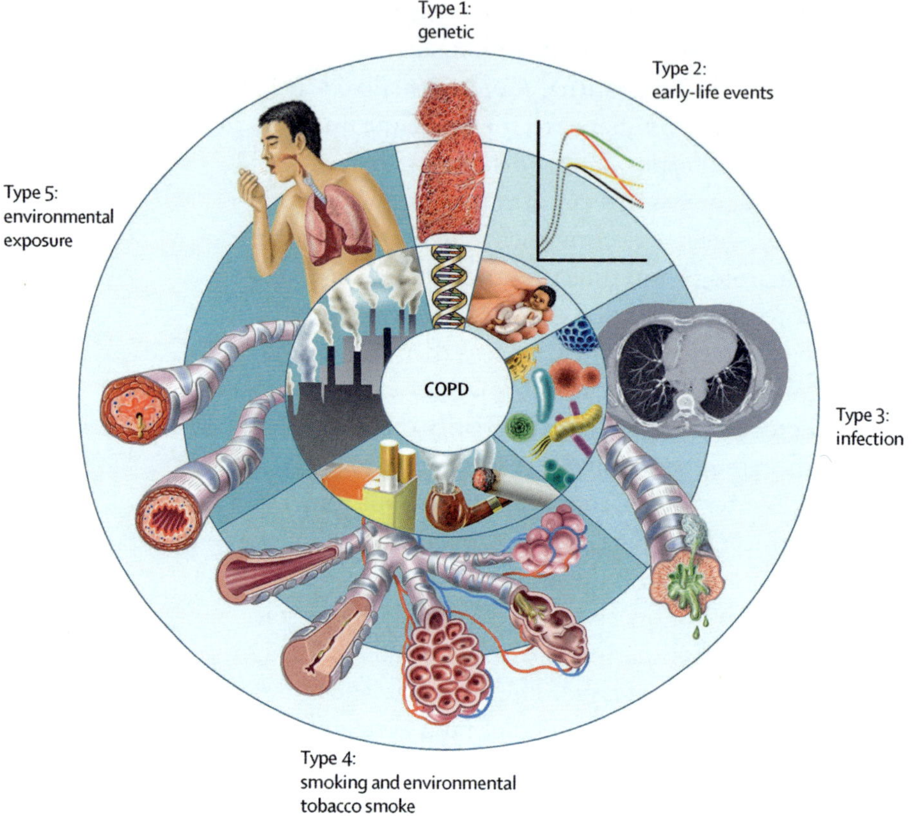

FIG. 4A

FIG. 4B Pathological manifestations of pancreatic B-cell tumors from Netter's *Ciba Collection of Medical Illustration*, vol. 4 (Netter 1965, 158, section v, plate 16)

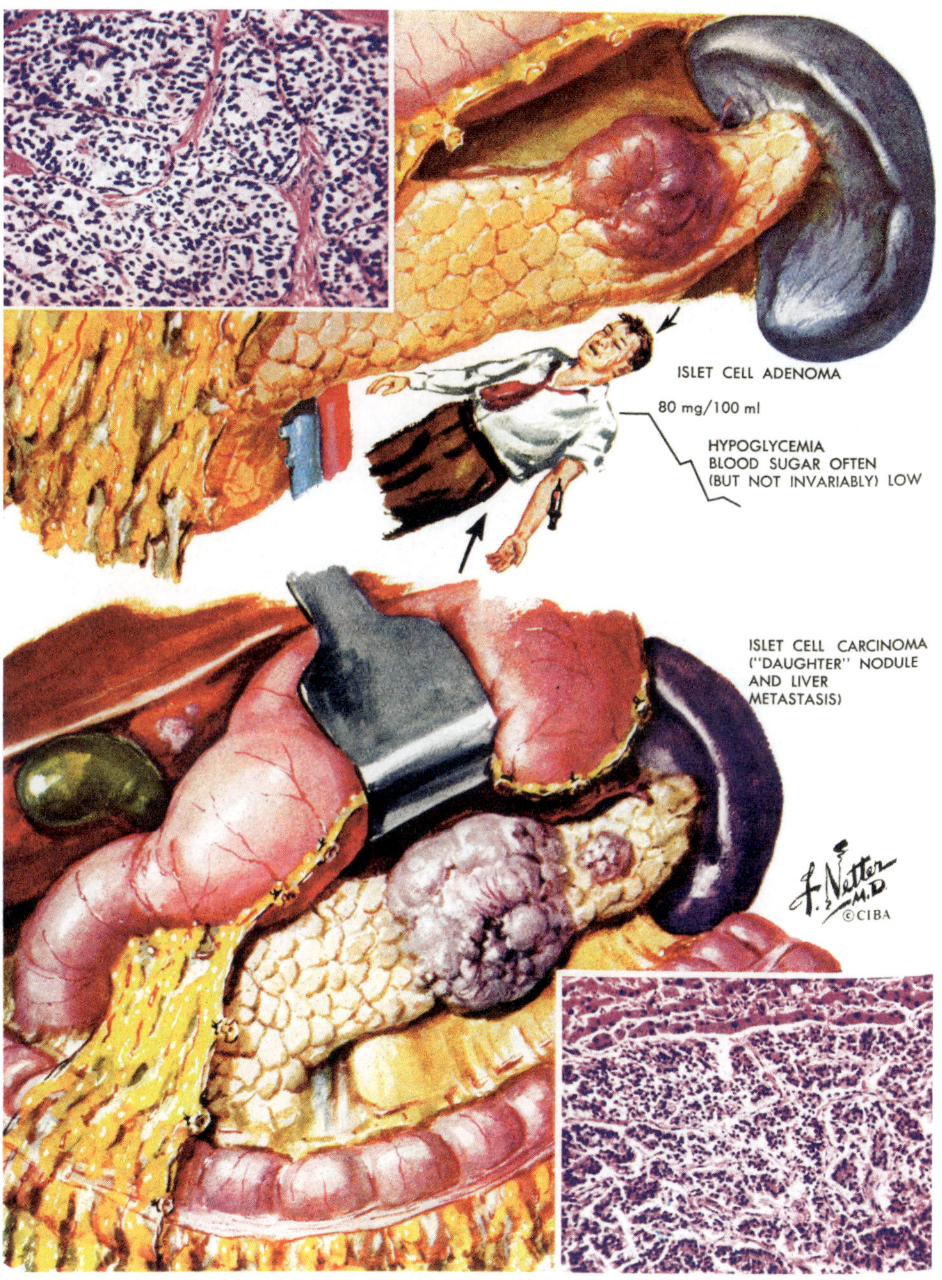

FIG. 4B

volumes of altogether more than 4,000 illustrations and reprinted late in his life as a six-volume set called *Atlas of Human Anatomy*, which became "the best-selling atlas in American medical schools" (Hansen 2006, 483).

Netter certainly did not invent the visualization of disease, but unlike images in the tradition of the anatomical or pathological atlas, he did not focus on the body and its organs as observed in the dissection theater. Instead, he highlighted anatomical or pathological details together with some human activity, thereby contextualizing the medical content with typical circumstances and blending nature with culture into knowledge. FIG. 4B This approach was meant to make it easier to memorize clinically relevant aspects or important systematic connections in medical knowledge. His signature was a functionalist approach also in a different sense. He liberated himself from strict conventions of complete anatomical comprehensiveness in order to achieve better legibility and "intuitive" understandability by focusing on visualizing the relevant details only. He prioritized the didactic function of visualization over its accuracy in terms of Daston and Galison's mechanical objectivity (2007). He did not use these terms, which were introduced into the academic debate only later, but he very consciously developed this style on principles shared by other medical illustrators:

> I have seen many beautifully rendered illustrations in which the artistic technique overpowers the message of the plate. In many cases, artistic restraint in the general portions of the illustration allows one to have a background against which to contrast the areas of focus through the use of increased detail, rendering, and contrast. (John A. Craig, quoted in Hansen 2006, 483)

His background in commercial illustration and his economic success thanks to the collaboration with the Ciba company (i.e., not an academic institution) may have helped him to establish the Netter approach, but from very early on in his career, he had been convinced that medical images function rather by their selectiveness than comprehensiveness:

> Strange as it may seem, the hardest part of making a medical picture is not the drawing at all. It is the planning, the conception, the determination of the point of view, and the approach which will best clarify the subject that take the most effort. (Netter 1949, quoted from Hansen 2006, 485)

As an illustrator, Netter did not just draw the specimen in front of him, and the drawing was not the difficult part. Instead, he had to face a series of representational decisions in order to "clarify" the image. For Netter, "naturalness" was the effect of careful planning and decision-making about "focus," "plane," and "point of view," as he explained:

> By focus, I mean the amount of the subject to be included in the picture. By plane, I mean the depth of the dissection. The artist must decide at what depth or plane of the body he will make his drawing. The term point of view is self-explanatory but must be considered very carefully in planning an illustration. (Netter 1949, quoted from Hansen 2006, 485)

Nothing, of course, was "self-explanatory" in Netter's images; on the contrary, precisely the "self-explanatory" was the effect of his mastery of visual craft and design.

Especially for the popular appeal of Netter's *Human Anatomy*, there is yet another important source, which in all likelihood can be described as the founding scene for a popular human anatomy with scientific standing: the German physician and science popularizer Fritz Kahn (1888–1968). Kahn did not collaborate with a pharmaceutical company but with a publishing house attached to a naturalists' society. Even in his early pieces for the German weekly *Berliner Illustrirte Zeitung*, Kahn had begun to demonstrate his extraordinary potential for developing visual strategies for which he would later become famous. A particularly spectacular example is his employment of the zooming-in technique that not only moves between scales of magnification but juxtaposes the entire human figure with a single muscle and its microstructures as fibers to a visually dramatized single image rather than a proper sequence. FIG. 5A, 5B In a similar vein, Kahn employed the blending of developmental time with representational space to a single image for explaining Haeckel's "law of ontogenesis," FIG. 5C taking the visualization of cell lineages and differentiation to cross-species comparison. Kahn's images clearly are fantastic, as they mix time and space with different representational modes for arriving at a single visual interpretation of biological form, function, and development.

Like Netter fifty years later, Kahn's images were regarded as so successful that the publishing house Kosmos commissioned the heavily illustrated multivolume set *Das Leben des Menschen* (The Life of Man, Kahn 1922–31) with the subtitle "Popular Human Anatomy, Biology, Physiology, and the Developmental Biology of Man" (our translation). With these books, Kahn perfected his style of visualization to employ technological analogies for explaining organs and their functions in images that carefully blended anatomical structure, physiological theory, and explanatory technical models to complex scenes of human "modern" life, i.e., contemporary culture with radio, dance, motor cars, cinema, machines, etc. (figures **5A**, **5B**, **6A**, and **6B**; see von Debschitz and von Debschitz 2017; Borck 2007).

Being an active member of the left-liberal culture in Berlin during the Weimar years and a practicing Jew, Kahn quickly realized that there was no future for him in Nazi Germany. He immigrated to the United States, where he would start a second career as popular science writer, though not quite as successful as in Germany. He managed to solicit a two-volume English translation of his German five-volume masterpiece under the new title *Man in Structure and Function* (Kahn 1943), thereby pinpointing the signature of his

FIGS. 5A–C Images from various publications by Fritz Kahn. **A** and **B**, comparison of early image in *Berliner Illustrirte Zeitung* (here as reused in *Man in Structure and Function*, Kahn 1943, 130) with later book cover (from Kahn 1922–1931, vol. 2) using the same motif of perfecting zooming in to a single, integrated image

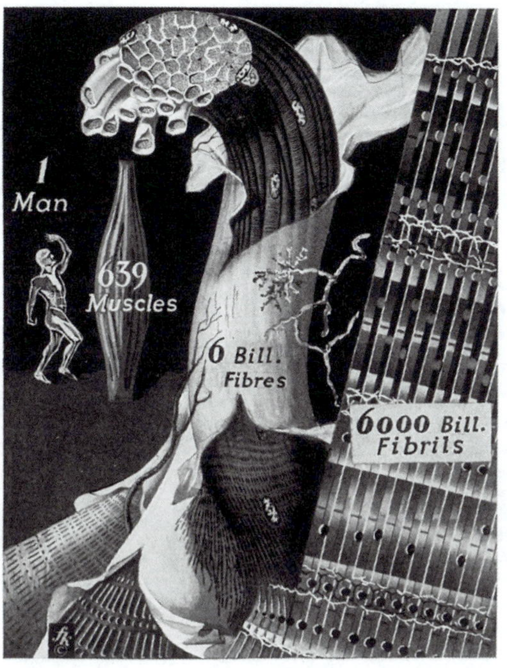

FIG. 5A

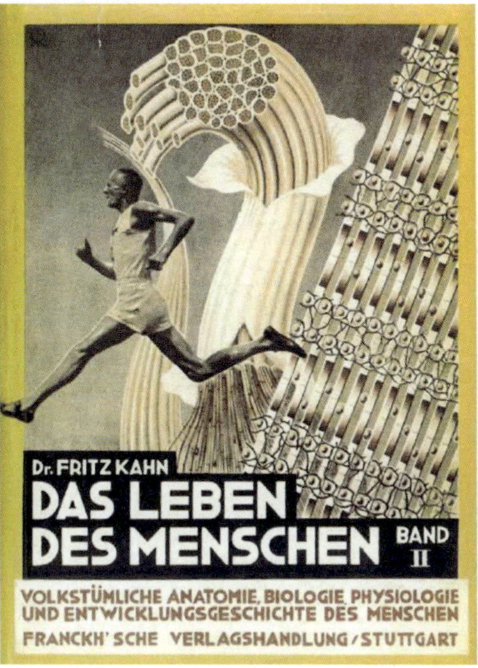

FIG. 5B

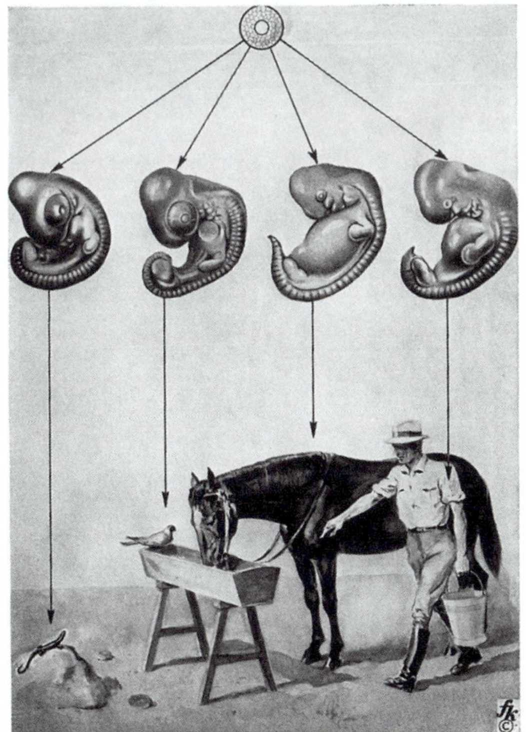

FIG. 5C

FIG. 5C Haeckel's law of the ontological recapitulation of phylogeny (from Kahn 1943, 33, fig. 26) in a similarly integrated single image combining different species (reptile, bird, horse, man)

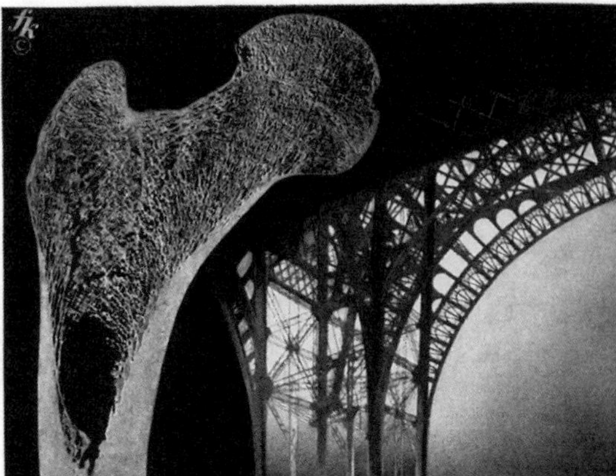

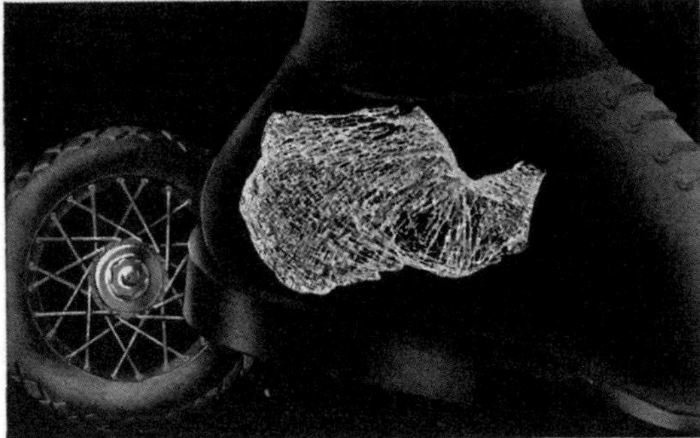

FIG. 6A

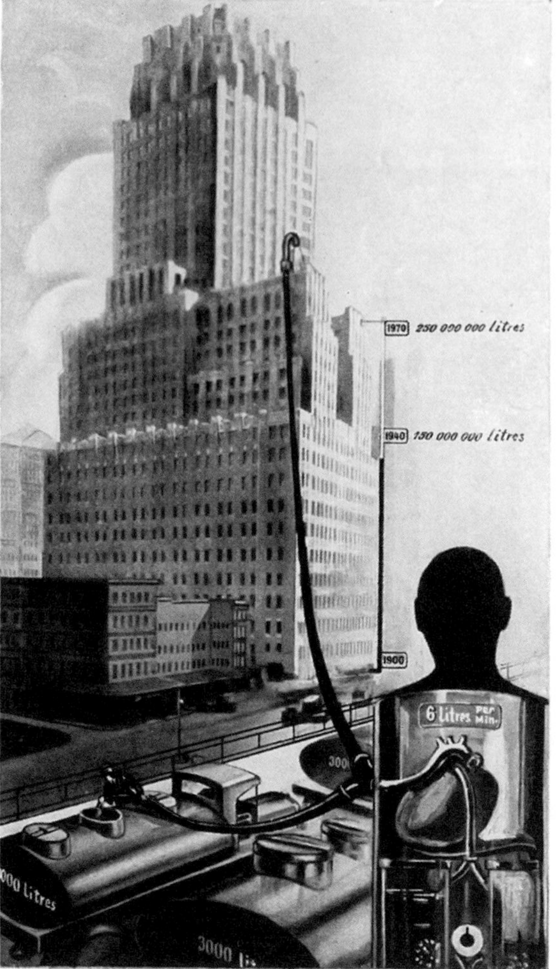

FIG. 6B

FIGS. 6A/B Images from Kahn, *Man in Structure and Function* (Kahn 1943, 60 and 180, figs. 42 and 121, respectively) visualization style. FIG. 6A, 6B Kahn pioneered a form of visualization that was scientifically correct and optically inspiring with its many references to modern culture, but which he especially developed for visualizing anatomy together with physiology. In contrast to Netter, Kahn focused on the healthy body and its functioning, though he regularly included chapters on diseases as examples of functional disturbances and to explain their pathophysiology. With his style, Kahn mediated between modern culture and the human body using one to explain the other and thereby familiarizing his audience with both.

There is no evidence of a personal contact between Netter and Kahn, but given Kahn's historical prominence it is almost impossible to imagine that Netter developed his typical style of visualization without familiarity with Kahn's images, while their different biographical and professional trajectories easily explain some of the visual differences. Netter was a professional illustrator, using his medical background for his decisions regarding selection and abstraction. Kahn, by contrast, was a physician with a liberal agenda who used his skills in conceptualizing visualizations (for many of his images he developed the visual idea only and relied on professional designers for the execution). His inspiration to rely on technological analogies and machine models for physiological functions shows him in the specific role of a popularizer of medical knowledge with an extraordinary attitude toward modern culture. If the Netter approach revolved around focus, plane, and point of view, Kahn embraced the political utopia of a healthier life achieved by an enlightening education about the body's functions (including liberal views on human sexuality). For achieving this, Kahn blended form and function, anatomy and physiology, morphology and process, where Netter concentrated on diseases and their pathology.

Both styles of visualization connect scientific knowledge with broader conceptions of nature, culture, and human life. They do so for didactic purposes. The images operate by embedding medical knowledge in daily life. FIGS. 5 AND 6 The image from the LifeTime Initiative FIG. 1 does not engage directly with these styles of didactic images, but we argue that their prominence in medical education contributes to its appearance as "natural." Abstraction and zooming in, so familiar since Kahn's revolutionary visualizations and Netter's three cardinal elements of focus, plane, and point of view, orchestrate the design decisions in the background of figure **1**.

5
Conclusion: Infographics and Imaginaries

Our contribution to this volume has focused on a single image [FIG. 1] from a biomedical article, meant to present a vision for biomedical research and practice to a broader scientific community. Our analysis suggests that the image is neither the visualization of scientific data nor a mere illustration of the text but makes a significant contribution to the articulation of the vision expressed in the article and lends rhetorical support to it. The combination of associations, scientific content, and legibility exhibited by the image is typical for the genre of infographics. We will discuss this notion in this final section in order to connect our observations on the LifeTime image with a more critical evaluation of the Initiative, thereby exploring potential significance for visual studies of science.

Scientific publications include images that exhibit a wide variety of functions. Some reproduce evidence, such as traces or inscriptions produced by instruments; some visualize data derived from quantifying such traces; some represent models derived from the data (Rheinberger 2023). Yet others show aspects of methods (e.g., schematic representations of experimental designs or research technologies). Accordingly, there is a growing discussion in visual studies of science on what such visualizations actually represent and how they take on a role of their own in the life sciences so that they can even be regarded as a form of experimentation (e.g., Coopmans et al. 2014). The image we discussed here [FIG. 1] plays none of these roles. Instead, it is an image that expresses a vision of future medicine by alluding to other types of images. Its role is to align a continuously transforming style of data-intensive, molecular biomedicine with an understanding of health and disease that combines cellular pathology with a long-term perspective on pathogenesis. This kind of visionary image is less frequently discussed in the visual studies of science, and the analysis of this particular exemplar might thus complement existing studies. Here, we suggest conceptualizing the image as a type of infographic that is geared not toward representing data but to communicating and interpretating complex information.

Infographics is not a new type of visualization; Charles Joseph Minard's famous visualization from 1869 of Napoleon's failed Russia campaign in 1811/12 is often regarded as the starting point of the genre. The designer Edward Tufte declared this to be "one of the best statistical graphics ever" (Tufte 2006, 122), because Minard combined comparison with contrast, causality, structure, and multivariate analysis to a completely integrated diagram, making it a piece of evidence in itself. Minard superimposed on a roughly topographical map of Europe, spanning from the French Empire's border on the left to Moscow on the right, a representation of the shrinking numbers of Napoleon's soldiers along their path toward Moscow in the upper half in brown and on their return in black beneath it. In the lower part of the map, he tracked the temperature of the respective days when the army reached a location by dotting a line from the name to the graph at the bottom.

Minard not only found a solution for integrating a temporal axis into the topographical representation of space and spatial relations; indeed, his map was a two-dimensional representation of a four- or five-dimensional space of knowledge. Minard conceived of a visual synthesis of a complex historical event—in fact, a single image for a disastrous decision resulting in a sheerly endless series of events until eventually close to nothing of Napoleon's massive army returned to its home territory. He achieved an integration of several layers of information into a coherent picture, a Latourian "immutable mobile" with autonomous epistemic potential. Before Minard's diagram, there was no way of representing these heterogeneous events "naturally" in

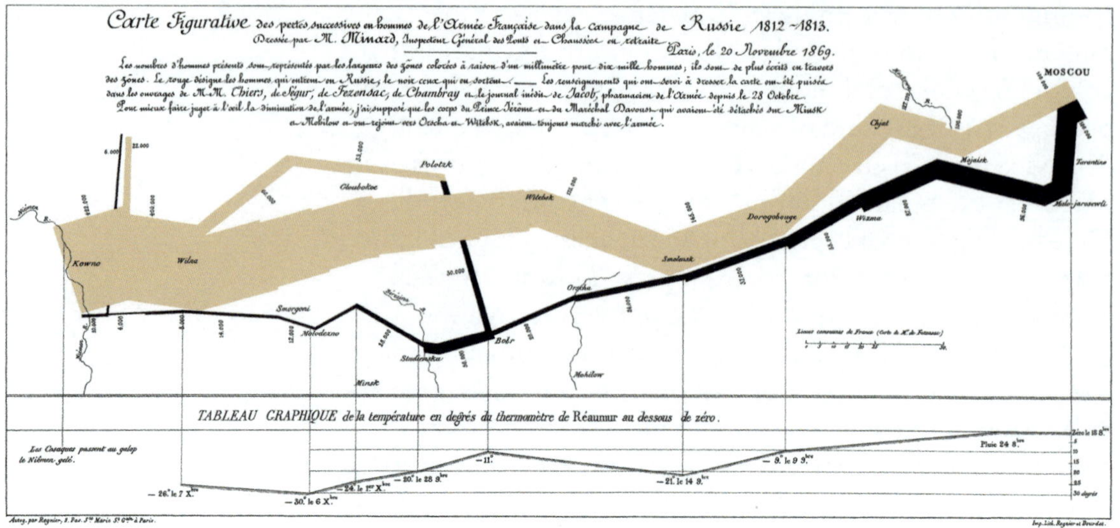

FIG. 7

FIG. 7 Charles Minard's map of Napoleon's defeat in Russia (published 1869) a two-dimensional plane, as this form of representation had to be conceived in the first place. The map's conventions had to be agreed upon, and a standard needed to be implemented. Today, this kind of graphic, representing the amounts of material or personnel as width of the arrow, is known as a "Sankey diagram," named after another graphical innovator.

In Section IV we showed how medicine has developed its own tradition of infographics that established new ways not only of integrating multidimensional medical knowledge, but of communicating a vision of the body in the medical realm to a broader audience by applying focus, selectiveness, abstraction, and the blending of visual languages. Infographics in this context might be seen as peripheral to knowledge making, as they seem to belong to science education or the communication of science to a wider public. However, in a context where scientists are increasingly specialized, while at the same time research policies and funding schemes demand ever larger interdisciplinary consortia of collaborators with vastly different backgrounds, infographics, as part of viscourses (Knorr-Cetina 1999), take on crucial roles in communication among researchers and coordination of scientists with stakeholders closely associated with their research, such as funders, university administrators, or patient groups. Such is the case with the LifeTime image. FIG. 1

Formally, this image is not a data visualization like Minard's map, FIG. 7 and yet, like the early infographic, it integrates not only the temporal dimension, here, of an individual's lifetime, with the spatial dimension, here, of the cellular body. As shown in Section III, through its visual metaphors and references it also contextualizes the visualization of the aging process in a conceptual space of cellular disease and in a research culture of molecular analysis. Like Minard's image it combines graphics with text, and like Netter's and Kahn's work, it achieves its rhetorical force from decontextualizing and recontextualizing physiological and pathological phenomena.

Unlike in Netter's and Kahn's images, the focus of the LifeTime image is not on the anatomical body with its functions and malfunctioning, nor on the body in its sociocultural situatedness in a world of modern technology, but on the cellular body as a bundle of individual trajectories, some of which assume a pathological path. If we look at figure **1A** again, at the left-side entry point, the blue tube-like lines enter the life stream as mostly "healthy cells." In the transparent box of life's incidents—internal stimuli and external factors from exposure to changing environments—only some of them reach "healthy aging," while others meet a less lucky fate. Thus, in addition to representing a specific way of cellular development going astray, i.e., pathological deviation, the clusters represent the possible fates of an entire organism, i.e., the human being or patient. Cellular fate and personal fate become one. Or, in the symbolism of the image, there is no person-level fate; there is only a cellular process that makes up a life.

The vision promoted by the image is that disease, whether primarily genetically or environmentally induced, can be detected close to its origin in the developmental process, and hence such deviation from the normal can be addressed, mitigated, and potentially corrected before the arrival of clinical symptoms. Thus, this vision of medicine promises that an individual's fate to become ill, which is determined by the fate of cells entering a disease trajectory, can be known, and ultimately medicine can intervene in the personal fate as located in the cell. Disease, then, is no longer destiny, but a person's health trajectory is controllable and changeable.

Returning to Canguilhem's discussion of the normal and the pathological, one might caution that organisms exhibit intrinsic variation and react dynamically to various stimuli. Whether the pathologically relevant variations can be detected long before the manifestation of clinical signs in an ocean of cellular reactions can be doubted. This is not the place to discuss the plausibility nor the ethics of the vision of interceptive medicine, but it should be clear that the notion of disease as fate, inscribed into the molecular signatures of our cells, and the idea that fate can be overcome by technologies for deleting or rewriting our cellular scripts neither appears achievable at this point, nor is it necessarily desirable.

The vision expressed in the image, as we pointed out, is located in the broader imaginary of personalized or precision medicine and in line with a broader biomedical shift in healthcare from environmental and social determinants of health to individualized disease, emerging toward the end of the twentieth century (Quirke and Gaudillière 2008). While the vision of LifeTime emphasizes increased temporal and spatial depth and resolution in the analysis of pathogenesis (and possibly dissolves classical conceptualizations of the pathological, as discussed earlier), on a social level it is continuous with earlier visions of molecularized and individualized medical surveillance and intervention. Hence, recurrent criticism of the social order that simultaneously supports and is created by biomedical technologies articulated from within medicine as well as in the humanities and social sciences apply here as well. Healthcare as envisioned by LifeTime risks:

1) increased (bio-)medicalization, i.e., the trend to place aspects of life into the realm of medicine that were not seen in that way before (Hofmann 2016; Clarke et al. 2003), in this case, life before the onset of disease;

2) inescapable overdiagnosis, i.e., the diagnosis of conditions that would not have caused harm when undetected, but still might trigger interventions connected to costs and potentially negative effects (Hofmann 2016), in this case, regarding deviant trajectories with a benign fate;

3) unbalanced interventionism, i.e., a focus on diagnosis and treatment, in this case, of cellular processes in the absence of illness, as a technological fix at the expense of prevention by means of addressing social and environmental determinants of disease (Tabery 2023);

4) commercialization, i.e., the push to translate medicine and research into business development, in this case involving the recruitment of increasingly younger people as potential patients and consumers in the economy of medical services and pharmaceutical products (Clarke et al. 2003).

What is important for us is to see how the image is not merely illustrating the text in the LifeTime article but co-creates the new articulation of the biomedical imaginary (Erikainen and Chan 2019; Meunier and Herzog 2023) to which this criticism pertains by purporting it as a rational enterprise that claims an objective approach to disease, based on automated procedures, big data, and AI technologies, rather than on a patient's illness or suffering as the starting point for medical intervention. It does so as much through its intricate use of visual metaphors expressing the underlying notion of pathological processes and by references to research technologies that can be marshalled to detect and intervene on them, as through its specific omissions. The most striking absence in the image is the environment in which the body develops and that influences the molecular relations within and across cells through epigenetic processes, microbiota, and other interfaces. Thus, the cellular processes themselves appear as the only available locus of intervention. Furthermore, the image eclipses the person through the abstract representation of bodies as clouds of cells, as mentioned above. Everything beyond the level of cells matters only insofar as it has an impact on the cellular level. Life is depicted here as a process but not as a biography. In this way, resilience achieved by viable social relations or the negative impacts of social processes, as emphasized by critics of biomedicine, are eclipsed here as well. At the very least, these omissions make the LifeTime image an interesting object for the visual studies of science as a locus for observing the intersection of social and political values on the one hand and epistemic values as reflected in methods and theoretical assumptions on the other hand.

As an exemplary infographic for visionary science, figure 1 communicates a vision of cell-based interceptive medicine within the socio-technological imaginary of precision medicine. The image exhibits an epistemic value system in the life sciences that has emerged gradually in the last seventy years and can be described in terms of molecularization and datafication. This scientific perspective has interacted in many ways with social agendas of individualization and market economies, i.e., the very sociopolitical context excluded in the biomedical perspective. The absence of the person with its biographical life, full of social circumstances and accidental environmental conditions, serves to make the claim that it does not matter how cells came to deviate, whether through an inherited mutation or exposure to environmental harm. The deviation will be detected through monitoring the body as a collection of cells, thus making the individual's life subject to institutionalized and marketized control. Overall, we show how in the case discussed visualization not only functions as a didactic addendum but also adds crucial plausibility and legitimacy to the project by representing the idea as something *imageable* (and not just *imaginable*) and hence achievable.

A

Althusser, Louis (1990) *Philosophy and the Spontaneous Philosophy of the Scientists & Other Essays*. Edited by Gregory Elliott. Translated by Ben Brewster. London: Verso.

B

Baedke, Jan (2013) "The Epigenetic Landscape in the Course of Time: Conrad Hal Waddington's Methodological Impact on the Life Sciences." *Studies in History and Philosophy of Science Part C: Studies in History and Philosophy of Biological and Biomedical Sciences* 44 (4, Part B): 756–73. https://doi.org/10.1016/j.shpsc.2013.06.001.

Baigrie, Brian Scott, ed. (1996) *Picturing Knowledge: Historical and Philosophical Problems Concerning the Use of Art in Science*. Toronto: University of Toronto Press.

Belsky, Drew Danielle (2022) "Illustrations Performed with Care: Enacting Accuracy in Medical Illustration." In *Making Sense of Medicine: Material Culture and the Reproduction of Medical Knowledge*, edited by John Nott and Anna Harris, 219–31. Bristol: Intellect.

Blasimme, Alessandro, and Effy Vayena (2016) "'Tailored-to-You': Public Engagement and the Political Legitimation of Precision Medicine." *Perspectives in Biology and Medicine* 59 (2): 172–88. https://doi.org/10.1353/pbm.2017.0002.

Blumenberg, Hans (2016) *Paradigms for a Metaphorology*. Translated by Robert Savage. Ithaca, NY: Cornell University Press.

Borck, Cornelius (2007) "Communicating the Modern Body: Fritz Kahn's Popular Images of Human Physiology as an Industrialized World." *Canadian Journal of Communication* 32 (3–4): 495–520. https://doi.org/10.22230/cjc.2007v32n3a1876.

Borck, Cornelius, ed. (2013) *Hans Blumenberg beobachtet: Philosophie, Wissenschaft und Technik*. Freiburg: Verlag Karl Alber.

Borck, Cornelius (2016) "How We May Think: Imaging and Writing Technologies across the History of the Neurosciences." *Studies in History and Philosophy of Science Part C: Studies in History and Philosophy of Biological and Biomedical Sciences* 57 (June): 112–20. https://doi.org/10.1016/j.shpsc.2016.02.006.

Borck, Cornelius (2017) "Vital Brains: On the Entanglement of Media, Minds, and Models." In *Vital Models: The Making and Use of Models in the Brain Sciences*, edited by Tara Mahfoud, Sam McLean, and Nikolas Rose, 233: 1–24. Cambridge, MA: Academic Press. https://doi.org/10.1016/bs.pbr.2017.06.005.

Borck, Cornelius (2022) "Tactile Vision, Epistemic Things and Data Visualization." *Berichte zur Wissenschaftsgeschichte* 45 (3): 415–27. https://doi.org/10.1002/bewi.202200032.

C

Canguilhem, Georges (1991) *The Normal and the Pathological*. Translated by Carolyn R. Fawcett. New York, NY: Zone Books.

Chappell, Lia, Andrew J. C. Russell, and Thierry Voet (2018) "Single-Cell (Multi)Omics Technologies." *Annual Review of Genomics and Human Genetics* 19: 15–41. https://doi.org/10.1146/annurev-genom-091416-035324.

Clarke, Adele E., Janet K. Shim, Laura Mamo, Jennifer Ruth Fosket, and Jennifer R. Fishman (2003) "Biomedicalization: Technoscientific Transformations of Health, Illness, and U.S. Biomedicine." *American Sociological Review* 68 (2): 161–94. https://doi.org/10.1177/000312240306800201.

Coopmans, Catelijne, Janet Vertesi, Michael E. Lynch, and Steve Woolgar, eds. (2014) *Representation in Scientific Practice Revisited*. Cambridge, MA: MIT Press.

D

Daston, Lorraine, and Peter Galison (2007) *Objectivity*. New York, NY: Zone Books.

Debschitz, Uta von, and Thilo von Debschitz (2017) *Fritz Kahn: Infographics Pioneer*. Cologne: Taschen.

Delehanty, Megan (2010) "Why Images?" *Medicine Studies* 2 (3): 161–73. https://doi.org/10.1007/s12376-010-0052-2.

Dröscher, Ariane (2014) "Images of Cell Trees, Cell Lines, and Cell Fates: The Legacy of Ernst Haeckel and August Weismann in Stem Cell Research." *History and Philosophy of the Life Sciences* 36 (2): 157–86. https://doi.org/10.1007/s40656-014-0028-8.

E

Erikainen, Sonja, and Sarah Chan (2019) "Contested Futures: Envisioning 'Personalized,' 'Stratified,' and 'Precision' Medicine." *New Genetics and Society* 38 (3): 308–30. https://doi.org/10.1080/14636778.2019.1637720.

H

Hansen, John T. (2006) "Frank H. Netter, M.D. (1906–1991): The Artist and His Legacy." *Clinical Anatomy* 19 (6): 481–86. https://doi.org/10.1002/ca.20358.

Hedgecoe, Adam (2004) *The Politics of Personalised Medicine: Pharmacogenetics in the Clinic*. Cambridge, UK: Cambridge University Press.

Heintz, Bettina, and Jörg Huber, eds. (2001) *Mit dem Auge denken: Strategien der Sichtbarmachung in wissenschaftlichen und virtuellen Welten*. Zurich: Edition Voldemeer.

Hentschel, Klaus (2014) *Visual Cultures in Science and Technology: A Comparative History*. Oxford: Oxford University Press.

Hofmann, Bjørn (2016) "Medicalization and Overdiagnosis: Different but Alike." *Medicine, Health Care and Philosophy* 19 (2): 253–64. https://doi.org/10.1007/s11019-016-9693-6.

J

Jasanoff, Sheila (2015) "Future Imperfect: Science, Technology, and the Imaginations of Modernity." In *Dreamscapes of Modernity: Sociotechnical Imaginaries and the Fabrication of Power*, edited by Sheila Jasanoff and Sang-Hyun Kim, 1–33. Chicago: University of Chicago Press.

Jones, Caroline A., and Peter L. Galison, eds. (1998) *Picturing Science, Producing Art*. New York, NY: Routledge.

K

Kahn, Fritz (1922-1931) *Das Leben des Menschen: Eine volkstümliche Anatomie, Biologie, Physiologie und Entwicklungsgeschichte des Menschen*, vols. 1–5. Stuttgart: Franckh'sche Verlagsbuchhandlung.

Kahn, Fritz (1943) *Man in Structure and Function*, vol. 1. Edited and translated by George Rosen. New York, NY: Alfred Knopf.

Kemp, Martin (1997) "Seeing and Picturing: Visual Representation in Twentieth-Century Science." In *Science in the Twentieth Century*, edited by John Krige and Dominique Pestre, 361–89. Amsterdam: Harwood.

Knorr-Cetina, Karin (1999) "'Viskurse' der Physik: Wie visuelle Darstellungen ein Wissenschaftsgebiet ordnen." In *Konstruktionen: Sichtbarkeiten*, edited by Jörg Huber and Martin Heller, 245–63. Vienna: Springer.

Kobak, Dmitry, and Philipp Berens (2019) "The Art of Using T-SNE for Single-Cell Transcriptomics." *Nature Communications* 10 (1): 5416. https://doi.org/10.1038/s41467-019-13056-x.

Konrad, Kornelia Elke, Harro van Lente, Christopher Groves, and Cynthia Selin (2017) "Performing and Governing the Future in Science and Technology." In *The Handbook of Science and Technology Studies,* 4th ed., edited by Ulrike Felt, Rayvon Fouché, Clark A. Miller, and Laurel Smith-Doerr, 465–93. Cambridge, MA: MIT Press.

L

Latour, Bruno (1986) "Visualisation and Cognition: Drawing Things Together." In *Knowledge and Society: Studies in the Sociology of Culture Past and Present*, edited by Henrika Kuklick and Elizabeth Long, 6: 1–40. Greenwich, CT: Jai Press.

Lynch, Michael, and Steve Woolgar, eds. (1990) *Representation in Scientific Practice*. Cambridge, MA: MIT Press.

M

McAllister, James W. (2013) "Reasoning with Visual Metaphors." *The Knowledge Engineering Review* 28 (3): 367–79. https://doi.org/10.1017/S0269888913000295.

Meunier, Robert (2022) "Approaches in Post-Experimental Science: The Case of Precision Medicine." *Berichte zur Wissenschaftsgeschichte* 45 (3): 373–83. https://doi.org/10.1002/bewi.202200020.

Meunier, Robert, and Christian Herzog (2023) "Omics and AI in Precision Medicine: Maintaining Socio-Technical Imaginaries by Transforming Technological Assemblages." *TATuP – Zeitschrift für Technikfolgenabschätzung in Theorie und Praxis* 32 (3): 48–53. https://doi.org/10.14512/tatup.32.3.48.

N

Netter, Frank H. (1949) "A Medical Illustrator at Work." In *Ciba Symposia (May–June)*, edited by Caspari Rosen, 10, 6: 1087–92. Ciba Pharmaceutical Products, Inc.

Netter, Frank H. (1965) *Endocrine System and Selected Metabolic Diseases: The Ciba Collection of Medical Illustrations*, vol. 4. New York, NY: Colorpress.

Nyhart, Lynn K. (2023) "Commentary: Visual Cultures, Publication Technologies, and Legitimation in the Life Sciences." *Berichte zur Wissenschaftsgeschichte* 46 (2–3): 283–93. https://doi.org/10.1002/bewi.202300025.

P

Pauwels, Luc, ed. (2006) *Visual Cultures of Science: Rethinking Representational Practices in Knowledge Building and Science Communication*. Hanover, NH: Dartmouth College Press.

Plass, Mireya, Jordi Solana, F. Alexander Wolf, Salah Ayoub, Aristotelis Misios, Petar Glažar, Benedikt Obermayer, Fabian J. Theis, Christine Kocks, and Nikolaus Rajewsky (2018) "Cell Type Atlas and Lineage Tree of a Whole Complex Animal by Single-Cell Transcriptomics." *Science* 360 (6391): eaaq1723. https://doi.org/10.1126/science.aaq1723.

Q

Quirke, Viviane, and Jean-Paul Gaudillière (2008) "The Era of Biomedicine: Science, Medicine, and Public Health in Britain and France after the Second World War." *Medical History* 52 (4): 441–52. https://doi.org/10.1017/S002572730000017X.

R

Rajewsky, Nikolaus, Geneviève Almouzni, Stanislaw A. Gorski, Stein Aerts, Ido Amit, Michela G. Bertero, Christoph Bock, et al. (2020) "LifeTime and Improving European Healthcare through Cell-Based Interceptive Medicine." *Nature* 587 (7834): 377–86. https://doi.org/10.1038/s41586-020-2715-9.

Rheinberger, Hans-Jörg (2023) *Split and Splice: A Phenomenology of Experimentation.* Chicago: University of Chicago Press.

S

Stanger, Ben Z., and Geoffrey M. Wahl (2024) "Cancer as a Disease of Development Gone Awry." *Annual Review of Pathology: Mechanisms of Disease* 19: 397–421. https://doi.org/10.1146/annurev-pathmechdis-031621-025610.

Steiner, Katharina, and Lukas Engelmann (2023) "Circulation as a Visual Practice." *Berichte zur Wissenschaftsgeschichte* 46 (2–3): 143–57. https://doi.org/10.1002/bewi.202300023.

Stolz, Daiana, Takudzwa Mkorombindo, Desiree M. Schumann, Alvar Agusti, Samuel Y. Ash, Mona Bafadhel, Chunxue Bai, et al. (2022) "Towards the Elimination of Chronic Obstructive Pulmonary Disease: A Lancet Commission." *The Lancet* 400 (10356): 921–72. https://doi.org/10.1016/S0140-6736(22)01273-9.

T

Tabery, James (2023) *Tyranny of the Gene: Personalized Medicine and Its Threat to Public Health.* New York, NY: Knopf.

Tang, Xiao-Yan, Shanshan Wu, Da Wang, Chu Chu, Yuan Hong, Mengdan Tao, Hao Hu, Min Xu, Xing Guo, and Yan Liu (2022) "Human Organoids in Basic Research and Clinical Applications." *Signal Transduction and Targeted Therapy* 7: 168. https://doi.org/10.1038/s41392-022-01024-9.

Topol, Eric J. (2014) "Individualized Medicine from Prewomb to Tomb." *Cell* 157 (1): 241–53. https://doi.org/10.1016/j.cell.2014.02.012.

Tsimberidou, Apostolia M., Elena Fountzilas, Mina Nikanjam, and Razelle Kurzrock (2020) "Review of Precision Cancer Medicine: Evolution of the Treatment Paradigm." *Cancer Treatment Reviews* 86 (June). https://doi.org/10.1016/j.ctrv.2020.102019.

Tufte, Edward R. (2006) *Beautiful Evidence.* Cheshire, CT: Graphics Press.

V

Virchow, Rudolf Ludwig Karl (1860) *Cellular Pathology.* Translated by Frank Chance. London: John Churchill.

W

Waddington, Conrad Hal (1957) *The Strategy of the Genes: A Discussion of Some Aspects of Theoretical Biology.* London: Allen & Unwin.

Weismann, August (1893) *The Germ-Plasm: A Theory of Heredity.* Translated by W. Newton Parker and Harriet Rönnfeldt. New York, NY: Charles Scribner's Sons.

Wellmann, Janina (2022) "History of Embryology: Visualizations through Series and Animation." In *The Palgrave Handbook of the History of Human Sciences*, edited by David McCallum, 259–90. Singapore: Springer Nature. https://doi.org/10.1007/978-981-16-7255-2_22.

Building Biosociality through Visualizations of Genome-Wide Sequencing Risk for an Online Patient Decision-Making Aid (DECIDE)

Adam Christianson, Ariane Hanemaayer, Sophia Martineck,
Alexandra Hamann, Jan M. Friedman, and Alison Elliott

Our chapter contributes to the visualization of disease by focusing on genome-wide sequencing (GWS) and risk. We examine how risk is communicated to patients using decision-making aids in genetic counseling. Following a sociological analysis of an existing aid, we worked collaboratively with a science communicator and an illustrator to revisualize an affective and connected experience that could be translated to prospective patients through a decision-making aid. Personal decision-making aids (PDAS) are often designed to inform patients about procedures, which can assist with their informed consent for testing and treatment options. PDAS are meant to improve patient knowledge and to allow people to use this knowledge alongside their values and preferences to make a choice that feels right for them. We contend that these visual aids play an important role in providing not only information but also the potential to address the affective elements of decision-making. In so doing, our PDA is informed by the biosocial premise that connection is beneficial to patients and families. Our PDA presents the patient with an illustrated (graphic-medicine-style) comic that demonstrates the interconnectedness of someone undergoing genetic testing with all the relationships, actual and potential, throughout the diagnostic odyssey.[1]

To do so, we focus on the affective dimensions of visualizations of risk related to genome-wide sequencing with the case study from a decision-making aid developed by two of the authors (Friedman and Elliott) and their colleagues (see Birch et al. 2016). Their research tool is used in a children's hospital in British Columbia, and it informs the work of a team of geneticists and genetic counselors as well as the patients and families that they treat there. Over the last decade, the tool has been tested for effectiveness in practice. Our team took a patient-reported result about low empowerment as an opening and opportunity to re-illustrate some of the information around risks and benefits in the online decision aid. The process of analyzing, redesigning, and illustrating a new aid was not only interdisciplinary but also inter-sectoral. The process involved a great deal of dialogue across disciplinary and professional boundaries, which included productive disagreements, confusion, reinterpretation, development of a common language, consolidation, and compromise to reach the state of the PDA presented here.

To spell out the process, we first introduce GWS and our case study of a patient decision-making aid. Next, we analyze how risk is visualized in the tool. Then, we draw on the sociological concept of biosociality to rethink how patients might feel empowered and connected through the knowledge that could be gained from genetic testing. The analysis informed a collaboration among clinicians, sociologists, scientific communication specialists, and illustrators. To visualize the interconnectedness of patients and families with medical specialists, we draw on the concept of biosociality. This concept aims to empower through affective connection and offers alternative ways of informing patients about the potential of genetic testing. We focus on biosociality, as it aims to connect people through feelings of hope. We conclude the chapter by discussing our process, potential limitations, and future directions.

1 While there is an implicit assumption that connection is desirable to patients and families, there is also the openness of informed consent embedded within the process of PDA use. Patients may, however, also use the PDA to inform their decision against undergoing the tests.

Genome-Wide Sequencing and Risk

Patients with rare genetic diseases often experience a lengthy journey to diagnosis. Commonly called a *diagnostic odyssey* in the clinical literature, this journey begins when patients or parents of underage patients identify a serious, unexplained sign, symptom, or group of clinical features that do not resolve quickly. The search for a diagnosis becomes an odyssey when conventional clinical knowledge, measures, and tests are not effective, and physicians turn to specialized molecular knowledge that can delve into the deep interiors of the body's submicroscopic processes to arrive at a diagnosis. As patients and their families search for a diagnosis, they embark on what often amounts to a multiyear gamut of consultations and tests (Carmichael et al. 2015). This process has quality-of-life implications for the patient and can be costly and time-consuming for clinics and health systems.

New advances in genome sequencing offer patients and families a realistic option for ending the diagnostic odyssey. Genome-wide sequencing (GWS) is a process by which the patient's whole genome (genetic code) is analyzed concurrently, often alongside the genomes of other family members. GWS has the potential to shorten a diagnostic odyssey and is sensitive enough that an analyst can identify single-nucleotide variants across six billion nucleotides in the human genome. It is, therefore, a powerful tool for identifying pathogenic variants (genetic changes that result in disease) that might be missed by analyzing genes one at a time. New technologies make GWS increasingly affordable (Sawyer et al. 2016; Wetterstrand 2022) and, in some instances, even cost-saving in the long term (Regier et al. 2024). For these reasons, GWS is becoming a routine diagnostic option for patients and families who are suspected of having a genetic disease.

In addition to improving the treatment or management of a disease, there are additional reasons that patients and families might elect to undergo GWS. Clinicians on our team observed that GWS results can assist with family planning, including both guiding future reproductive options[2] and providing patients

2 Our own team addressed genetics, and its legacies related to eugenics, in our discussion. It was also discussed at length at the workshop in 2022. Recently, renewed interest in the media has exposed histories of forced sterilization of people with genetic diseases (e.g., Associated Press 2023). While these ethical dilemmas and historical contexts go beyond the scope of our paper, the genetic counselor and clinician on our team noted that they take patient autonomy as central to their work.

and families with a greater understanding of their condition, thus improving their quality of life through knowledge and access to societal resources they may need (Lingen et al. 2016; Makela et al. 2009). While GWS may be a cost-efficient way to end a patient's diagnostic journey, clinicians are dedicated to the idea that patients and families should carefully consider the risks and meanings associated with undertaking the test and receiving the results. While genetic testing is minimally invasive and comes at minimal physical risk to the patient, the consequences of undergoing genetic testing can be significant.

Further to ending the diagnostic odyssey, our team wanted to illustrate additional benefits to undertaking GWS. For example, the counseling process associated with GWS often helps people connect to others with similar conditions, and they are often connected to supports they would not have accessed otherwise, such as access to early childhood programs, developmental evaluation, or educational assistants at school. People also commonly express pride in how their genetic information forwards science (Birch et al. 2016). In our collaborative process, we focused on this experience of connection, which builds upon the literature on biosociality.

Diagnosing genetic conditions could also have negative outcomes. There are social, financial, medical, and psychological risks associated with undergoing GWS. For example, obtaining a diagnosis can have a psychological impact on the patient and family, especially if the condition found is incurable. Discovering a heritable gene could also affect the insurability of the patient's extended family, depending on the legal context where testing is completed. Further, learning and communicating a genetic condition has connotations that touch on the morals implicit in a person's reproductive choices, such as the valuation of (dis)ability (i.e., ableism), and the practical impacts of discrimination a person or family may experience. However, diagnoses are often elusive, even with GWS. About 35 to 50 percent of patients undergoing GWS can expect to receive a diagnosis. Those who do not receive a diagnosis may drop out of care or may mistakenly be advised or conclude their condition is not genetic, which may have dire consequences for the patient and their family. In these cases, the diagnostic odyssey may continue.[3] Because GWS examines more than 20,000 genes, it is also possible that testing will identify genetic variants that have nothing to do with the problems that led to the testing but still have serious implications. These genetic variants, known as incidental findings (IF), may indicate susceptibility to additional illnesses (e.g., cancer), with similar implications for the extended family. Moreover, patients risk uncovering variants of unknown significance (VUS), which may add further uncertainty. Both IF and VUS can extend and complicate a patient's diagnostic odyssey in unexpected ways.

Our team did not always agree about what is a negative outcome or possible risk to GWS. For example, the clinicians understood insurability as a major risk for some patients, whereas ending the odyssey was seen as a benefit. The sociologists, alternatively, believed that the possibility of not getting answers (a diagnosis) could be seen as a risk associated with getting the results of GWS, but, similarly, knowledge of VUS could also be distressing because of the uncertainty involved. Where the team did agree was on the importance of recognizing all these possible feelings through our illustrated graphics and maintaining the emphasis on connection in the final comic. We now turn to a discussion of the PDA that our project extends and adds to.

3 We focus on the risk associated with choosing whether to undertake GWS, with the aim of ending the diagnostic odyssey. There are other risks associated with the results of obtaining a negative GWS. For example, families (and physicians) could think that negative GWS means that the patient's disease is not genetic, which is not always the case. This misconception could have negative or unintended consequences for the patient and family. For example, a genetic diagnosis could later lead to treatment, even if not immediately available, as biomedicine and pharmacology improve over time.

DECIDE

Due in part to the high demand for genetic counselors, researchers in British Columbia (and elsewhere) identified the need for a computer-based tool to facilitate and optimize genetic counseling for GWS (e.g., Birch 2015). DECIDE (Decision & E-Counseling for Inherited Disorder Evaluation), our case study, was developed by a team of researchers at the University of British Columbia between 2014 and 2019. DECIDE aims to "guide adult patients or parents of affected children toward a decision about whether or not to have diagnostic GWS" (Adam et al. 2019, 11). It accomplishes this by providing video and textual information as well as illustrations about genetic testing and the benefits and risks associated with GWS. Patients are provided with a private invitation link to complete this virtual tool on their own time before meeting with a physician or genetic counselor, at which point the patient can have an informed discussion. The tool introduces patients to the possibility of consenting to the test and whether they also want to be informed about incidental genetic findings and VUS (Adam et al. 2019, 11).

DECIDE is a computerized patient decision aid (PDA). A PDA is an evidence-based approach to risk communication in which probabilities, treatment outcomes, and options are presented in a patient-friendly manner (Charles et al. 2005). Conventionally, decision-making aids present pictographic representations of probabilities alongside text to improve health numeracy and knowledge (Peters et al. 2007). Interactives frequently accompany these representations to help the patient weigh their values, preferences, and goals for health. PDAS are useful in contexts where individual patients face multiple or complex decisions that are challenging for clinicians to resolve based on clinical experience or knowledge alone (Montori et al. 2015). PDAS aim to enhance shared decision-making, making them an appealing complement to conventional genetic counseling (Sheehan and Sherman 2012; Adam et al. 2019). In addition to applying principles of PDA design, the DECIDE tool capitalizes on "nudge" techniques[4] to "maximize the odds that people will make high-quality decisions" about their decision to undergo GWS (Birch et al. 2016, 1303). By getting patients to focus on the most pertinent information related to the test and by simplifying the more effortful weighing of benefits and risks that a patient is expected to perform when making a decision, the tool aims to encourage decision-making without interfering with patient autonomy or misinforming the patient (Bansback et al. 2014).

A study assessing the clinical value of DECIDE found that the tool was as effective as conventional genetic counseling in

4 "Nudge" emerged as a term in the decision-making medical literature in 2008. In a book by Thaler and Sunstein (2008), an architecture of presenting choices about one's health is exposed through a number of experiments. The idea behind these techniques is to set up the decision space (either material or ideal) in such a way that people are meant to make the healthy choice. In the original experiments, this included things like putting fruit beside cake in a lunch buffet, as people know that fruit is the healthier choice and are more likely to choose that instead of the sweet treat. In DECIDE, the tool was informed by nudge techniques insofar as it assisted the user in a visualization of the decision space. It ranks the user's choices according to their values, so that they can make the decision about taking the test according to these values. So, it does not necessarily guide a particular choice but rather sets up the choice about whether to take the test according to the elicited responses from the user.

informing the user's basic knowledge of diagnostic GWS and its possible consequences (Adam et al. 2019). The tool was developed based on the findings of a systematic review of the GWS genetic counseling literature and multiple qualitative research projects with patients undergoing GWS, in addition to guidance from patients' families, genetics health professionals, and e-learning and decision scientists (Birch et al. 2016, 1300). The tool was beta- and usability-tested with parents of children with developmental delays or intellectual disabilities (Birch et al. 2016). It was later tested with parents of children with early-onset epilepsy of unknown cause (Adam et al. 2019). Participants in the above pilot study felt their knowledge about GWS increased significantly after using the tool. However, this study found that patients felt only slightly more "empowered" after engaging with the tool (Adam et al. 2019, 12). Empowerment is defined as the "degree to which a patient or parent believes that he or she [sic] has decisional, cognitive, and behavioral control, emotional regulation, and hope" (Adam et al. 2019, 12). Drawing on concepts in the sociology of medicine, we propose that the small improvement in patient empowerment could be related to the degree to which patients feel they understand how the results of the GWS test will be meaningful to them. In connection with this hypothesis, we focus on the concept of biosociality, as it aims to connect people through feelings of hope.

Our Approach to the Analysis

The comic represents an experimental cross-disciplinary attempt at empowering people who consider undergoing GWS; it is meant to complement the DECIDE tool by supporting their affective dimensions through visualization of the biosocial principles of connection and relationships. Our intervention is a product of a collaboration between a genetic physician (Friedman), a genetic counselor (Elliott), two sociologists (Hanemaayer and Christianson), and a team of medical illustrators (Hamann and Martineck). The authors collaborated to develop a series of cartoon vignettes aimed at building on the existing messaging in DECIDE by empowering people to think differently about their genetic risks and feelings of hope. This process was emergent, with Hanemaayer acting as the dialogical intermediary and organizer. Our analysis was done iteratively, and illustrations were designed and revised through regular conversation.

To identify the ways that biosociality could be emphasized, we applied concepts from sociology to deconstruct the DECIDE tool. Christianson and Hanemaayer analyzed DECIDE, drawing on the concepts of styles of thought, technologies of the self, and biosociality. This process involved ascertaining the ways in which the aid represented how an individual who is considering taking the test is enjoined to act (make a decision) under a given style of thought. Typically, a style of thought is derived from political economy and idealizes a person from a given collective who aims to secure their interests (Foucault 2000a; Paul Rabinow and Rose 2015). We applied style of thought by examining how risk is communicated in DECIDE. This concept illuminates the underlying assumptions about risk and how it should be calculated. Because it was developed, in part, to identify how risk is calculated as a technology of prudential individualism characteristic of advanced liberal societies, this concept was fit for purpose. It allowed the team to understand what kinds of calculations were implicitly expected of the user, and how users were idealized to manage those same risks (Garland 2003; Hunt 2003).

With respect to how we analyzed risk communication, we examined how potential outcomes were transformed into objective or subjective risks in DECIDE through words and images. The sociologists operationalized various forms of risk according to previous literature (i.e., Hunt 2003; Rose 1999). Objective risks were associated with the quantification of dangers, cultural anxieties, or an array of other potential hazards by an authority, ideally using established, rigorous, and scientific methods. These risks were contrasted with the subjective, personal, and often biased interpretations of dangers, cultural anxieties, and other potential hazards the individual perceives to be true (cf. Garland 2003). Contemporary medical decision-making often involves negotiations between the subjective interpretations of risk and the hazards interpreted by authorities. Personal interpretations of risk are often contrasted with scientific explanations for risk, and those can include moral, ethical, economic, and political problems relating to the health system or the state (Hunt 2003). We add a note here about our collaborative writing process. Questions about the political, ethical, and moral dimensions of science were a small place of disagreement among the team members. Where sociologists saw the infusion of values (e.g., morals) in scientific practices and explanations, this view was not fully shared by the clinicians. For example, science may operationalize political variables and study their impact on scientific research or even healthcare delivery, whereas sociologists viewed science as a social practice, which makes it intertwined with the social (i.e., moral, political, and ethical) dimensions of institutions.

The evidence-based medicine (EBM) decision-making paradigm conceptualizes risk calculus in two ways: a health decision needs to be correct under formalized assumptions (Djulbegovic 2021). Typically, this means a decision must be supported by the best available evidence such that rational persons would agree the decision is sound. Appraising the risk of an intervention based on this knowledge is called a "conclusion" and is often inferred from the results of systematic reviews on a given condition (Djulbegovic and Guyatt 2015; Sackett et al. 1996). These techniques of evidence synthesis rely on epidemiological reasoning and biostatistical methods. EBM privileges knowledge that comes from robust studies and evidence syntheses, as such methods are the most amenable to generating a consensus among rational actors and are, therefore, by their estimation, the closest approximation of truth possible (Djulbegovic and Guyatt 2015; Djulbegovic, Guyatt, and Ashcroft 2009).

Conclusions pertain to risk to the extent that they describe the objective dangers of undergoing a medical procedure. It is common to differentiate between actual risks and a patient's perceptions in discussions about risk (for challenges in doing so, see Djulbegovic 2021). When EBM defines objective risk, it refers to a rationalized program of action an individual is recommended to undertake that has been established scientifically using the best available data. These are differentiated from the risks a person perceives, which are plans of action considered expertly unverified, of personal importance, and often secondary to the objectively verifiable risks within the EBM paradigm (cf. Goldenberg 2006). The genetic counselor's role with respect to GWS is to discuss possible social and psychological implications of a genetic test, to explain clearly what the test can and cannot measure, and what this might mean for the patient and their family.

We approached DECIDE as a means of securing the health of individuals by encouraging them to make decisions that align their values with the appropriate conclusion. PDAS were developed within EBM to facilitate shared decision-making by helping patients think about the evidence of an intervention relative to their subjective values and preferences. In other words, we approach PDAS as a technology derived from EBM that attempts to encourage a way of acting and thinking that conforms with the principles of EBM. Indeed, the PDA joins other established technologies in EBM, such as clinical practice guidelines and evidence hierarchies.[5] Clinical practice guidelines and evidence hierarchies are both meant to assist clinical decision-making on the part of the physician, primarily. PDAS provide information to patients to help them with their decisions, and these materials are based on the best medical evidence.

In this respect, PDAS can be analyzed as a specific kind of "social technology." Foucault terms *technologies of the self* the technologies that "permit individuals to effect by their own means or with the help of others a certain number of operations on their own bodies and souls, thoughts, conduct, and way of being, so as to transform themselves in order to attain a certain state of happiness" (Foucault 2000b, 225). Technologies of the self, in our case, allow individuals to evaluate a potential intervention for themselves using the assumptions and ideas

5 Mykhalovskiy (2003) has described EBM as a "fundamentally text-mediated" approach to creating systemic and individual changes in medicine (see also Mykhalovskiy and Weir 2004).

through which the PDA is presented. In a sense, the knowledge from PDAs ideally provides the practical knowledge needed to make decisions that are in their best interest. As discussed above, the aim of PDAs is to engage in self-reflexive deliberation, which is consistent with what Hunt calls the ethical enterprise of the self in advanced liberal societies (2003, 172). Decision-making aids are not usually designed to compel people to make a particular decision but invite the user to imagine themselves relative to a predetermined set of values, personal preferences, and the current evidence—to encourage them to select the best decision *for themselves* (Bluhm 2009). The images were created in a way to enable the identification of the user with the "you" character in our comic. Our aid is meant to encourage people who decide to take the test to see themselves as connected to others; this is not to say that those who do not take the test are making the wrong decision, but rather that our comic is intended for that specific audience of test-takers.

The increasing reliance on PDAs in medical decision-making represents the changing landscape of EBM. Proponents increasingly recognize that evidence is necessary but insufficient on its own to make a good healthcare decision. More recently, proponents have differentiated between a conclusion and a decision. Decisions are context-dependent and made in consideration of the patient's values and preferences and include the consequences of specific actions in specific circumstances (Djulbegovic 2021; Djulbegovic and Guyatt 2015; Djulbegovic, Guyatt, and Ashcroft 2009). Objective evidence and subjective values and preferences are necessary to make an informed health decision, and aligning the patient's subjective perceptions with the objective risks is a challenge in healthcare decision-making. Unfortunately, the EBM paradigm has been routinely criticized for recalcitrance toward integrating subjective knowledge. Objective knowledge is privileged over context-specific knowledge (Greenhalgh 2012), and moral or values-based knowledge is often narrowly conceived as patient choices (Bluhm 2009). More recently,

Hanemaayer (2022) has addressed a challenge of integrating patient experience in the clinic, having identified the constraints imposed on decision-makers to follow guidelines based on objective evidence (see also Hanemaayer 2019), a process Christianson (2024) has applied to biomedically informed decision-making.

Decisions that rest on moral and subjective knowledge, which is particular to the patient, may trump action based on the best available evidence. EBM tends to objectify patient decisions by charting their decisions to systems in the brain. This is a major modification of the EBM paradigm that reflects the *molecularization* of medical decision-making. Since the mid-twentieth century, medicine has been influenced by two distinct ways of thinking about health. One style of thought is more closely associated with epidemiology, and the other is more closely associated with biomedicine. The molecularized style of thought associated with biomedicine allows scientists and patients alike to visualize health and illness at submicroscopic levels. The scope of the clinical gaze, or epidemiological style of thought, emerged in the nineteenth century, and, according to Rose (2007b), ends at the surfaces of organs and flows of blood, for example, within the body. This gaze informed clinical practice and was later amplified by epidemiology (and EBM), as it allowed physicians to differentially diagnose a disease based on inferences derived from knowledge of its distribution within a population.

In the case of patients and families who use DECIDE, what differentiates a diagnostic odyssey from traditional clinical diagnosis is the degree of specialized biomedical knowledge required. Biomedical knowledge offers new possibilities for perceiving the causes of disease as well as disease risk, and some scholars have raised worries about the direct mapping of the self to these processes. To paraphrase Rabinow (1996), genetics and molecular biology introduce a figure of the human who is predominantly constituted by their genetic code. Rose (2007a; 2007b) has argued that biomedicine introduces a new way of reasoning about the self and one's place in society.

Biomedicine enables the visualization of the processes that cause illnesses that are unobservable to the naked eye and that epidemiology can only approximate. The "deep spaces [of the mind and self have] begun to flatten out, to be displaced by a direct mapping of personhood, and its ills, upon the body or brain, which then becomes the principal target for ethical work" (Rose 2007b, 13). As Rose suggests, the supplantation of the clinical gaze with one derived from biomedicine has broader implications for the sociology of healthcare decision-making. Pykett and colleagues (2017) have discussed how the integration of biomedical knowledge into policy and practice privileges a new economic model of the individual. This individual is characterized by a game of split agencies: concurrently expected to act as the rational economic and prudential actor while simultaneously subject to the internal processes of their brain and body.

This novel economic model of the individual may reduce individual autonomy in two ways. Firstly, it draws on sociocultural understandings of the brain and genetic code as determinants of the self. Rabinow (1996) and Pykett et al. (2017) have discussed how their respective fields largely discredit the idea that individuals are reducible to their neurochemistry or genetic code. As we discuss below, the notion of a genetic code can have normalizing implications that inscribe a sense of fatalism. Our team sought to empower patients to feel confident and hopeful in their decision about whether or not to undergo GWS. It was important to emphasize how individuals are part of a complex system of relations in which their genes are only a small part.

Because of the centrality in which people place genes as a source of self-knowledge, patient decision-making aids do more than inform patients about a treatment. As Bombard et al. (2014) note, patients inscribe genetic testing with a "magic" founded on a belief that genetic testing has unique scientific power and, therefore, greater truth-value about themselves, and with greater emotional significance than other testing or information they receive. Likewise, in developing DECIDE, Birch et al. (2016) found that patients are motivated to undertake GWS because it offers them knowledge about their family and their child(ren). This finding is consistent with research about patients, who often feel that the results of genetic research are their personal information. Patients in these studies feel strongly about acquiring that information because that knowledge is constitutive of their identity (e.g., Bollinger et al. 2012; Tabor et al. 2012) and of their child's identity (Aldridge et al. 2021). How knowledge about one's genes is transmitted has deeper implications for one's sense of self than might be the case for other medical information.

Our approach to PDA development takes up the challenges expanded upon in this volume, in which we extend visualization beyond conventional understandings of what is seen to consider how people are invited to imagine and feel. Rose (1999) uses the term "techniques of visualization" to encompass the strategies people use to imagine themselves in relation to others and compel others to act in one way or another. Key to this is the importance of language as a tool to invite people to imagine themselves in and join alliances of rule (Rose, O'Malley, and Valverde 2006). In a related strain, Mel Chen (2012) has expanded on the ways language affects people through the way language and imagery invite people to feel—an affect—while also delimiting their ability to respond—an effect of language and visualizations.

Our intervention is informed by Chen's (2012) "biopolitics of animacy" and builds upon the work of Christianson (2024). Animacy is the quality of agency or liveliness accorded to an object in linguistics (Yamamoto 1999; Chen 2012). Chen illustrates how power can be exerted through micro-modifications in language and communication. Chen's contention is that the construction of livelihood carries affective potency that animates non-humans and de-animates people. Building on Butler's (2005) work on personal accounts of the self and feminist methods (cf. Doucet and Mauthner 2008), Christianson (2024) has argued for attention to pronoun use as an index of animacy. He has argued that how people are positioned in what Foucault (2012) calls "prescriptive texts" can inform an understanding of idealized power relations that individuals are called to inhabit. His method extends Doucet and Mauthner's (2008) process of subject tracing to consider the potency of the pronoun "you" over less potent pronouns like they/she/he and individualizing pronouns. Given that language and visualizations can influence the way a person can understand themselves and their choices, our team took care to center the patient as the most powerful agent in the GWS decision-making process, which is framed as a continuation of the diagnostic odyssey. The decision-maker is present in each panel, encouraging the reader to reflect on each stage of the process.

Another way that our team sought to empower patients was by thinking through the collectivizing effects of risk communication. We consider risk a technology linked to the ethical enterprise of the self, which is characteristic of an advanced liberal society. The notion of risk permits people to act as enterprising yet prudent individuals by providing them with the means to appraise their conduct reflexively relative to a consequence. To paraphrase Hunt (2003), the concept of risk capitalizes on the status of scientific authorities to transform subjective anxiety into real risk. This transformation empowers people to take action to improve themselves or manage that anxiety by providing a sense of direction grounded in an external authority while preserving their freedom to choose a life that suits them (see also Garland 2003). Without this objectification, Hunt (2003) argues, people are left with a lingering sense that something ought to be done without a definitive course of action.

Using these sociological concepts, we examined the strengths and weaknesses of DECIDE in encouraging people to think about themselves as molecular subjects. We aimed to empower the person deciding whether to undergo GWS to feel confident about its role in helping them understand themselves. We drew on Rose and Novas's (2005) contention that people who identify themselves predominantly in biological terms can make social change through their involvement in "biosocial" groups. Key to this process is the deployment of *hope* as a mode of collectivizing individuals in order to bring a shared biological future into being (Novas 2006, 291).

The aid was developed from the existing DECIDE tool and rewritten to visualize empowerment and biosociality, and to communicate subjective risks in this framework. Our aim was to assess and build on the current strengths of DECIDE by providing information that increases individual people's feelings of hope and control over their genetic health by considering the practical and moral knowledge (phronesis) DECIDE transmits. Phronesis, or practical knowledge, is a useful concept for understanding the "how of power" that links objective knowledge to the practice of using knowledge in context (Flyvbjerg 2001). Integrating phronesis into clinical decision-making supports the ideals of patient-centered medicine, which aims to integrate patient values and preferences into clinical decision-making. Building on Hunt's (2003) work on the practicality of risk, Hanemaayer (2022) has shown that the method of "sympathetic understanding" can provide an effective basis for physicians and patients to assess the meanings associated with complex clinical decisions. Our intervention was to integrate practical and effective knowledge into DECIDE's discussions of risk. We aimed to promote discussions of risk that capitalize on the unique capacities of genetic knowledge to encourage reflexivity and promote patient empowerment (through hope) and confidence (through biosociality).

Other pragmatic considerations were taken to ensure the accessibility and accuracy of the new aid. The text was verified for simple English accessibility using artificial intelligence (AI) to ensure it was easily readable by adults with at least a sixth-grade reading level. Each member developed and verified the text for accuracy of messaging. Hanemaayer then worked with Christianson, Hamann, and Martineck to ensure the images reflected the text, and then another round of member checking was performed with each member. The following discussion highlights the outcome of our analysis and the changes made by the team.

The Objective Benefits and Risks of GWS

When people discuss risk, it is common to distinguish between negatively coded "risks" (here, meaning hazards) and positively coded "benefits." Distinguishing between risks and benefits in this way is somewhat of a conflation of specific material outcomes, the valuation of those outcomes, and the objectification of those outcomes through probabilities and, as we discuss, other illustrations. We use "risk" to index the various ways these elements intersect in communication about benefits and risks. One of the strengths of DECIDE is that it accurately and accessibly communicates the epidemiological benefits and risks of undergoing GWS. DECIDE objectifies benefits and risks in two ways. First, it presents the reader with objective risks. For the purposes of this analysis, objective risk is defined as a measure of the likelihood, exposure, and magnitude of a danger established using rigorous, standardized scientific methods. This process of objectifying risk makes a danger appear "real" and is often used to enjoin people to act reflexively (Garland 2003; Hunt 2003).

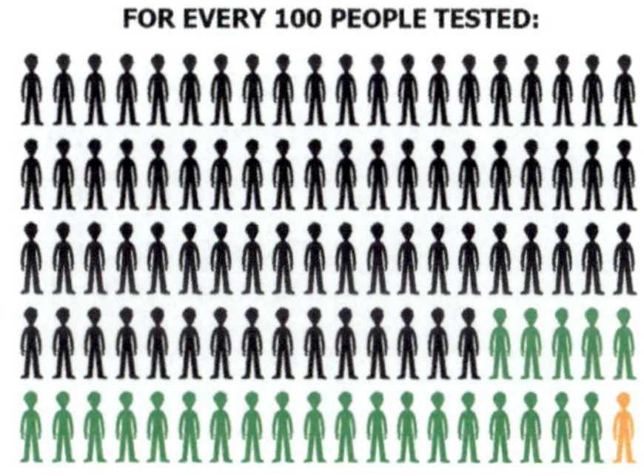

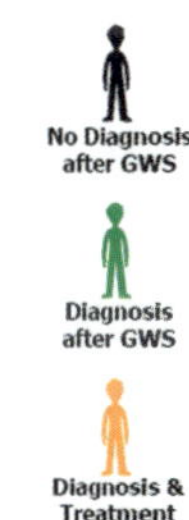

FIG. 1 Cates plot diagram representing the chance of a diagnosis and treatment from genome-wide sequencing. It's worth noting that without GWS, all other available testing is only likely to provide a diagnosis in no more than 20 percent of patients. GWS presents patients with a higher likelihood of diagnosis. GenCOUNSEL, DECIDE app. https://dcida2.cheos.ubc.ca/#/decision_aid/decide/intro?curr_intro_page_order=1 (Accessed: October 8, 2023) URL only accessible with permission. Reproduced with permission from GenCOUNSEL

FIG. 1

Building on EBM methodologies, DECIDE presents patients with the objective likelihood that a test will be informative. This benefit is presented numerically in DECIDE (GenCOUNSEL 2023): "Between 25 and 50 people will get a diagnosis for every 100 people who are tested. The exact numbers depend on the condition being tested. About 1 or 2 people in every 100 who get tested will get a treatment or change in management." The social scientists in our team interpreted this statement as potentially signaling to the patient the probability of obtaining the benefits of a precise diagnosis, which is consistent with an epidemiological style of thought. FIG. 1

In this example, the person using DECIDE is encouraged to reflect on the objective likelihood of getting a diagnosis after undertaking GWS. The patient is encouraged to expect the odds of receiving a diagnosis to be roughly less than half. DECIDE can be made more empowering by enhancing how risks and outcomes are communicated. Firstly, we might consider how the person using the aid is expected to visualize themselves when thinking about this image. The reader is encouraged to imagine themselves relative to an indeterminant mass of people. They may be the "one who may get treatment" (GenCOUNSEL 2023), but this is not clear. They might also be among those "who will get a diagnosis." While this is a valuable way of communicating risks, it is de-animating. Yamamoto (1999) notes that locating a person as an indistinguishable part of a group reduces individuation, which reduces a person's ability to see and understand themselves as having agency. It also depersonalizes the reader's relationship to this group, who are patients like them.

To enhance patient empowerment, we aimed to help the person using the aid to imagine themselves in a community fostered by the journey regardless of the diagnosis. Our team aimed to communicate biosociality by encouraging the reader to see themselves as immersed in webs of relationships arising from their diagnostic journey. We wanted to convey how one's search for a possible genetic explanation will bring them into contact with experts and others like them all around the world who can help them understand themselves and bring meaning to their condition. We illustrated how genetic testing could create supportive communities, often internationally, through networks fostered by teams of genetic specialists. FIG. 8 In panel 5, the reader is encouraged to visualize themselves as part of a community rather than an abstract population. This community is then reintroduced in panels 9 and 10 to demonstrate how these groups can empower the reader, even if the test is unproductive. Panel 10 also encourages the reader to think about the link between their genetic information and future scientific discoveries, a known motivator for many people undertaking GWS (Birch et al. 2016).

The second way we aim to change how benefits and risks are communicated is by highlighting the implications of different outcomes apart from diagnosis. The kinds of diagnoses patients might receive vary, and as the text in the decision aid explains, results from genome-wide sequencing are not always straightforward. We all have lots of different DNA variants, and we are still learning how to completely understand them. You might get three main types of results. First, we might find a genetic change or DNA variant, which can cause medical concerns. Second, we might not find any DNA variants that seem to be causing the problems. The third possibility is that we find something that looks unusual, but we don't know what it means. We call this a variant of uncertain significance, or VUS. Sometimes, we can do more tests to try to figure out what a VUS means, but other times, we just don't know. As we get more information in the future, we may be able to clarify the meaning (GenCOUNSEL 2023).

Benefits and risks are considered objective when the conventions of counting and categorizing them are sufficiently well-established, widespread, and uncontested (Garland 2003, 56). However, the system of counting and categorizing variants of concern is none of these. GWS often involves identifying one or two pathogenic variants from a larger group of usually benign or unrelated variants. The interpretation of these variants often pushes analysts to the limit of current knowledge (Elliott and Friedman 2018). From the patient's and their family's perspective, the risk of undertaking GWS is challenging to understand because analysts may be unsure about what they find.

To inform patients of these known unknowns, DECIDE presents a series of uncertainties associated with undergoing GWS. FIG. 2 In this instance, the reader is confronted with three possibilities, two of which do not result in knowing if there is a genetic cause for the condition, either because there is no known variant present in the genomes tested or because the variant identified is not associated with any known illness that would allow the geneticist to conclude that there is a genetic cause.

In contrast to the likelihood of getting a diagnosis, no statistical likelihoods are presented for the risk of getting an incidental finding or VUS, which is due to the variation of tests, labs, methods of analysis, disease, and other factors. Thus, from the perspective of the person using the tool, it could be unclear what kinds of results they expect and what those results may mean to them in relation to their diagnostic odyssey.

As it pertains to risk, epidemiology relies on conventions of counting individuals and determining the incidence of a given pathology across a population. However, GWS is preoccupied with, to paraphrase Rose (2007b), the deep interiors of the individual to the extent that it maps the specific genome of the complex, dynamic, and heterogeneous biological elements that make up an individual.[6] As we will discuss further below, this highly personalized biomedical way of thinking about risk diverges from EBM's tendency to abstract to the population.

Our team worked to communicate risks by focusing on how people might react to learning about a VUS or incidental finding. Care was taken to center the individual and highlight what they might see and feel when they are thinking about their risk. As an intended complement to existing educational materials, our comic aims to amplify the subjective experiences associated with the risks and benefits already communicated effectively in DECIDE. When read alongside the Cates plot developed for DECIDE, panel 6 encourages the person using DECIDE to visualize themselves receiving the results and what this could mean to them. The images include the possibility of treatment and the sense of confusion and concern that might accompany the results. The DECIDE user is reminded throughout that any concerns they might have should be discussed with their genetic counselor to encourage connection with a health team.

6 How variants are recognized also involves biostatistical methods and an epidemiological style of thought, which is one of the ways these two styles of thought overlap. While we do not address this in this chapter, it is significant to note that the dominant style of thought, the epidemiological one (which underpins EBM), is informing the molecular gaze. The clinical aspects of diagnosis remain epidemiological. The molecular aspects tend to remain in the biomedical, although the two are related in thought as well as institutional spaces.

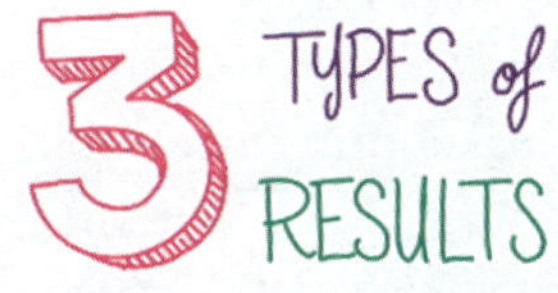

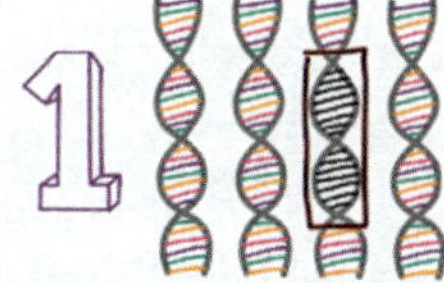

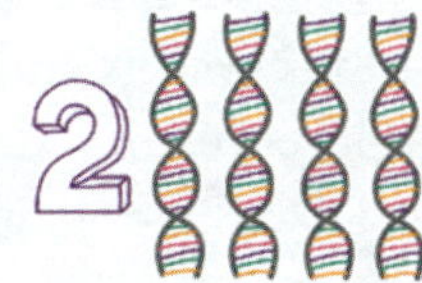

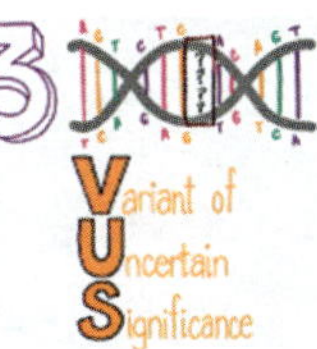

FIG. 2

Issues you considered in your decision about GWS

	Reasons for GWS	Reasons against GWS
Most important issues to you	• **Knowledge / explanation** • **Treatment / management** • **Feeling in control / acceptance**	• **Labelling and judging** • **Result regret**
Less important issues to you	N/A	• Incidental Findings (IF) worry
Unsure	• Family planning • Helping others / science	N/A

FIG. 3

FIG. 2 Types of results a person might get from GWS. GenCOUNSEL, DECIDE app. https://dcida2.cheos.ubc.ca/#/decision_aid/decide/intro?curr_intro_page_order=1 (Accessed: October 8, 2023). URL only accessible with permission. Reproduced with permission from GenCOUNSEL

FIG. 3 Representation of issues, values, and preferences. Reproduced from DECIDE. Types of results a person might get from GWS. GenCOUNSEL, DECIDE app. https://dcida2.cheos.ubc.ca/#/decision_aid/decide/intro?curr_intro_page_order=1 (Accessed: October 8, 2023). URL only accessible with permission. Reproduced with permission from GenCOUNSEL

The Subjective Benefits and Risks of GWS

Some benefits and risks are less clearly visualized in DECIDE. A perennial issue in evidence-based medical communication is a limited understanding of what is commonly called "patient values and preferences." An index of all non-clinically relevant components of a medical decision, including patient values and preferences, has been framed as an important but tertiary component of medical decision-making (cf. Djulbegovic and Guyatt 2017). The subjugation of patient values and preferences is reflected in the tendency of an individual's mode of valuing risk to be framed as a *perception* of risk, distinct and secondary to the scientifically established objective risks. While EBM increasingly acknowledges the importance of personal, contextual, and values-based decision-making, the full integration of this perspective remains elusive.

PDAS reflect a recent attempt in EBM to balance subjective and objective considerations when making a personal medical decision. Like most PDAS, DECIDE encourages patients to reflect on an array of personal "issues" that might arise from GWS. These include psychosocial factors, such as the feelings of control, worry, or regret patients might feel when receiving a test result; contextual issues pertaining to the healthcare system, particularly insurability; and cultural and personal issues, such as reproductive planning and reducing feelings of blame. The user is then asked to rate the importance of such issues using a Likert scale. The outcome of this activity is then presented to the user as a two-by-two table, such as, FIG. 3 in which the pros and cons are automatically sorted according to the relative importance of each issue, as ranked by the user.

Subjective benefits and risks, while presented as "issues" and represented in a narrative format using quotes from families who have undergone the test, are nonetheless benefits or risks associated with undergoing GWS. The user of the aid is invited to objectify these risks so that they can visualize *their* values and preferences alongside the scientifically established risks mentioned. Hence, DECIDE also objectifies subjective risks, albeit without explicit pictographic

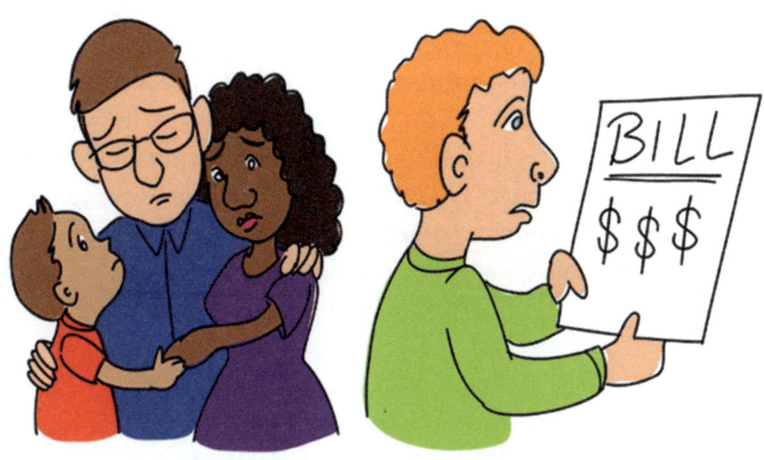

FIG. 4

FIG. 4 Visualization of the risks of incidental findings in DECIDE. GenCOUNSEL, DECIDE app. https://dcida2.cheos.ubc.ca/#/decision_aid/decide/intro?curr_intro_page_order=1 (Accessed: October 8, 2023). URL only accessible with permission. Reproduced with permission from GenCOUNSEL

representations of how the user might feel. Again, they are encouraged to reflect on people *like them* but not necessarily to envision themselves.

While users are encouraged to reflect on their values and preferences, the affective dimension of decision-making is not explicitly visualized in DECIDE. A notable inversion of the risks presented above, the only instance where risks pertaining to patient values and preferences are explicitly visualized pictographically is when discussing incidental findings. FIG. 4

In this instance, the user of the aid is advised that incidental findings might affect an entire family and weigh on the minds of loved ones. Worries about the difficulty of obtaining extended health or life insurance in the future is visualized alongside this information about how the user may be negatively affected.

To help people see the meaningful implications of different outcomes, we aimed to illustrate how the decision-maker might feel relative to different outcomes of GWS. Panels 7–10 illustrate the contextual and value-based costs and benefits a patient may consider. We focused on the benefits of *getting* a diagnosis in panels 7 and 8 and the risks of receiving a VUS in panels 9 and 10. Building on Rose and Novas's (2005) work on hope, we gesture to a more hopeful future in which genetic knowledge is linked to resources and community rather than the burden of added costs and stigma that may come with a diagnosis. Importantly, to underscore patient autonomy, each panel stresses that these hopes and anxieties should be discussed thoroughly with the genetic counselor.

From Moralization to a Moral Economy of Hope

Finally, we analyzed the normative information transmitted alongside knowledge about genetics. DECIDE transmits information about genetic variations in an accessible format to improve health literacy about GWS, consistent with the principles of PDA design (Charles et al. 2005; Peters et al. 2007). The tool provides an accessible way of understanding genetic variation and expression by way of a musical metaphor, which is animated alongside the following explanation:

> Think of the human body as a piece of music. Music is made up of notes that tell people how to play the song. . . . In music, the order of notes needs to be correct to play the song, and in our bodies the order of DNA needs to be correct for development, function, and growth to happen the way it is supposed to. Sometimes, when we play music, certain notes are missed or played at the wrong time. Sometimes, this sounds like a mistake; other times, it just sounds a little different. Likewise, with DNA, parts can be lost or changed—something we call a "variant." (GenCOUNSEL 2023)

Having a metaphor for genetic variation (a book, a blanket, music) has been shown in several studies to help people understand genetic variation in a way that is not pejorative (e.g., Sexton

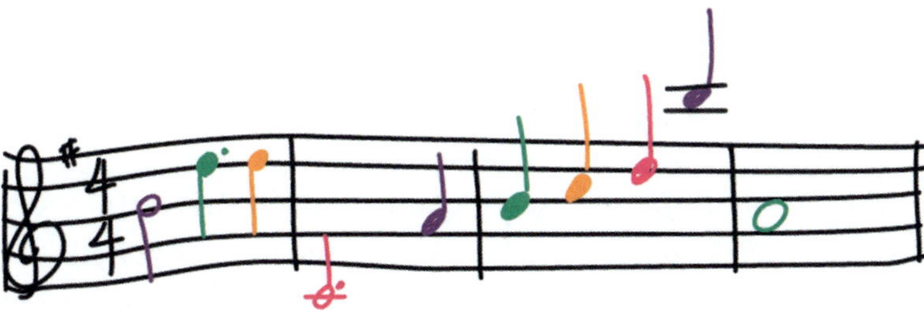

FIG. 5

FIG. 5 Genetic variation as misplayed notes. GenCOUNSEL, DECIDE app. https://dcida2.cheos.ubc.ca/#/decision_aid/decide/intro?curr_intro_page_order=1 (Accessed: October 8, 2023). URL only accessible with permission. Reproduced with permission from GenCOUNSEL

and James 2022; Pinheiro et al. 2017). However, using metaphors also risks conveying cultural connotations that undermine the explanation. Implicit in this text and accompanying images is an understanding of the self and the kinds of ethical work the text encourages. The self is an expression of one's genetic code, represented as a piece of music. FIG. 5 Correct biological function is an expression of this code or the reading of that code. Deciding to undertake GWS can provide information about those variants or "errors" in the code, which can help people understand their condition and, ultimately, themselves.

While knowledge about one's genetic code may offer information about oneself, the patient and family could be ambivalent about the kinds of ethical work they ought to undertake based on this knowledge, even within the tool. The literature identifies risks and benefits, including notions like regret and self-blame (Birch et al. 2016; Adam et al. 2019), which are also reflected in the narratives patients are encouraged to reflect on:

> Until I got a diagnosis for her, I always had in the back of my mind that something I did in pregnancy caused the problem. (GenCOUNSEL 2023)

> I don't know if I could handle it if it turned out she got this from my genes. (GenCOUNSEL 2023)

In these quotations, we can see the subjective benefits and risks of knowing one's genetic self. While on the one hand, learning that an illness has a genetic etiology might absolve one of the guilt that the illness was caused by a parent's behavior (e.g., during pregnancy), another quote illustrates the risk of knowing that the illness was hereditary, reflecting a genetic error passed down by one or both parent(s). In this respect, the values of the people determining whether to get GWS are pitted against their preferences. This PDA provides the parent with conflicting, albeit necessary, information. While a parent's goal may be to end their child's diagnostic odyssey, ideally leading to treatment, this may raise questions about an uncertain future and the ability to manage the child's condition.

The musical metaphor may play a role in these notions of self-blame and regret. It could evoke deterministic images of gene transmission and expression, as it visualizes symptoms as an expression of errors. While the accompanying text notes

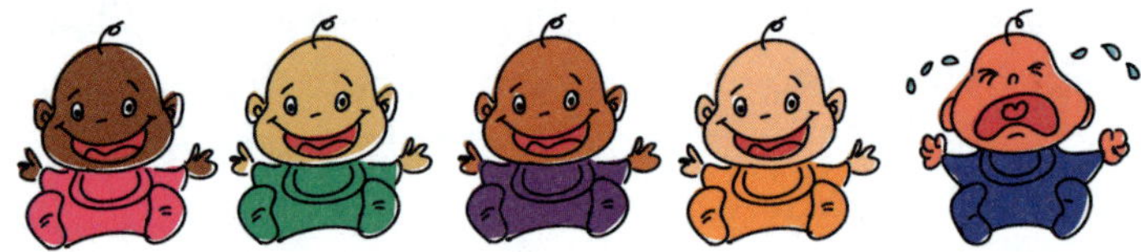

FIG. 6

FIG. 6 Genetic variations make babies cry. GenCOUNSEL, DECIDE app. https://dcida2.cheos.ubc.ca/#/decision_aid/decide/intro?curr_intro_page_order=1 (Accessed: October 8, 2023). URL only accessible with permission. Reproduced with permission from GenCOUNSEL

that genetic variation can be heard as errors or just a "little different," only the errors are visualized. FIG. 5 This is compounded when a gene variant is equated with a baby crying. FIG. 6 While this is an inaccurate representation of the science of genetics, which is far more nuanced and complex, it resonates with cultural understandings of heredity. The risk of regret and self-blame is related to uncertainty about the parent's genes or behaviors. These narratives raised concerns about the cause of the patient's disease or disability, which could be, in this case, made more dire by the molecular style of thinking that underpins this metaphor.

We propose alternative visualizations by working with causal language to provide an explanation that ends the diagnostic odyssey and avoids the risk that those who underwent GWS might feel regret or self-blame. Building on the work of Rose (2007a), Rose and Novas (2005), and Rabinow (1996), the new images highlight the artifice of genetic medicine. Rabinow (1996) was among the first to acknowledge that the subject position developed in biomedicine disentangles biology from notions of fate.[7] The fact that people make decisions about how to act on their bodies based on genetic knowledge means, contrary to the often ethological proposition that underlies genetic knowledge, that people can actively enact changes on themselves based on genetic knowledge through deliberate acts of choice. As Bombard et al. illustrate, genetic knowledge was a deciding factor in a patient's decision to undergo chemotherapy, though the results often offered no objective "clear course of action ... patients generally interpreted the results to mean whatever they wanted them to mean, aligning them with their pre-existing treatment preferences" (2014, e208). While this is framed as a limitation, we can capitalize on this knowledge to encourage patient empowerment. Building on the work of Rose (2007a) and Rose and Novas (2005), we expand on the interpretive flexibility of genetic risk to highlight how the indeterminacy of genetic knowledge is no longer limited to a clean binary between normality and pathology but one in which biology is untethered from destiny and in which there is a multiplicity of ways of choosing how to be human from a range of possible futures (Rose 2007b, 40; see also Clarke and Wallgren-Pettersson 2019).[8]

We aimed to increase patient empowerment by encouraging the reader to adopt an active position in which they viewed themselves as occupying a dynamic role in a complex system of relations in which their genes are only a small part. The explanation of genetic variation was minimized so that the users of the aid could focus on themselves and the process. Panels 1–4 of figure 8 retool the story of genetic variation and genetic testing to foreground the process without a metaphor.

7 We direct the reader to Borck and Meunier's chapter on interceptive biomedicine in this volume, "Imaginary Imaging."

8 Genetics has also been working to decouple from essentialist understandings. This has happened through genomic education (Duncan et al. 2024), new textbooks for medical education (Donovan et al. 2024), and classroom approaches (Donovan et al. 2024).

The team initially experimented with other metaphors before deciding against using them at all. Building on Rose (1999), we determined that because metaphors act as imperfect translators, they often rely on conventional understandings that cause certain failures in translation. Christianson (2024) has illustrated how these failures in translation can foster unexpected ambivalences, which lead to patients dropping out of care. Our approach acknowledges that patients are increasingly health-literate, especially in conditions that affect them. Panels **1–4** present essential information about genetics and contextualize that information with the emotion or affective state of an imagined patient undergoing the process. The intent here is to center the decision-maker, often a parent of a child with a medically unexplained condition, undergoing the genetic testing part of their diagnostic odyssey.

Discussion and Conclusion

Our aim is for the reader to visualize themselves as an empowered individual who is more than their genes, with dynamic relations and concerns, and who is a potential member of a biosocial community. This comic situates the decider in a complex process that extends well beyond GWS, preparing them to expect to play multiple roles. It highlights how they might feel at key moments in the process and encourages them to reflect on their concerns and to ask for more information. It casts the relationships between patients and specialists as non-hierarchical, in which genetic specialists form a team with the patient and their family. As a complement to the DECIDE tool, this cartoon may well help patients to feel hope in the face of genetic insecurities, but this hypothesis is yet untested.

This chapter presented an analysis of a current tool, an application of sociological concepts of risk, styles of thought, animacy, and biosociality to inform the illustration of a comic that could be integrated into the current PDA. At present, the images of graphic medicine symbolize proof that collaborations between the social sciences, biomedicine, science communication, and graphic medicine are valuable and can inform alternative ways of conceiving risk. However, our team has yet to test this concept in practice, and we hope to obtain funding to do so with our clinician collaborators in the future. For example, one of our major revisions to DECIDE has been to drop the musical metaphor for an accessible and literal depiction of the testing process. This change was made on theoretical grounds and will need to be tested for efficacy in transmitting the concept alongside DECIDE or as a stand-alone informatic. We have attempted to foster a moral economy of hope by reframing information already transmitted in an existing decision-making aid. We intend to empower patients to feel more confident in making complex health decisions, using concepts in the sociology of anxiety and risk (Hunt 2003). Whether these images do improve the users' affective experiences around decision-making in a way that makes them feel connected to a biosocial community requires further investigation. The comic will also require further group testing with patient groups, patient activists, and patients to ensure it resonates with their values and preferences.

This tool was developed for parents as the most likely decision-makers for a child with a suspected genetic disease as part of a more comprehensive decision-making process. While this was our focus, the effects of genetic testing extend well beyond the individual. Future research could consider dedicated tools for children and family members and may also consider the ethics of informed consent for health decisions that extend beyond the patient. It is not our intention, however, to suggest that these tools would substitute for the human relationships of the clinic. Aids are meant to complement clinical practice but not replace it. Genetic counseling is a significant part of the communication and decision-making process and the biosocial relationships facilitated by genomic medicine.

Specific to the artistic collaboration process, one constraint was translating social and scientific principles into images. One of the most challenging aspects of the translation process involved styling the subject. Our attempt to encourage personal self-reflection came across two roadblocks. First, we found it an ongoing challenge to differentiate the patient and the persons impacted by the decision from the individual making the decision. While, commonly, patients make their own decisions and accept the personal risks of undergoing treatment, genetic testing is often done on and for others, such as on a child with neurodevelopmental or physical disabilities. The subject of this intervention was shifting and multiple, reflecting a more interconnected and relational subject than the medium seemed to permit.

One limitation that warrants further research is the tension between personalization and representation. Our initial attempts at representing the subjects in the aids without cues to gender or race resulted, in retrospect, perhaps obviously, in an alien appearance. FIG. 7 These undermined the affective dimension we wanted to foster. But communicating these aspects inevitably drew on hegemonic representations of race, gender, and sexuality, which may also, inevitably, alienate some people. Similar tensions in representation have been cited in discussions of sexual orientation, e.g., with regard to gingerbread persons (Jourian 2015). The problem of urging people to see themselves will become stronger as the personalization of medicine homes further in on narrower risk groups and conditions. Striking a balance between humanization and biased representations may be a future challenge for personalized medicine.[9] Our comic extends Epstein's (2008) critique of diversification or balkanization of healthcare research to patient outreach and education materials. As treatments become specialized for a specific community, group, or indeed the individual, educational materials may encounter challenges around how the "you" that a tool addresses can be represented.
We might reflect on whether it is possible or desirable to illustrate a person's independence from the webs of interconnection in which they are constituted.Our sociological analysis has approached the tool as a product of medical knowledge that aims to assist in decision-making, which could impact a family's life. Given our theoretical commitments, PDAs themselves have been thought to inscribe power into the capacity of individuals

9 With improvements in technology, graphic medicine may be further personalized, such as designing one's avatar prior to reading the comic. Artificial intelligence can render new forms of art quickly, and this may be a further limitation to the comic form in future.

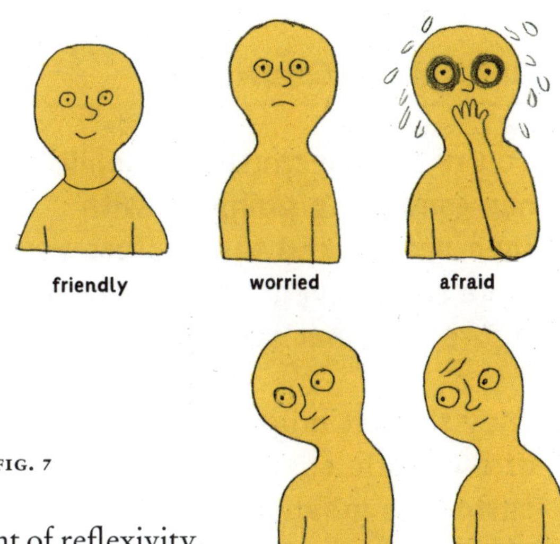

FIG. 7

to choose to accept risks. From the standpoint of reflexivity, future research could assess our assumptions and their integration into the tool. Questions could be raised about how power is inscribed through our illustrations. Moreover, one might question whether the reinscription of power reflective of shared decision-making is possible or desirable. While the authors have written elsewhere (Hanemaayer 2019; 2022; Christianson 2024) that decision-making guidelines and aids can have antithetical effects and consequences that affect their intended aims, our collaboration raises questions about the individualizing nature of clinical decisions. A transdisciplinary collaboration has illuminated the various objectives of the team: the clinicians have aimed to improve their ability to provide patients with the information and treatment they need to live their lives, the illustrators have aimed to communicate complex ideas in accessible and fruitful ways, and sociologists have concerned themselves with the implicit assumptions within the decision aids. Our collaborations have had their odysseys, which have raised further questions about the circumstances within which families need to make such decisions, how the arts can be impactful and empower patients through representations of connectedness and hopeful affect, and how clinical knowledge can be used to amplify the biosociality of the human condition.

GENOME SEQUENCING

You're here because your child has something going on with their health, and the doctors you have seen haven't been able to figure out what's wrong.

They think it might be because of a genetic change. This cartoon is meant to teach you about something called genome sequencing. It's a way to look at all the information in your genes to learn about your health.

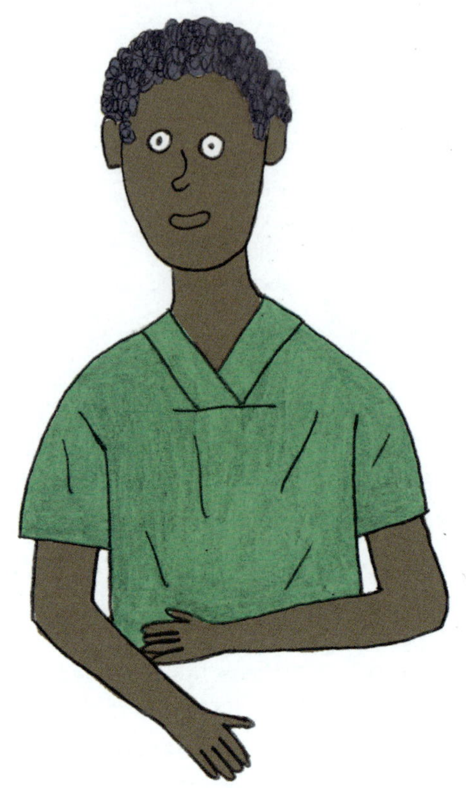

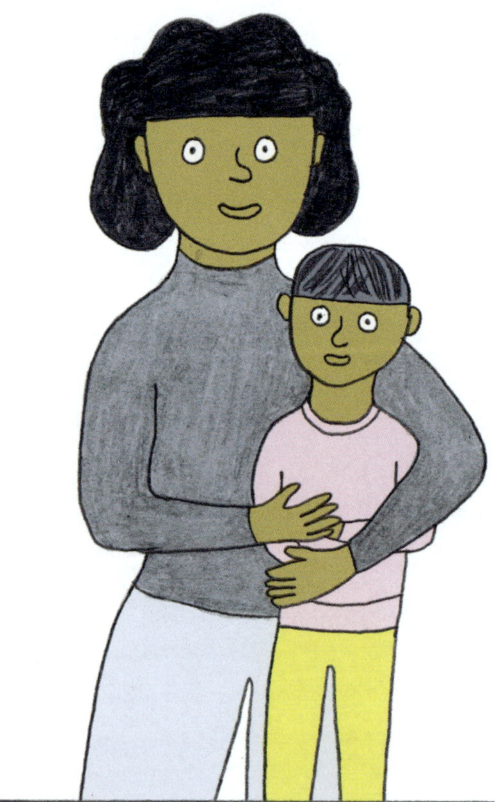

Before you talk with a genetic counsellor, this cartoon can help you understand more about genome-wide sequencing. That way, when you meet with your counsellor, you'll be ready to talk about whether it's a good choice for you.

Together, we can discuss more about what genome sequencing means for your child and your family's health, your values and personal preferences.

1

FIG. 8, PANELS 1–10

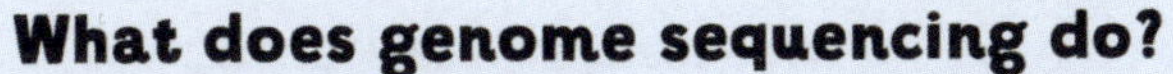

What does genome sequencing do?

DNA is made out of a combination of four molecules called **A, C, G** and **T**.

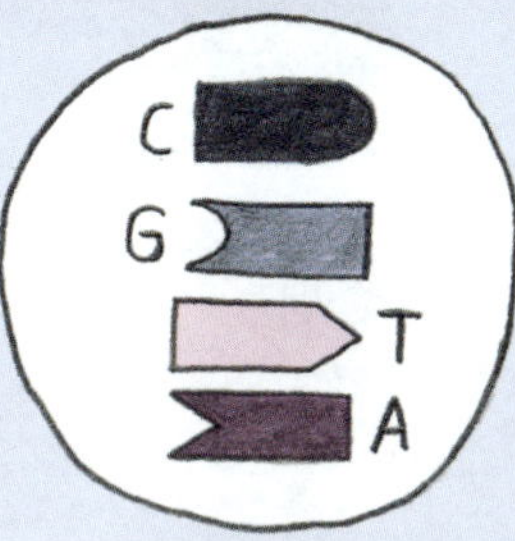

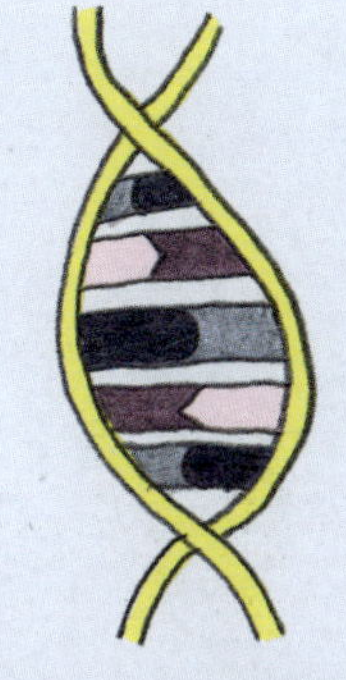

gene sequence

The whole set of **DNA** in our body is called the **genome**.

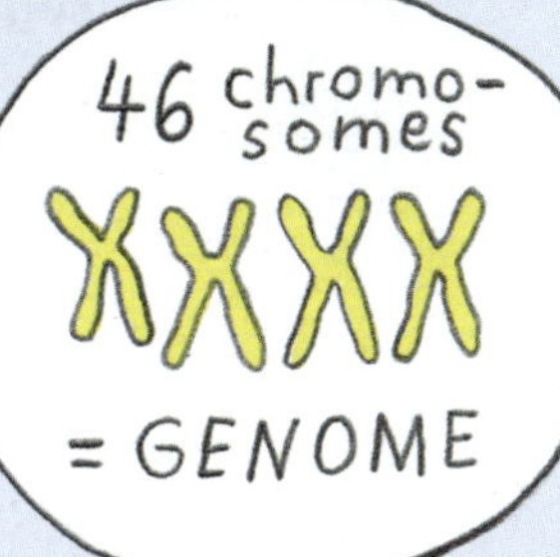

Each of us has a very personal set of genes that makes us a unique person.

Each of our **46 chromosomes** is made up of one very long DNA molecule.

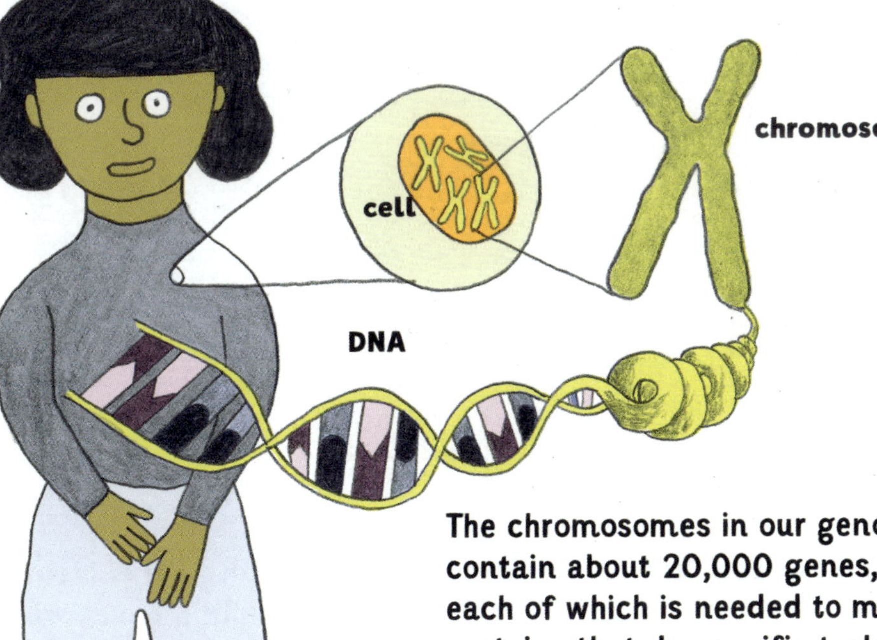

The chromosomes in our genome contain about 20,000 genes, each of which is needed to make proteins that do specific tasks in our bodies.

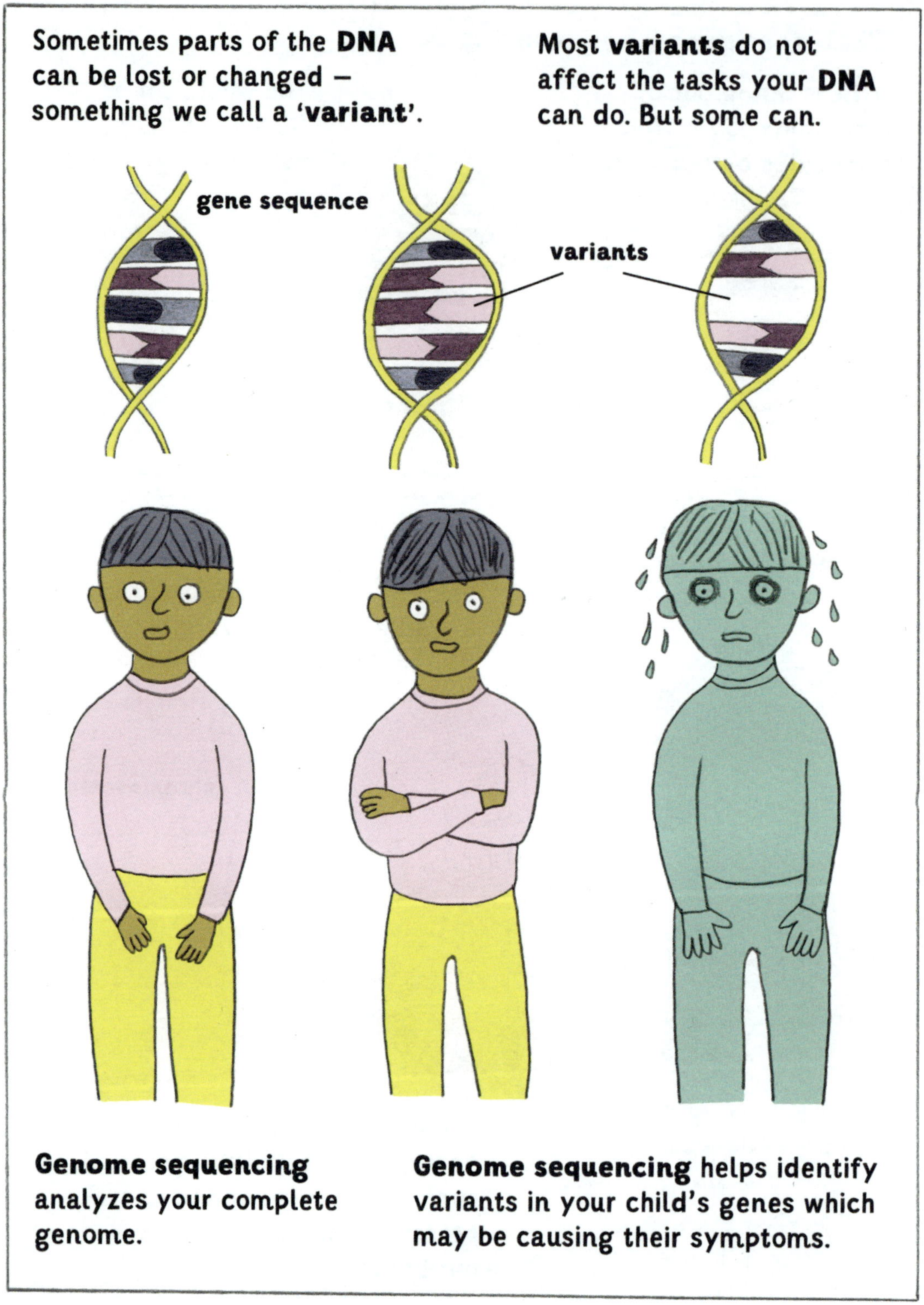

Sometimes parts of the **DNA** can be lost or changed – something we call a '**variant**'.

Most **variants** do not affect the tasks your **DNA** can do. But some can.

gene sequence

variants

Genome sequencing analyzes your complete genome.

Genome sequencing helps identify variants in your child's genes which may be causing their symptoms.

3

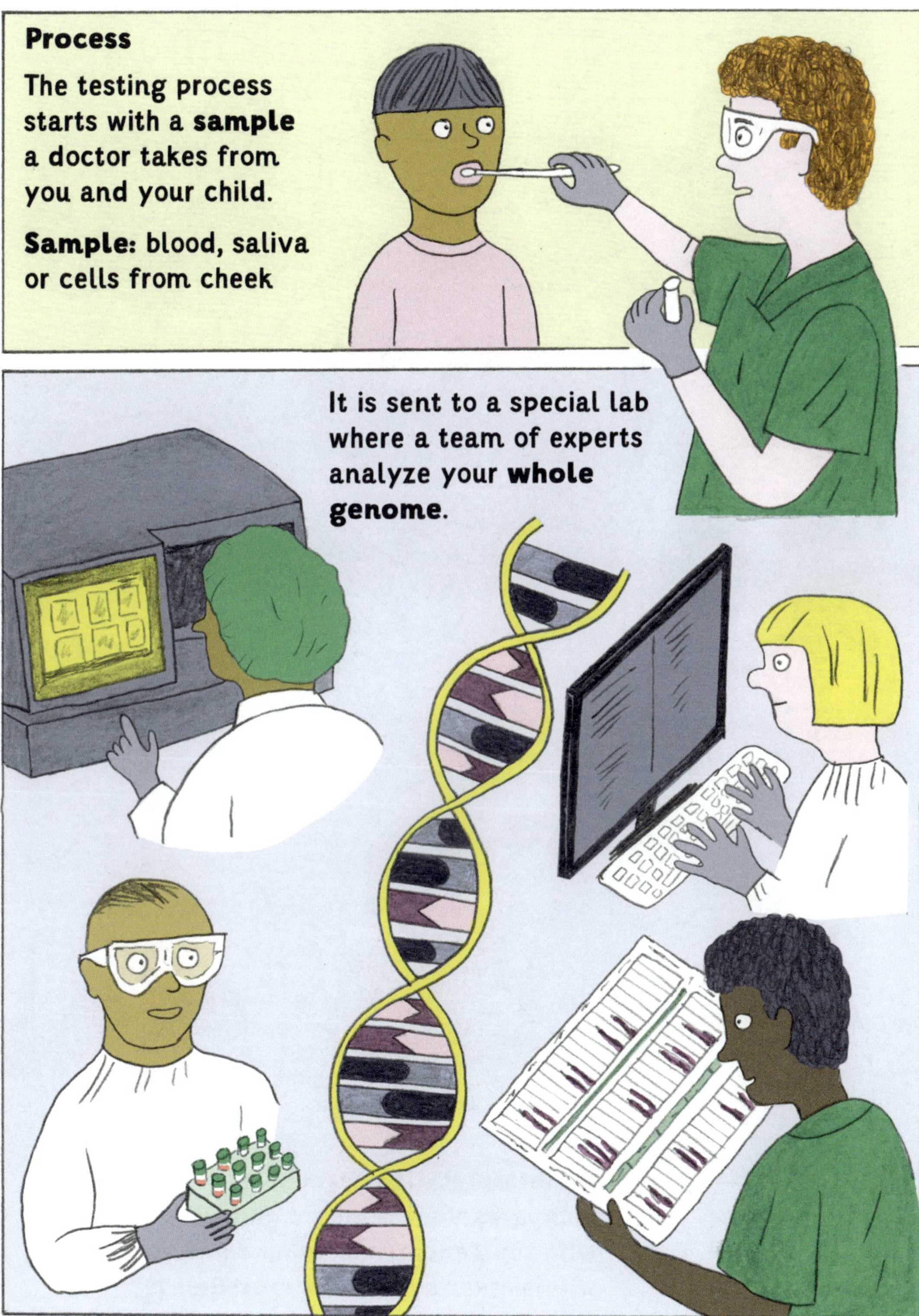
Process
The testing process starts with a **sample** a doctor takes from you and your child.
Sample: blood, saliva or cells from cheek
It is sent to a special lab where a team of experts analyze your **whole genome**.

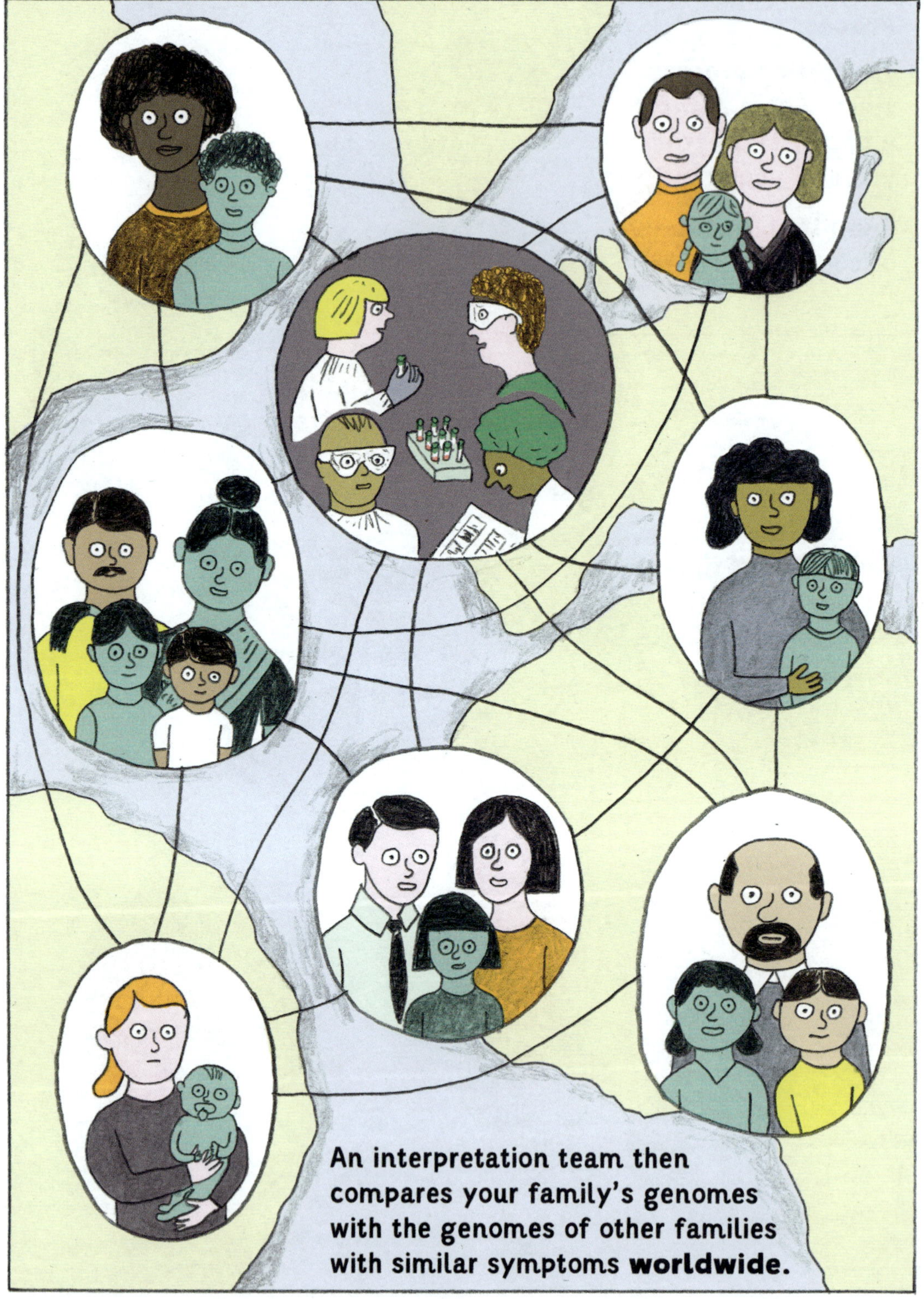
An interpretation team then compares your family's genomes with the genomes of other families with similar symptoms **worldwide**.
5

Results
There are different types of results:
1) You might get a diagnosis, which means that a genetic variant explains why your child is sick.
Only 35–50 out of 100 people who take the test get a diagnosis.
The result sometimes helps to improve your child's treatment.

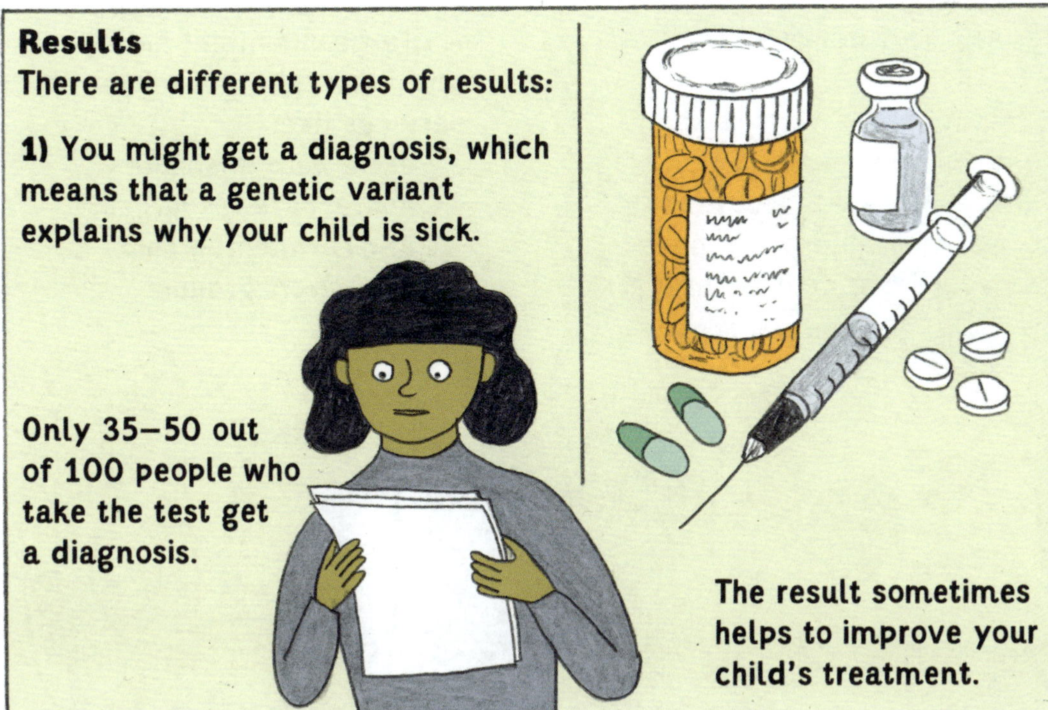

2) The interpretation team might find a variant of uncertain significance.

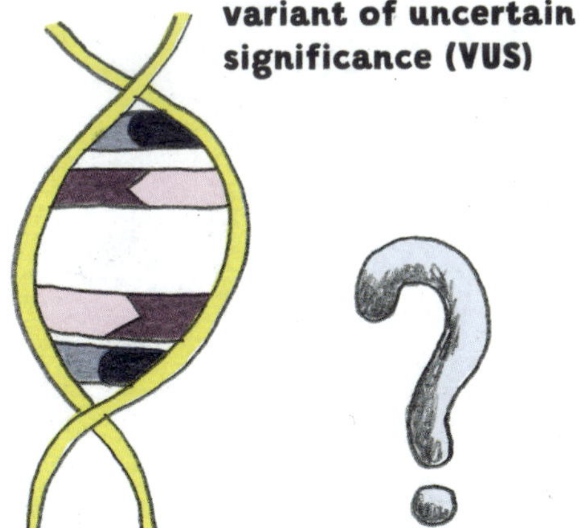

A VUS does not mean there is no genetic cause, and it doesn't mean there is one. They just don't know.

3) The interpretation team might also find variants responsible for health conditions unrelated to the reason you took the test.

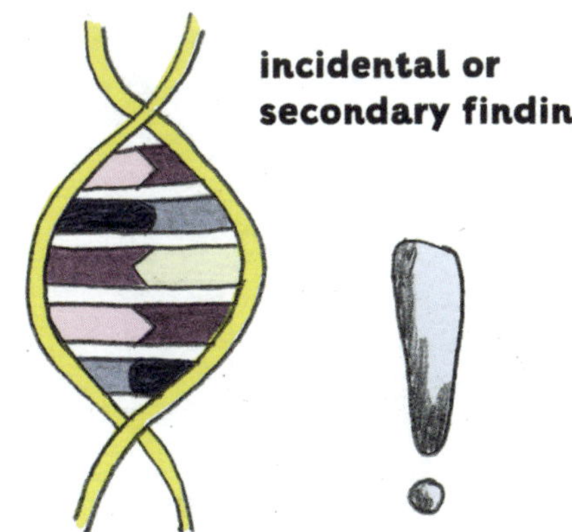

These findings tell you about other conditions you or your family might have in the future.

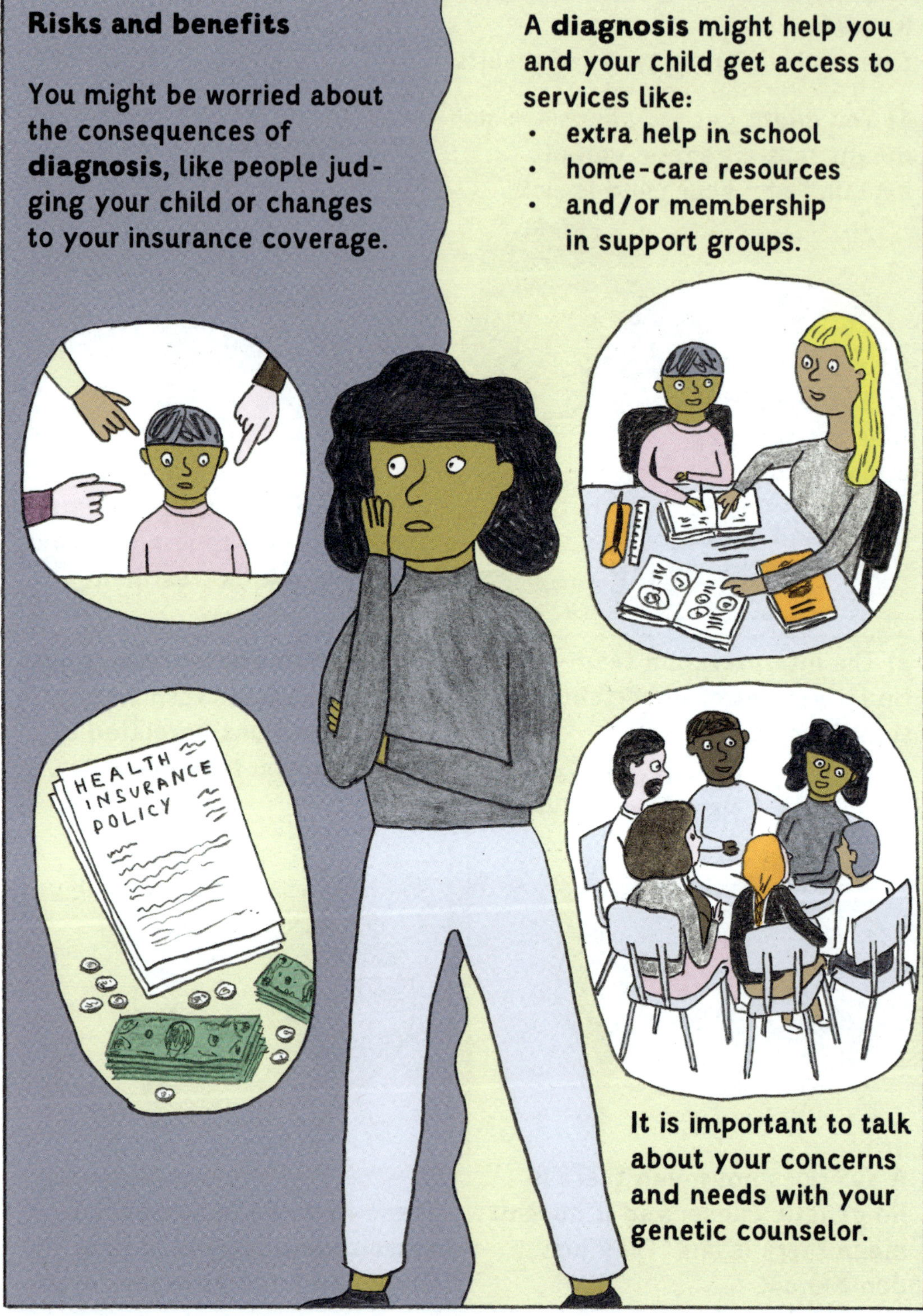
Risks and benefits
You might be worried about the consequences of diagnosis, like people judging your child or changes to your insurance coverage.
A diagnosis might help you and your child get access to services like:
• extra help in school
• home-care resources
• and/or membership in support groups.
HEALTH INSURANCE POLICY
It is important to talk about your concerns and needs with your genetic counselor.
7

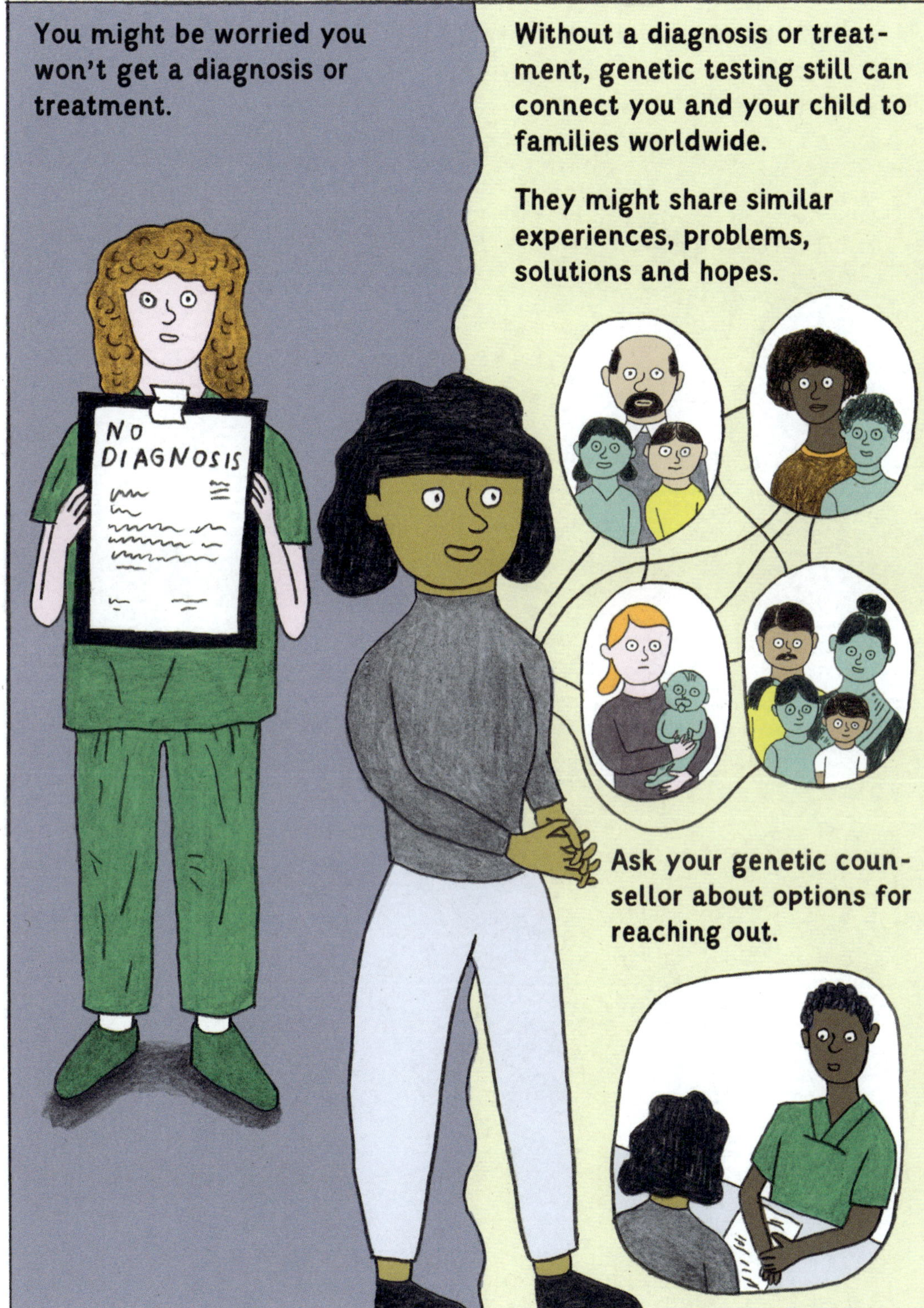
You might be worried you won't get a diagnosis or treatment.
NO DIAGNOSIS
Without a diagnosis or treatment, genetic testing still can connect you and your child to families worldwide.
They might share similar experiences, problems, solutions and hopes.
Ask your genetic counsellor about options for reaching out.

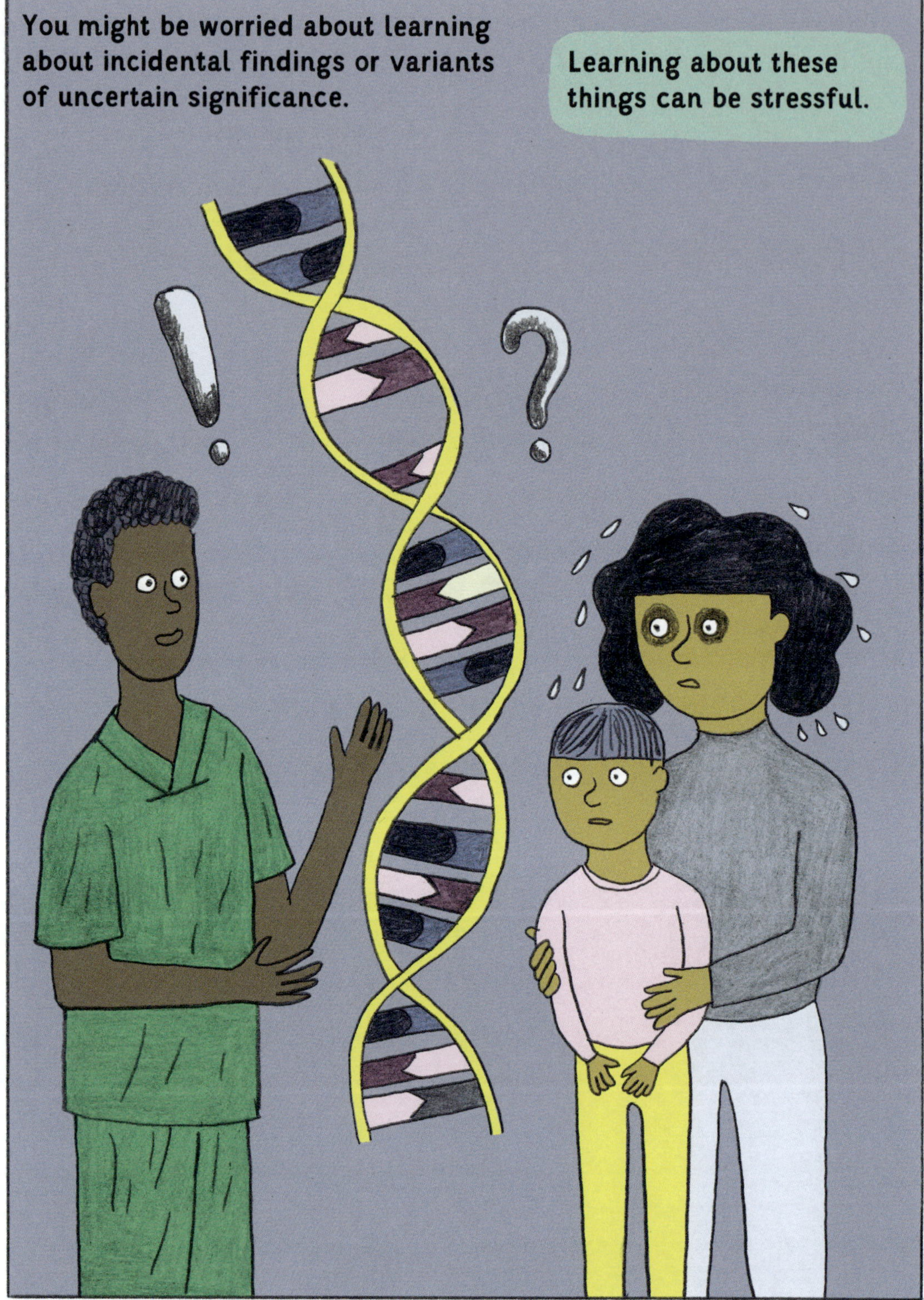
You might be worried about learning about incidental findings or variants of uncertain significance.
Learning about these things can be stressful.
9

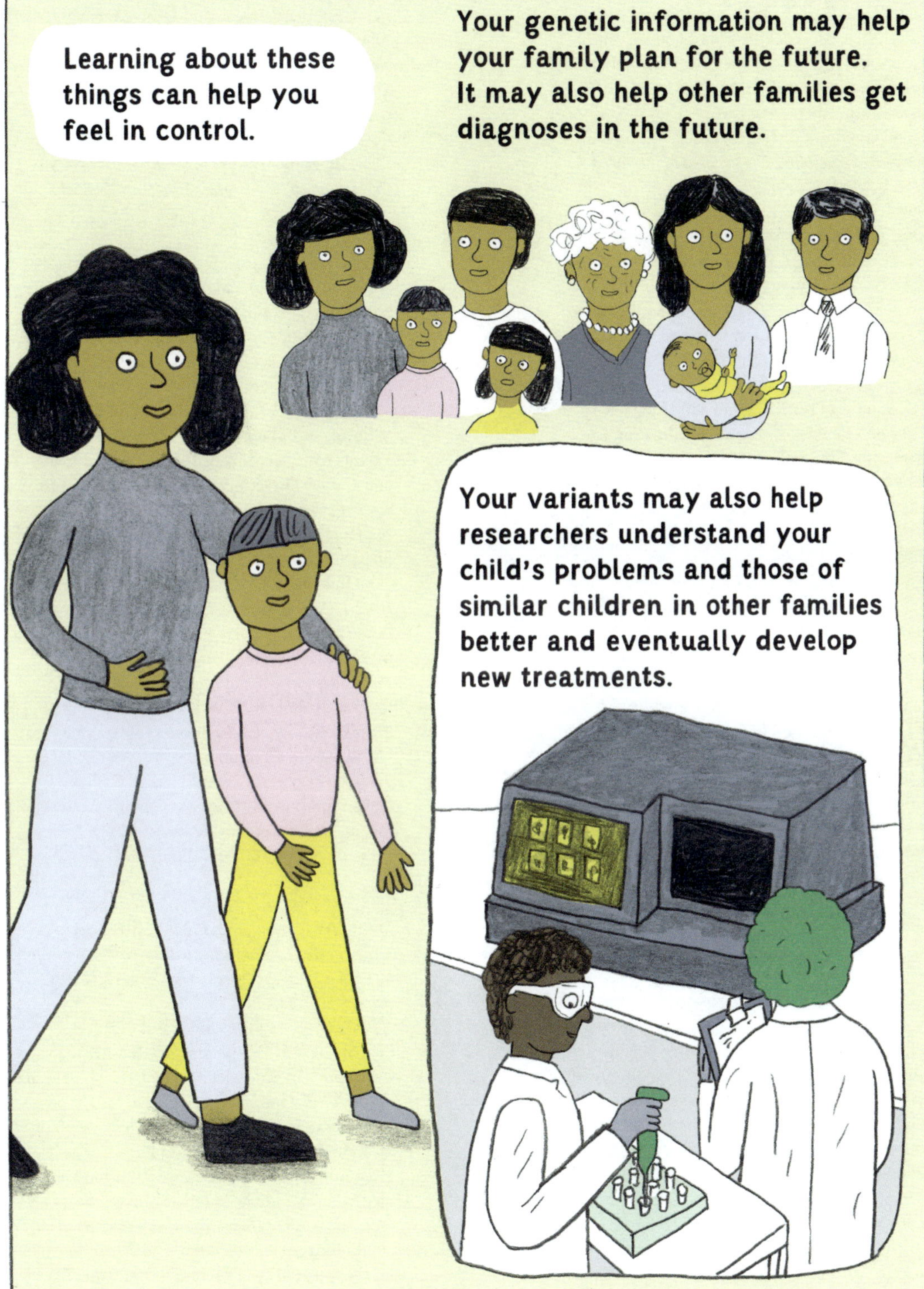
Learning about these things can help you feel in control.
Your genetic information may help your family plan for the future. It may also help other families get diagnoses in the future.
Your variants may also help researchers understand your child's problems and those of similar children in other families better and eventually develop new treatments.

A

Adam, Shelin, Patricia H. Birch, Rachel R. Coe, Nick Bansback, Adrian L. Jones, Mary B. Connolly, Michelle K. Demos, Eric B. Toyota, Matthew J. Farrer, and Jan M. Friedman (2019) "Assessing an Interactive Online Tool to Support Parents' Genomic Testing Decisions." *Journal of Genetic Counseling* 28 (1): 10–17. https://doi.org/10.1007/s10897-018-0281-1.

Aldridge, Caitlin E., Horacio Osiovich, Harold Hal Siden, RAPIDOMICS Study, GenCOUNSEL Study, and Alison M. Elliott (2021) "Rapid Genome-Wide Sequencing in a Neonatal Intensive Care Unit: A Retrospective Qualitative Exploration of Parental Experiences." *Journal of Genetic Counseling* 30 (2): 616–29. https://doi.org/10.1002/jgc4.1353.

Associated Press (2023) "California Tries to Find 600 Victims of Forced Sterilization for Reparations." https://www.theguardian.com/us-news/2023/jan/05/california-reparations-forced-sterilization (Accessed: November 5, 2024).

B

Bansback, Nick, Linda C. Li, Larry Lynd, and Stirling Bryan (2014) "Development and Preliminary User Testing of the DCIDA (Dynamic Computer Interactive Decision Application) for 'Nudging' Patients towards High Quality Decisions." *BMC Medical Informatics and Decision Making* 14 (August): 62. https://doi.org/10.1186/1472-6947-14-62.

Birch, Patricia H. (2015) "Interactive E-Counselling for Genetics Pre-Test Decisions: Where Are We Now?" *Clinical Genetics* 87 (3): 209–17. https://doi.org/10.1111/cge.12430.

Birch, Patricia H., S. Adam, N. Bansback, R. R. Coe, J. Hicklin, A. Lehman, K. C. Li, and J. M. Friedman (2016) "DECIDE: A Decision Support Tool to Facilitate Parents' Choices Regarding Genome-Wide Sequencing." *Journal of Genetic Counseling* 25 (6): 1298–1308. https://doi.org/10.1007/s10897-016-9971-8.

Bluhm, Robyn (2009) "Evidence-Based Medicine and Patient Autonomy." *International Journal of Feminist Approaches to Bioethics* 2 (2): 134–51. https://doi.org/10.3138/ijfab.2.2.134.

Bollinger, Juli Murphy, Joan Scott, Rachel Dvoskin, and David Kaufman (2012) "Public Preferences regarding the Return of Individual Genetic Research Results: Findings from a Qualitative Focus Group Study." *Genetics in Medicine: Official Journal of the American College of Medical Genetics* 14 (4): 451–57. https://doi.org/10.1038/gim.2011.66.

Bombard, Y., L. Rozmovits, M. E. Trudeau, N. B. Leighl, K. Deal, and D. A. Marshall (2014) "Patients' Perceptions of Gene Expression Profiling in Breast Cancer Treatment Decisions." *Current Oncology* 21 (2): e203–11. https://doi.org/10.3747/co.21.1524.

Butler, Judith (2005) *Giving an Account of Oneself*. New York, NY: Fordham University Press. https://doi.org/10.2307/j.ctt13x01rf.

C

Carmichael, Nikkola, Judith Tsipis, Gail Windmueller, Leslie Mandel, and Elicia Estrella (2015) "'Is It Going to Hurt?': The Impact of the Diagnostic Odyssey on Children and Their Families." *Journal of Genetic Counseling* 24 (2): 325–35. https://doi.org/10.1007/s10897-014-9773-9.

Charles, Cathy, Amiram Gafni, Tim Whelan, and Mary Ann O'Brien (2005) "Treatment Decision Aids: Conceptual Issues and Future Directions." *Health Expectations: An International Journal of Public Participation in Health Care & Health Policy* 8 (2): 114–25. https://doi.org/10.1111/j.1369-7625.2005.00325.x.

Chen, Mel Y. (2012) *Animacies: Biopolitics, Racial Mattering, and Queer Affect*. Durham, NC: Duke University Press. https://doi.org/10.1215/9780822395447.

Christianson, Adam (2024) "Barriers: A Critical Examination of Pre-Exposure Prophylaxis Non-Compliance." London: Goldsmiths, University of London.

Clarke, Angus J., and Carina Wallgren-Pettersson (2019) "Ethics in Genetic Counselling." *Journal of Community Genetics* 10 (1): 3–33. https://doi.org/10.1007/s12687-018-0371-7.

D

Djulbegovic, Benjamin (2021) "Ethics of Uncertainty." *Patient Education and Counseling* 104 (11): 2628–34. https://doi.org/10.1016/j.pec.2021.07.025.

Djulbegovic, Benjamin, and Gordon H. Guyatt (2015) "Evidence-Based Medicine and the Theory of Knowledge." In *Users' Guide to the Medical Literature: A Manual for Evidence-Based Practice*. Edited by Gordon H. Guyatt, D. Rennie, M. O. Meade, and D. J. Cook, 3rd edition, 63–68. McGraw-Hill Education. https://jamaevidence.mhmedical.com/content.aspx?bookid=847§ionid=69031459.

Djulbegovic, Benjamin, and Gordon H. Guyatt (2017) "Progress in Evidence-Based Medicine: A Quarter Century On." *The Lancet* 390 (10092): 415–23. https://doi.org/10.1016/S0140-6736(16)31592-6.

Djulbegovic, Benjamin, Gordon H. Guyatt, and Richard E. Ashcroft (2009) "Epistemologic Inquiries in Evidence-Based Medicine." *Cancer Control* 16 (2): 158–68. https://doi.org/10.1177/107327480901600208.

Donovan, Brian M., Awais Syed, Sophie H. Arnold, Dennis Lee, Monica Weindling, Molly A. M. Stuhlsatz, Catherine Riegle-Crumb, and Andrei Cimpian (2024) "Sex and Gender Essentialism in Textbooks." *Science* 383 (6685): 822–25. https://doi.org/10.1126/science.adi1188.

Donovan, Brian M., Monica Weindling, Jamie Amemiya, Brae Salazar, Dennis Lee, Awais Syed, Molly Stuhlsatz, and Jeffrey Snowden (2024) "Humane Genomics Education Can Reduce Racism." *Science* 383 (6685): 818–22. https://doi.org/10.1126/science.adi7895.

Doucet, Andrea, and Natasha S. Mauthner (2008) "What Can Be Known and How? Narrated Subjects and the Listening Guide." *Qualitative Research* 8 (3): 399–409. https://doi.org/10.1177/1468794106093636.

Duncan, R. G., R. Krishnamoorthy, U. Harms, M. Haskel-Ittah, K. Kampourakis, N. Gericke, M. Hammann, M. Jimenez-Aleixandre, R. H. Nehm, M. J. Reiss, and A. Yarden (2024) "The Sociopolitical in Human Genetics Education." *Science* 383 (6685): 826–28. https://doi.org/10.1126/science.adi8227.

E

Elliott, Alison M., and Jan M. Friedman (2018) "The Importance of Genetic Counselling in Genome-Wide Sequencing." *Nature Reviews Genetics* 19 (12): 735–36. https://doi.org/10.1038/s41576-018-0057-3.

Epstein, Steven (2008) *Inclusion: The Politics of Difference in Medical Research*. Chicago Studies in Practices of Meaning. Chicago, IL: University of Chicago Press. https://press.uchicago.edu/ucp/books/book/chicago/I/bo5414954.html.

F

Flyvbjerg, Bent (2001) *Making Social Science Matter: Why Social Inquiry Fails and How It Can Succeed Again*. Translated by Steven Sampson. Cambridge, UK: Cambridge University Press. https://doi.org/10.1017/CBO9780511810503.

Foucault, Michel (2000a) "Governmentality." In *Michel Foucault: Power*. Edited by J. D. Faubion, 3: 201–22. New York: Penguin Books.

Foucault, Michel (2000b) "Technologies of the Self." In *Michel Foucault: Ethics*. Edited by Paul Rabinow, 223–52. New York: Penguin Books.

Foucault, Michel (2012) *The History of Sexuality*. vol. 2: *The Uses of Pleasure*. New York: Penguin Books.

G

Garland, David (2003) "The Rise of Risk." In *Risk and Morality*. Edited by Richard V. Ericson and Aaron Doyle, 165–92. Green College Thematic Lecture Series. Toronto: University of Toronto Press. https://doi.org/10.3138/9781442679382.

GenCOUNSEL, DECIDE APP, accessed October 8, 2023, URL only accessible with permission.

Goldenberg, Maya J. (2006) "On Evidence and Evidence-Based Medicine: Lessons from the Philosophy of Science." *Social Science & Medicine* 62 (11): 2621–32. https://doi.org/10.1016/j.socscimed.2005.11.031.

Greenhalgh, Trisha (2012) "Why Do We Always End up Here? Evidence-Based Medicine's Conceptual Cul-de-Sacs and Some Off-Road Alternative Routes." *Journal of Primary Health Care* 4 (2): 92–97. https://doi.org/10.1071/HC12092.

H

Hanemaayer, Ariane (2019) *The Impossible Clinic: A Critical Sociology of Evidence-Based Medicine*. Vancouver: University of British Columbia Press. https://doi.org/10.59962/9780774862097.

Hanemaayer, Ariane (2022) "The Ethic of Responsibility: Max Weber's Verstehen and Shared Decision-Making in Patient-Centred Care." In *The COVID Pandemic: Essays, Book Reviews, and Poems*. Edited by Therese Jones and Kathleen Pachucki, 179–93. Cham: Springer Nature Switzerland. https://doi.org/10.1007/978-3-031-19231-9_16.

Hunt, Alan (2003) "Risk and Moralization in Everyday Life." In *Risk and Morality*. Edited by Richard V. Ericson and Aaron Doyle, 165–92. Green College Thematic Lecture Series. Toronto: University of Toronto Press. https://doi.org/10.3138/9781442679382.

J

Jourian, T. J. (2015) "Queering Constructs: Proposing a Dynamic Gender and Sexuality Model." *The Educational Forum* 79 (4): 459–74. https://doi.org/10.1080/00131725.2015.1068900.

L

Lingen, M., L. Albers, M. Borchers, S. Haass, J. Gärtner, S. Schröder, L. Goldbeck, R. von Kries, K. Brockmann, and B. Zirn (2016) "Obtaining a Genetic Diagnosis in a Child with Disability: Impact on Parental Quality of Life." *Clinical Genetics* 89 (2): 258–66. https://doi.org/10.1111/cge.12629.

M

Makela, Nancy L., Patricia H. Birch, Jan M. Friedman, and Carlo A. Marra (2009) "Parental Perceived Value of a Diagnosis for Intellectual Disability (ID): A Qualitative Comparison of Families with and without a Diagnosis for Their Child's ID." *American Journal of Medical Genetics, Part A* 149 (11): 2393–2402. https://doi.org/10.1002/ajmg.a.33050.

Montori, Victor M., G. Elwyn, P. Devereaux, Sharon E. Straus, R. Brian Haynes, and Gordon Guyatt (2015) "Decision Making and the Patient." In *Users' Guide to the Medical Literature: A Manual for Evidence-Based Practice*. Edited by Gordon H. Guyatt, D. Rennie, M. O. Meade, and D. J. Cook, 3rd edition, 63–68. London: McGraw-Hill Education. https://jamaevidence.mhmedical.com/content.aspx?bookid=847§ionid=69031459.

Mykhalovskiy, Eric (2003) "Evidence-Based Medicine: Ambivalent Reading and the Clinical Recontextualization of Science." *Health* 7 (3): 331–52. https://doi.org/10.1177/1363459303007003005.

Mykhalovskiy, Eric, and Lorna Weir (2004) "The Problem of Evidence-Based Medicine: Directions for Social Science." *Social Science & Medicine* 59 (5): 1059–69. https://doi.org/10.1016/j.socscimed.2003.12.002.

N

Novas, Carlos (2006) "The Political Economy of Hope: Patients' Organizations, Science and Biovalue." *BioSocieties* 1 (3): 289–305. https://doi.org/10.1017/S1745855206003024.

P

Peters, Ellen, Judith Hibbard, Paul Slovic, and Nathan Dieckmann (2007) "Numeracy Skill and the Communication, Comprehension, and Use of Risk-Benefit Information." *Health Affairs* 26 (3): 741–48. https://doi.org/10.1377/hlthaff.26.3.741.

Pinheiro, Ana P. M., Rachel H. Pocock, Margie D. Dixon, Walid L. Shaib, Suresh S. Ramalingam, and Rebecca D. Pentz (2017) "Using Metaphors to Explain Molecular Testing to Cancer Patients." *The Oncologist* 22 (4): 445–49. https://doi.org/10.1634/theoncologist.2016-0270.

Pykett, Jessica, Rhys Jones, and Mark Whitehead (2017) "Introduction: Psychological Governance and Public Policy." In *Psychological Governance and Public Policy: Governing the Mind, Brain and Behaviour*, 1–20. Routledge Research in Place, Space and Politics. New York, NY: Routledge/Taylor & Francis Group.

R

Rabinow, Paul (1996) *Essays on the Anthropology of Reason*. Princeton, NJ: Princeton University Press. https://doi.org/10.2307/j.ctv1fkgd8r.

Rabinow, Paul, and Nikolas Rose (2015) "Biopower Today." In *Biopower: Foucault and Beyond*. Edited by Vernon W. Cisney and Nicolae Morar, 297–325. Chicago, IL: University of Chicago Press. https://press.uchicago.edu/ucp/books/book/chicago/B/bo20133023.html.

Regier, Dean A., Rosalie Loewen, Brandon Chan, Morgan Ehman, Samantha Pollard, Jan M. Friedman, Sylvia Stockler-Ipsiroglu, Clara van Karnebeek, Simone Race, Alison M. Elliott, Nick Dragojlovic, Larry D. Lynd, and Deirdre Weymann (2024) "Real-World Diagnostic Outcomes and Cost-Effectiveness of Genome-Wide Sequencing for Developmental and Seizure Disorders: Evidence from Canada." *Genetics in Medicine: Official Journal of the American College of Medical Genetics* 26 (4): 101069. https://doi.org/10.1016/j.gim.2024.101069.

Rose, Nikolas (1999) *Powers of Freedom: Reframing Political Thought*. Cambridge, UK: Cambridge University Press. https://doi.org/10.1017/CBO9780511488856.

Rose, Nikolas (2007a) "Molecular Biopolitics, Somatic Ethics and the Spirit of Biocapital." *Social Theory & Health* 5 (1): 3–29. https://doi.org/10.1057/palgrave.sth.8700084.

Rose, Nikolas (2007b) *The Politics of Life Itself: Biomedicine, Power, and Subjectivity in the Twenty-First Century*. Princeton, NJ: Princeton University Press. https://www.jstor.org/stable/j.ctt7rqmf.

Rose, Nikolas, and Carlos Novas (2005) "Biological Citizenship." In *Global Assemblages: Technology, Politics, and Ethics as Anthropological Problems*. Edited by A. Ong and S. J. Collier, 439–63. Oxford: Blackwell Publishing. https://doi.org/10.1002/9780470696569.ch23.

Rose, Nikolas, Pat O'Malley, and Mariana Valverde (2006) "Governmentality." *Annual Review of Law and Social Science* 2: 83–104. https://doi.org/10.1146/annurev.lawsocsci.2.081805.105900.

S

Sackett, David L., William M. C. Rosenberg, J. A. Muir Gray, R. Brian Haynes, and W. Scott Richardson (1996) "Evidence Based Medicine: What It Is and What It Isn't." *BMJ* 312 (7023): 71–72. https://doi.org/10.1136/bmj.312.7023.71.

Sawyer, S. l., T. Hartley, D. A. Dyment, C. l. Beaulieu, J. Schwartzentruber, A. Smith, H. M. Bedford, G. Bernard, F. P. Bernier, B. Brais, D. E. Bulman, J. Warman Chardon, D. Chitayat, J. Deladoëy, B. A. Fernandez, P. Frosk, M. T. Geraghty, B. Gerull, W. Gibson, R. M. Gow, G. E. Graham, J. S. Green, E. Heon, G. Horvath, A. M. Innes, N. Jabado, R. H. Kim, R. K. Koenekoop, A. Khan, O. J. Lehmann, R. Mendoza-Londono, J. L. Michaud, S. M. Nikkel, L. S. Penney, C. Polychronakos, J. Richer, G. A. Rouleau, M. E. Samuels, V. M. Siu, O. Suchowersky, M. A. Tarnopolsky, G. Yoon, F. R. Zahir, FORGE Canada Consortium, Care4Rare Canada Consortium, J. Majewski, and K. M. Boycott (2016) "Utility of Whole-Exome Sequencing for Those Near the End of the Diagnostic Odyssey: Time to Address Gaps in Care." Edited by FORGE Canada Consortium and Care4Rare Canada Consortium. *Clinical Genetics* 89 (3): 275–84. https://doi.org/lin.

Sexton, Adrienne, and P. A. James (2022) "Metaphors and Why These Are Important in All Aspects of Genetic Counseling." *Journal of Genetic Counseling* 31 (1): 34–40. https://doi.org/10.1002/jgc4.1463.

Sheehan, Joanne, and Kerry A. Sherman (2012) "Computerised Decision Aids: A Systematic Review of Their Effectiveness in Facilitating High-Quality Decision-Making in Various Health-Related Contexts." *Patient Education and Counseling* 88 (1): 69–86. https://doi.org/10.1016/j.pec.2011.11.006.

T

Tabor, Holly K., Jacquie Stock, Tracy Brazg, Margaret J. McMillin, Karin M. Dent, Joon-Ho Yu, Jay Shendure, and Michael J. Bamshad (2012) "Informed Consent for Whole Genome Sequencing: A Qualitative Analysis of Participant Expectations and Perceptions of Risks, Benefits, and Harms." *American Journal of Medical Genetics, Part A* 158 (6): 1310–19. https://doi.org/10.1002/ajmg.a.35328.

Thaler, R. H., and C. R. Sunstein (2008) *Nudge: Improving Decisions About Health, Wealth, and Happiness*. New Haven, CT: Yale University Press.

W

Wetterstrand, K. A. 2022. "DNA Sequencing Costs: Data from the NHGRI Genome Sequencing Program (GSP)." National Institutes of Health. https://www.genome.gov/about-genomics/fact-sheets/DNA-Sequencing-Costs-Data.

Y

Yamamoto, Mutsumi. 1999. *Animacy and Reference: Slcs.46*. Amsterdam: John Benjamins Publishing Company. https://benjamins.com/catalog/slcs.46.

Seen but Not Heard

Awa Naghipour, Joana Atemengue Owona,
and Golnar Kat Rahmani

A Transdisciplinary Approach to Visualizing Intersectional Discrimination in German Healthcare

Awa Naghipour

Overview

Our overall aim with this project is to further awareness of experiences of intersectional discrimination in German healthcare contexts and make them accessible to a variety of audiences. This project was co-created in an evolving transdisciplinary process from September 2023 to April 2024. Qualitative, participatory research elements were employed by 1) conducting semi-structured interviews with three individuals holding multiple attributes that render them susceptible to discrimination and 2) each individual explicitly choosing one quote on which to put emphasis and move forward with. This was followed by a two-step artistic realization to three-dimensionally visualize the selected key sentences employing 1) a translation of the selected quote to musical notations and 2) inscribing the musical notations onto a lead installation using embossing and debossing as stylistic and conceptual elements. A leaflet, titled *How Not to Gaslight*, FIG. 8 was designed to continue the conversation with interacting audiences. This scientifically informed artistic approach and realization was collaboratively shaped by the authors' perspectives from medical science, clinical experience, sociopolitical engagement, artistic practice, and graphic design, integrating elements of experimental sound composition, fine arts, and sculpting.

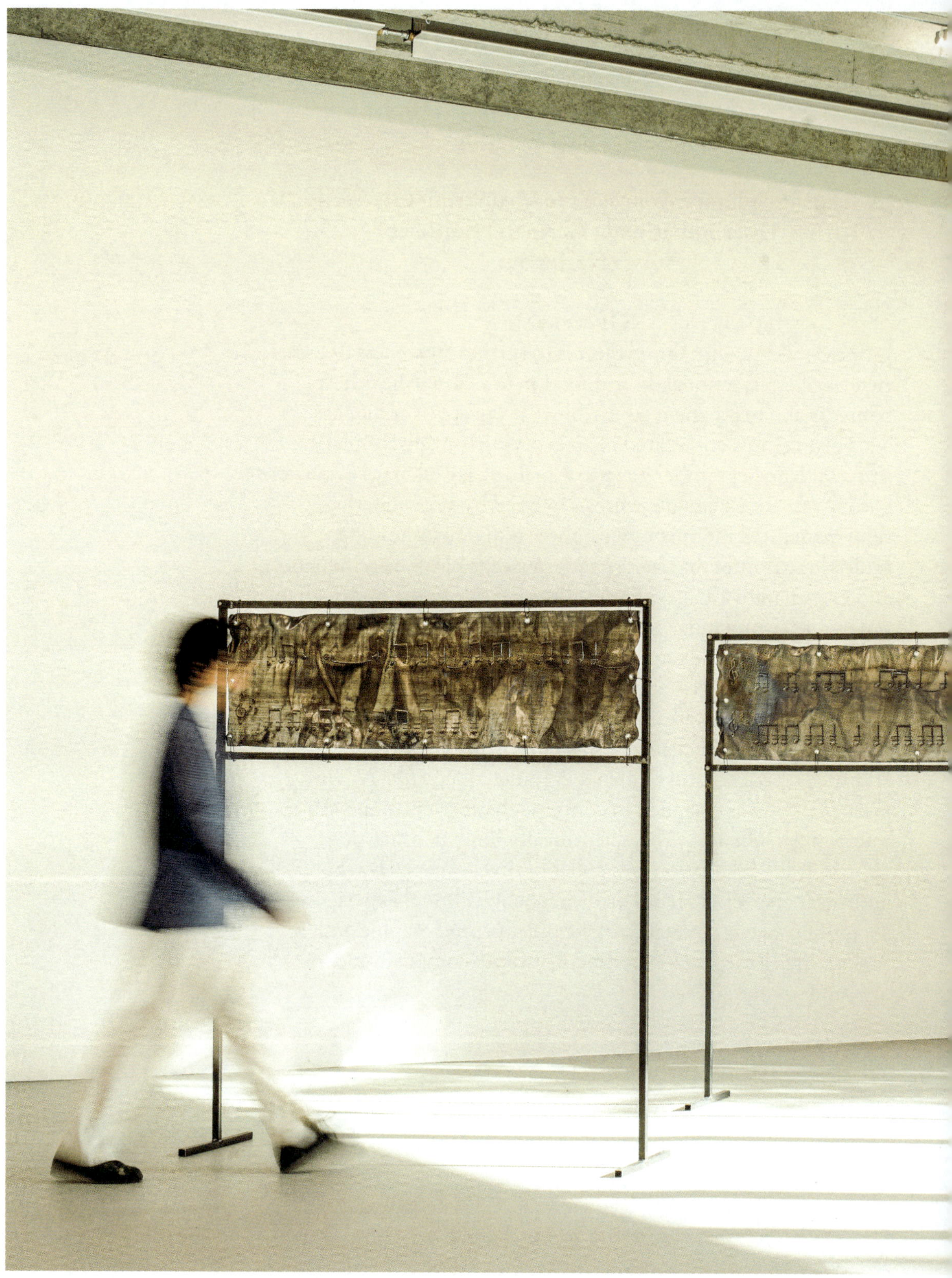

FIG. 1

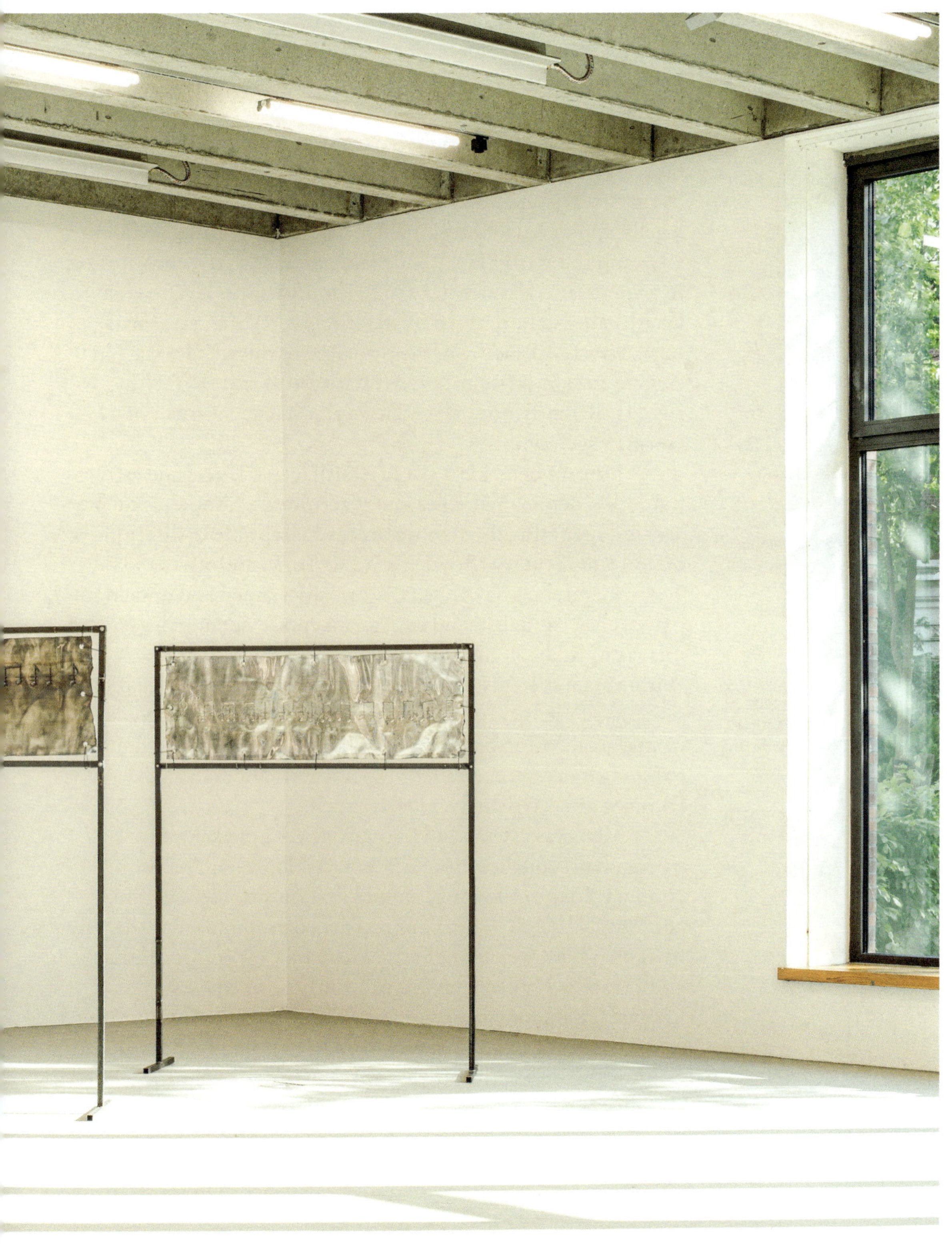

FIG. 1 Awa Naghipour, Joana Atemengue Owana, Golnar Kat Rahmani, *Seen but Not Heard*, installation view, 2024. Photo: Joana Atemengue Owona

Introduction

The right to equitable healthcare implies that every human being, regardless of their sex/gender,[1] race,[2] ethnicity, sexual orientation, socioeconomic status, ability, or further marginalizing characteristics, should have access to and be treated equitably by healthcare institutions and professionals (Bartig et al. 2021; OHCHR and WHO 2008). This right has been declared and legally stipulated in the global Declaration of Human Rights in 1948 and the World Health Organization's (WHO) constitution in 1946 (OHCHR and WHO 2008). On a national level, a right to health can also be derived from Article 2 (2) of the German Basic Law (GG) and from the principle of the welfare state in Article 20 (1) GG (Reimer 2021; Bartig et al. 2021). Yet, this right is currently not realized for a significant segment of German society.

Human beings consist of multifaceted layers and attributes that define their roles and place them among societal hierarchies, rendering them more or less susceptible to discrimination and inequity (Bowleg 2012; OHCHR and WHO 2008). These hierarchies have been historically shaped and upheld by patriarchal, capitalist, and racist concepts, evident in legacies of misogyny and colonialism (Bowleg 2012; Hankivsky 2014). Within such systems, each individual navigates complex intersections of identity, experiencing varying degrees of privilege or marginalization based on factors including (but not limited to) sex/gender, race, ethnicity, socioeconomic status, and ability (Bowleg 2012; OHCHR and WHO 2008).

Medical systems and knowledge are not exempt from patriarchal, capitalist, structurally racist logic—quite the contrary. In the following, we will first outline the scientific conceptual basis to which our project corresponds. For this, in a brief overview, we highlight two main foci—1) androcentrism and 2) racism—which have significantly molded medical knowledge and practice to exclude dissenting identities and lived realities outside a certain norm,[3] and to uphold practices of oppression therewith (Bowleg 2012). We then explore intersectionality as a framework to help us understand and analyze

1 Using "sex/gender" instead of "sex and gender" is an intentional choice to emphasize the interrelationship between the terms "sex" and "gender" and their underlying concepts, characterizing what van Anders describes as "whole people/identities" (2015, 1181). Authors such as Hyde and colleagues propose using the "/" in between "gender" and "sex" instead of "and" to underscore the "close interconnection" between the terms, thereby challenging a binary categorization and use of the terms (2019, 33).

2 We emphasize that race is a socially constructed category, historically rooted in racist ideology to justify oppression, and we reject any interpretation or reification of race as a proxy for biological traits—a misconception widely perpetuated, particularly in medical sciences (Heinz et al. 2014).

3 As Sebring summarizes, "Medicine, as a practice and as a profession, has largely been developed by and for a very specific kind of body: the wealthy, white, able-bodied, heterosexual, cissex, endosex and cisgender male subject" (2021; drawing on Gkiouleka et al. 2018; Shildrick 1997).

interlocking systems of oppression affecting multi-marginalized groups within the healthcare context. Next, we outline our scientifically informed, multistep artistic approach to visualizing discrimination of individuals holding layered social identities in the German healthcare system. In a closing artist statement, we further elaborate on our artistic choices and execution.

Background

Androcentrism, the Gender Data Gap, and Sex/Gender as Modifiers of Health and Disease

The so-called gender data gap in medical knowledge has evolved over a centuries-long androcentric skew in knowledge production. As Londa Schiebinger poignantly concludes, "Even in studies where women were included, the male body typically represented the normal human; the female body has traditionally been studied as a deviation from that norm" (2000, 1172; referring to Rosser 1994). That sex/gender can play a pivotal role in influencing health, longevity, disease occurrence, diagnosis, therapy, and outcome as well as preventative behavior has been described extensively (Tannenbaum et al. 2019; Stefanick and Schiebinger 2020; Mauvais-Jarvis et al. 2020; Heise et al. 2019; Oertelt-Prigione and Regitz-Zagrosek 2012). Mauvais-Jarvis et al. (2020) recently summarized the manifold influences sex/gender can have on health and disease, far beyond the nowadays fortunately widely known myocardial infarction. Myocardial infarction can manifest itself with more than just the "typical"[4] chest pain, especially in females; further non-specific symptoms such as nausea, vomiting, abdominal pain, and pain in the jaw, neck, and shoulders can occur. This misconception has often led to later diagnosis and therapy with inferior outcomes over decades (Haider et al. 2020; Mauvais-Jarvis et al. 2020). But the examples go further than that: smoking proves to be a stronger risk factor for stroke in women than in men, and women show differing therapeutic needs after menopause onset in chronic pulmonary disease and are prone to have a prolonged course of

4 The use of "typical" in quotation marks references the frequently employed term in medical textbooks and guidelines, which reflects a cis-male norm. In contrast, symptoms from individuals presented from outside this norm, such as women, are often described as "atypical."

disease in pulmonary influenza A infections due to persisting inflammation, to name a few lesser-known facts (Mauvais-Jarvis et al. 2020). This list could be extended endlessly. The longer a sex/gender-sensitive and disaggregated research practice is performed, the more insights on multifaceted influences we gain (Peters and Woodward 2023; Brady et al. 2021).

Devaluation and denial of lived realities of marginalized genders against the cis-male[5] norm have a long history, dating back to Hippocrates's positing that the womb was the origin of all diseases (Tasca et al. 2012). To this day, marginalized genders, notably women labeled hysterical, often confront dismissal as, for instance, their pain is attributed to psychological rather than somatic origins (Samulowitz et al. 2018; Stefanick and Schiebinger 2020; Tasca et al. 2012; Becher and Oertelt-Prigione 2022).

Sex/gender-sensitive scientific and medical practice aims to bridge this gap to equalize a to-date unilateral, fragmentary biomedical body of knowledge that does not yet do justice to a sex/gender-diverse population (Tannenbaum et al. 2019). This implies not only considering women but reflecting on biases and stereotypes toward all gender identities and realities. It further means scrutinizing widely held beliefs of allegedly female- or male-specific or -typical diseases and calls for a critical deconstruction of a dichotomous concept of sex/gender toward an expansion of sex/gender concepts and realities outside the binary (DuBois and Shattuck-Heidorn 2021). Overall, overcoming an androcentric and binary framework in scientific methodology and medical practice means that cis as well as trans, inter, and nonbinary gender realities are by default equally prioritized in medical research and practice (Hahne 2024; DuBois and Shattuck-Heidorn 2021).

5 Cis indicates that the sex assigned at birth (by examining the genitals) equates to one's gender identity.

Racial Biases and Colonial Continuities

As multifaceted individuals, other differentiating factors, such as experiencing racism or not, can influence lived realities. Racial biases persist in daily medical assessment and care, especially the disproportionate underestimation and undertreatment of pain among individuals of color. This topic has been more extensively studied in the US, in particular among Black and African American patients. The term to describe the phenomenon around racism and pain is called the racial pain bias (Meghani, Byun, and Gallagher 2012; Hoffman et al. 2016; Waytz, Hoffman, and Trawalter 2015; Dore et al. 2014; Mathur et al. 2014; Staton et al. 2007). Hoffman et al. conducted two studies in which they 1) investigated whether laypeople and medical professionals held false beliefs regarding biological differences between Black vs. White[6] people rooted in colonial ideology, such as "black people's skin is thicker than white people's skin," and 2) examined if an association between false belief and inaccurate pain assessment and treatment could be observed in medical staff (2016, 4297). They concluded in their findings in a sample of 92 laypeople and 222 medical students and residents that "beliefs about biological differences between blacks and whites—beliefs dating back to slavery"—still exist (Hoffman et al. 2016, 4300). Fifty percent of medical staff endorsed the stated false beliefs. Further, for both populations, those beliefs were "associated with the perception that black people feel less pain than do white people." The medical professionals who believed the false statements were prone to bias in pain assessment and inadequate treatment recommendations (Hoffman et al. 2016, 4300).

In addition to interpersonal levels of discrimination, institutional and structural manifestations of racism in medical care prove relevant. So-called race correction in clinical algorithms based on long-held false convictions of race as a proxy for genetic and biological traits have been recently re-examined by Vyas, Eisenstein, and Jones in 2020, ranging from algorithms for lung function tests, estimated kidney function, and urinary tract infections in children (Akintemi and Roberts 2022). Ostensibly objective clinical assessment tools such as pulse oximeters have shown to be inaccurate in assessing hypoxemia (low oxygen levels in the blood), detecting hypoxemia three times less in Black than in White patients due to pulse oximeters being less apt to measure accurately on darker skin (Sjoding et al. 2020). These manifold examples plastically illustrate the ongoing interindividual, institutional, and structural racism

6 Capitalizing "White" to align with "Black" is a conscious choice. As American historian Nell Irvin Painter states, "The capital W stresses 'White' as a powerful racial category whose privileges should be embedded in its definition." Capitalizing the "W" situates "'Whiteness' within the American ideology of race, within which 'Black,' but not 'White,' has been hypervisible as a group identity. Capitalizing all our races—'Black,' 'Brown' and 'White'—simply makes this ideology visible for all" (Painter 2020). The Center for the Study of Social Policy emphasizes "that it is important to call attention to White as a race as a way to understand and give voice to how Whiteness functions in our social and political institutions and our communities" and therewith hold White people and institutions accountable for their role in sustaining racism (Nguyễn and Pendleton 2020).

embedded in medical assessment and care (Bailey et al. 2017). Germany, however, lags behind in providing a differentiated picture of the local situation.

No Racism in German Healthcare?

To date, data on racism in healthcare settings is scarce in Germany. As exemplified in the previous section, most evidence on racial bias in medical practice, e.g., disadvantages in access to and quality of healthcare, higher disease burden, and mortality (e.g., maternal mortality) derives from US-American studies (Bailey et al. 2017; Hoffman et al. 2016; Vyas, Eisenstein, and Jones 2020; Sjoding et al. 2020; Bartig et al. 2021). Tendencies and relevant evidence are not unrestrictedly transferable to the German context and need further contextualization to local conditions, ideally through locally developed and executed study designs (Bartig et al. 2021; Ateş et al. 2023; Aikins et al. 2021). This is especially crucial given Germany's particular history of colonialism and the Nazi regime, which includes distinct forms of racism against Sinti and Roma, anti-Slavism, antisemitism, and anti-Muslim racism (Foroutan et al. 2022).

The Country of Poets and Thinkers Lacks Pertinent Vocabulary

Two studies have significantly advanced knowledge on racism in Germany in recent years. The 2023 "Racism and Its Symptoms – Report of the National Monitoring of Discrimination and Racism with a Focus on Health" (Ateş et al. 2023) and the "Afrozensus 2020" (Aikins et al. 2021) have shed light on the experiences of racialized populations across societal areas including healthcare. They are the two recent pivotal studies in Germany that analyze racist dynamics in the healthcare context by conducting a survey among the affected population on a grander scale.

"Afrozensus" is the first German study directly involving the "Afro-German," "afro-diasporic," and "Black" population, all self-attributed identities by the participants. The survey was entirely community-based, from the scientific team to the sample population. The German Centre for Integration and Migration Research (DeZIM) surveyed further marginalized populations and distinguished "Black," "Asian," and "Muslim" individuals (Ateş et al. 2023). The main findings of the selected studies are elaborated in the following. The "Afrozensus" portrayed findings of 6,000 participants stating their experiences of racist discrimination in 14 areas of life, including healthcare. In the healthcare subsection, two-thirds of the participants disclosed not having been taken seriously in healthcare encounters, and 73–74 percent stated that they had been discriminated against due to their skin color or attributed ethnicity. The "Racism and its Symptoms" report by DeZIM summarizes that the majority of people who stated to have had negative experiences in healthcare contexts were women (Ateş et al. 2023). Especially women of color, 68 percent of Muslim and 67 percent of Black women stated to have experienced more unjust and worse treatments than others in their healthcare encounters, pointing at intersectional dynamics.

The experience of discrimination in healthcare has been described to serve as a distinct risk factor, evoking less healthcare utilization and hence delayed diagnosis and therapy, potentially leading to the chronification of diseases (Bartig et al. 2021; Pascoe and Richman 2009). In the 2023 report, every seventh Black woman, every eighth Muslim woman, and every eighth Asian woman reported having delayed medical treatment or avoided treatment altogether in the past twelve months due to concerns of being discriminated against, not being taken seriously, or receiving poor treatment (Ateş et al. 2023). On an organizational level, data shows a lower probability of receiving a doctor's appointment when a name of Nigerian or Turkish origin is given in comparison to a name of German origin, despite using identical wording in the request. Further, patients with academic titles were more likely to be favored than those without academic titles, revealing classist dynamics (Ateş et al. 2023). Both studies emphasized the need for prioritization of the serious and harmful topics of racist and multi-discriminatory practices perpetuated by the German healthcare system and the lack of awareness and data in current research and policy (Ateş et al. 2023; Aikins et al. 2021).

One aspect of the scarcity of data to describe and precisely differentiate those affected by racism and those who are not is the lack of distinguished vocabulary in Germany (Bartig et al. 2021; Yeboah 2017). The term "migration background" is widely used in German data collection (Bartram et al. 2023). It legally defines all individuals themselves or with at least one parent born without German citizenship (Statistisches Bundesamt 2024). In addition to being vague, the term insufficiently distinguishes between populations that face racism and thus has been repeatedly criticized (El-Mafaalani 2023; Yeboah 2017).

Both portrayed studies and the continuous significant work on racism and (especially mental) health of certain researchers have surely enhanced and progressed the ongoing process of finding more precise vocabulary to analyze the German population affected by racism (for additional insights see Foroutan et al. 2022 and Lazaridou et al. 2023). Nevertheless, further development in terms of more nuanced research methodology and its comprehensive implementation and institutionalization is yet to be carried out. While the existence of racism in the German healthcare context is clearly undeniable, gaps in evidence persist, and a more granular analysis of local conditions is still needed.

Further, it is crucial to acknowledge single-axis analysis to be insufficient to recognize human beings as a whole, holding a diverse set of attributes to comprise a complex identity and societal contextuality. Attributes such as sex/gender do not solely exist in a vacuum but are embedded in psychosociocultural conditions, layered with, e.g., age, ability, ethnicity, socioeconomic status, and education. These diverse realities can have implications on health and disease, access to the healthcare system, and the quality of healthcare provided (Heise et al. 2019; McGlothen-Bell et al. 2023; Crear-Perry et al. 2021). To facilitate an in-depth understanding of the interplay of the layers of identity and oppression, an intersectional framework can be helpful (Hankivsky and Christoffersen 2008; Hankivsky et al. 2010; Bowleg 2012; 2021).

Intersectionality: From Practice to Framework and Vice Versa

Intersectionality emerged from Black feminist activism (Truth 1851; Combahee River Collective 1977; Bowleg 2012), and the term was first described in a scholarly way by Kimberlé Crenshaw in the 1980s (Crenshaw 1989). To put it simply, intersectionality offers a framework to equally and simultaneously consider multiple axes of oppression affecting multi-marginalized persons and communities. Equivalent to Crenshaw's analysis of discriminatory hiring practices' unique impact on Black women in comparison to White women or Black men (Crenshaw 1989), Black women encounter challenges in healthcare that do not equate to those of White women or Black men. Drawing from US-based data showing maternal mortality disproportionately affecting Black women (GBD 2015 Maternal Mortality Collaborators 2016) or recent developments in the Covid-19 pandemic's multiplying of disease burden and outcomes connected to intersecting axes of socioeconomic status, race, ethnicity, and employment in care professions (Andrasfay and Goldman 2021; Arias and Tejada-Vera 2023), it is quite evident that intersecting layers of discrimination result in unique and amplified barriers to adequate healthcare access and treatment globally (Hankivsky and Christoffersen 2008).

Olena Hankivksy, an expert on intersectionality in health research and global health, comprehensively describes intersectionality as "an understanding of human beings as shaped by the interaction of different social locations" and places these interactions "in a context of connected systems and structures of power" (2022, 2). These can correspond to macrostructural determinants within the concept of social and structural determinants of health, as described by Dahlgren and Whitehead (1991), encompassing areas such as law, policy, and economic regulations. Through such dynamic interactions, "interdependent forms of privilege and oppression shaped by colonialism, imperialism, racism, homophobia, ableism, and patriarchy are created" (Hankivsky 2014, 2).

7 Black, Indigenous, people of color.

A leading scholar on intersectionality in social and behavioral sciences as well as in health equity research, Lisa Bowleg punctuates the interconnectedness of the individual experience to structural levels of oppressive systems when she proposes "a central consideration of intersectionality" to be "how multiple social identities at the individual level of experience (i.e., the micro level) intersect with multiple-level social inequalities at the macro structural level" (2012, 1269). Bowleg then goes on to connect the personal experience of a middle-class Latina lesbian at the intersections of gender, race, ethnicity, and sexual orientation to the structural manifestations of heterosexism and racism in healthcare practice (2012).

Although intersectionality has been discussed and applied in the scholarly fields of law, politics, and social sciences, its transfer to public health and medicine has been slow-going (Bowleg 2012; Ogungbe, Mitra, and Roberts 2019). As Bowleg stated in 2012, "Public health's commitment to social justice makes it a natural fit with intersectionality's focus on multiple historically oppressed populations. Yet despite a plethora of research focused on these populations, public health studies that reflect intersectionality in their theoretical frameworks, designs, analyses, or interpretations are rare" (2012, 1267). Especially qualitative (Abrams et al. 2020) but also quantitative (Guan et al. 2021; Bauer et al. 2021) research methods have emerged to try to incorporate intersectionality as a framework within public health. Nevertheless, Bowleg later reflects that it has yet to be determined how to adequately translate a concept that initially derived from critical practice to the medical, scientific realm without losing its depth, structural criticism, and politically transformative core (2021).

Intersectionality is deeply rooted in sociopolitical work, grounded in decades-long BIPOC[7] feminist social movements (Truth 1851; Combahee River Collective 1977; Bowleg 2012; Collins 2015; Hankivsky 2014). Therefore, highlighting and valuing lived experiences should be an inherent part of aiming toward a healthcare practice that is sensitive to intersectional discrimination. This involves maintaining an underlying critical consciousness of how to interweave scholarship and lived experiences, ensuring that lived experiences are intrinsic to the knowledge produced. The core tenets of intersectionality evoke its capacity to be critical, political, and aimed at power structures to transform societal contexts of oppression. It is neither simply an addition of identity layers, nor is it just a tool to describe disparities, which makes its transfer to conventional health sciences challenging (Guan et al. 2021). Targeting inequity and hence delineating the interdependence of individual levels of discrimination to institutional and structural levels of oppression is key (Bowleg 2012; 2021; Poteat 2021). Centering lived experience therefore functions as an indicator to dissect underlying structures of inequity, which then need to be addressed to evoke transformative change.

Methodology and Material

To underscore intersectional realities in German healthcare contexts, we developed a scientifically informed artistic process aimed at furthering awareness of these experiences and underlying issues. In the following, the methodological approach, artistic choices, material, and results are explained in more detail.

Interviews

> Interviewing gives us access to the observations of others. Through interviewing we can learn about places we have not been and could not go and about settings in which we have not lived. . . . We can learn about all the experiences, from joy through grief, that together constitute the human condition. Interviewing gives us a window on the past. . . . Interviewing rescues events that would otherwise be lost. The . . . sorrows of people . . . leave no record except in their memories. And there are, of course, no observers of the internal events of thought and feelings except those to whom they occur. Most of the significant events of people's lives can become known to others only through the interview (Weiss 1994, 1–2).

The inclusion criteria for the participants were defined as:

1) Multilayered social identities, as in co-occurrence of multiple axes of discrimination. The minimum consisted of identifying as a marginalized gender (not a cis male, e.g., female, trans, inter, nonbinary, gender-fluid) and BIPOC (not as White).
2) Having experienced discrimination in German healthcare contexts.

Recruitment of Participants

In contrast to predominantly androcentric, White narratives, we chose to speak to individuals who have experienced intersectional discrimination in the healthcare system in Germany. Since the conversation on experiences of discrimination in the healthcare setting proves to be a sensitive topic, we decided to extend the invitation to participants via trusted colleagues and friends as well as their environments. Due to the short timeline of the overall project, we aimed to find at least two and a maximum of five interview participants. We intentionally communicated that we as project collaborators ourselves hold different layers of marginalization within our social identities, to provide potential participants an idea of the (non-White, non-cis-male) setting in advance. The interview was announced to be 45 minutes long with a possible extension to 60 minutes if the situation required. We offered the verbal languages German, English, and Farsi as well as the option to interview in person, via video call, phone call, or voice messaging, or in written form. We remained open to suggestions that the participants felt most comfortable with and that were customized to their circumstances. Anonymization and artistic modification of shared quotes were communicated.

Interview Protocol

We employed semi-structured interviews to gather in-depth narratives from participants. The semi-structured format was chosen to ensure reproducibility and key topics to be covered in the conversation while allowing participants to express their thoughts and experiences freely and flexibly (Zhang, Chang, and Du 2021). We designed and conducted the interviews with great care and conscious effort toward reflexivity to reduce bias or influence over participants' responses. The guide consisted of open-ended questions to provide explicit room for the participants to share and emphasize their narrative focal points and core experiences. To prepare the participants for the vulnerable topic to be discussed and allow for customization and amendments, we shared the questions well in advance. Furthermore, we distinctly communicated that all questions and topics were optional and open to be personalized as much as needed to create a sense of control and agency in the upcoming conversation. Informed consent was secured.

The interview consisted of a total of nine sections. In the introduction, the outline and aim of the project were described, and a common ground was offered by introducing the project instructors as also holding multilayered social identities. All following questions were formulated as open-ended questions allowing for an in-depth exploration and elicitation of the participants' thoughts and experiences. The second section introduced the topic of layered identities and discrimination at large, asking for the participants' definition of their sense of identity in their historical and cultural context as well as their understanding of the term "discrimination." The third section addressed discriminatory practices specifically related to their identity in the context of the German healthcare system. The fourth section asked if scenarios occurred in which the participant felt disregarded or not taken seriously. If so, the section further explored potential consequences arising from those experiences. The fifth section's main theme was access barriers to healthcare facilities and included communication as one aspect. The sixth section explored coping strategies and resources developed therefrom. The seventh section asked for ideas from the participant on how, in their opinion, an improvement of the current situation should be approached. The eighth section targeted hopes and worries about the future of the healthcare system and explored what a system would look like in which the participant would feel safe and justly cared for. The closing segment offered to add anything that was not touched upon and the option to formulate a direct demand for the leaflet *How Not to Gaslight* (described in the "Results" section).

Key Sentence

After the interview, a participatory approach was set by asking the participants to select a key sentence. The key sentence was characterized as a significantly important aspect for the participant within their overall experience of being discriminated against in the healthcare context. To offer the least restriction, the participants were encouraged to set any thematic emphasis preferred.

Musical Notations

The rationale behind translating spoken words into resonant musical notations lies in the association with marginalized voices being overlooked when hierarchically positioned as inferior in social dynamics. In Paul Wingfield's interpretation and analysis of the work on speech-melodies by Czech composer Leoš Janáček (late nineteenth to early twentieth centuries), speech is described to embody "both external and internal 'realities' or 'truths,'" and as Janáček himself formulated, speech is the "embodiment" of thought or emotion (1992, 282). We drew on these impulses in our artistic approach to make our interlocutors' experiences legible to a broader audience, in a way that resonated beyond traditional narration. The key sentence chosen by each participant, initially recorded in audio format, served as the basis. The melodic pattern and vocal pitch were determined by ear and subsequently mapped onto the piano as a reference instrument. This process aligns with methods as described and employed by Jewish-American composer Steve Reich in his earlier work in the late 1980s using voice recordings and translating them into musical notations for string instruments to compose his piece *Different Trains* in

1988: "Reich selected small speech samples that had a marked melodic contour and then wrote them down as accurately as possible in musical dictation" (Puca 1997, 550). Melodic variabilities of the different voices, as well as the rhythm and speed of the spoken word, were accounted for and reflected in different melodies. An external composer affirmed the readability and logic behind the mapping of the spoken word into musical notations.

In the mapping process, we consciously removed some of the traditional features of musical notations, such as the staff, to critically comment on elitist utilization of music theory as an art of the educated bourgeois, used to distinguish by deliberately excluding others. The explicit choice not to use "x" as a symbol to indicate spoken word and rather to utilize the musical notation of complex tonal sound derived from the intention to grasp the multiple layers behind emotions, history, and depth of the narrative beyond the spoken word.

Results

Three people reached out to be interviewed. After receiving a thorough description of the project details and the use of their data, all participants consented to participation. Each participant read the interview protocol in advance, and there were no requests for changes or sections to be left out. The interviewees opted for German-language discussions. We ensured participants that only one self-chosen quote out of the interview, a demand for the leaflet, and their layers of social identity would be included in this project; therefore, only this information is disclosed.

Layers of Social Identity

Participant 1 described their layers of social identity as 27 years old, identifying as a woman but as a loose category not within a binary understanding of gender, an Afro-German person of color, pansexual, neurodivergent, and having psychiatric comorbidities. (Quote 1; racism in healthcare)

Participant 2 described their layers of social identity as 35

8 Original quote in German: "Also ich hab' generell nicht viel Vertrauen, dass mir mit erlebtem Rassismus im medizinischen Kontext geholfen wird, oder dass er als solcher überhaupt anerkannt wird."

9 Original quote in German: "Sie haben aber ADHS, Sie können nicht acht Stunden am Tag im Kurs sitzen und zuhören und lernen."

10 Original quote in German: "So jetzt reicht's aber, Sie müssen jetzt endlich mit diesem Schmerz lernen zu leben, weil alle Frauen machen das und alle Frauen erleben das."

11 https://www.natelewisart.com.

years old and identifying as a cis woman of color. (Quote 2; ADHD) Participant 3 described their layers of social identity as genderqueer and of color, with family experience of displacement in fleeing another country to come to Germany, being socialized in Germany, and having a five-year-old child. (Quote 3; women in pain)

Quotes

The self-selection of the most meaningful and relevant passages of the interview yielded the following quotes to build upon in the further process of the project:

Quote 1, Participant 1:

> "So, in general, I don't have much confidence that I would be helped with racism in the medical context. Or that it would be recognized as such."[8]

Quote 2, healthcare professional to Participant 2:

> "But you have ADHD. You are incapable of sitting in a course for eight hours, listening and learning."[9]

Quote 3, healthcare professional to Participant 3:

> "Now that's enough. You need to finally learn how to live with the pain because all women do and all women experience pain."[10]

Translation to Musical Notations

The translation of the quotes to musical notations was performed as explained in the methods section "Musical Notations," which yielded three compositions. These quotes were prepared for translation to the lead sculpture. The process of applying the technique of embossing and debossing of musical notations was informed by the earlier work of artist Nate Lewis,[11] who participated in the workshop from which this edited volume results. We used embossing and debossing to insinuate the hierarchical expression of the portrayed, facilitating the embodiment of dominance/inferiority, the interplay of power and vulnerability, and offering plasticity to the asymmetrical relationship between healthcare professionals and patients

12 Gaslighting refers to the dismissal of a person's perception and lived reality; placed in medical context, it is referred to as medical gaslighting. Dusenbery states, "When medicine denies the reality of your bodily experience, it is a deeply invalidating form of gaslighting" (2017, 295). Sebring further elaborates: "Important to understanding the reasoning behind medical gaslighting is the ideologies that uphold medicine and science as the be-all-and-end-all; the ultimate source of objective, indisputable knowledge and truth. Western medicine as we know it today is a colonial enterprise that upholds logic, reason and science above lived experience" (2021, 1957).

in the setting of medical care (Freeman and Stewart 2019).

Lead Sculpture

To produce the lead sculptures, the metal was meticulously embossed and debossed by hand, while the reduced sheets of notations were used as a template. Each piece of lead ranged in size from 1.30 meters to 1.50 meters in width, and 45 centimeters in height. For installation purposes, the resulting sheets were framed by handcrafted steel stands, each with a height of 1.80 meters, and fixed onto the steel compositions using wire and eyelets, allowing the lead to be visible from both sides.

Leaflet

To provide a direct, accessible, and practical approach to the topic and to open up the possibility of carrying on this critical, transdisciplinary practice, we developed a leaflet that accompanied the installation and volume. The leaflet, with the title *How Not to Gaslight*,[12] contained a representational quote from the participants, which they explicitly shared for the purpose of directing them at healthcare professionals and/or the healthcare system as a whole. It further included an invitation to contact the project directly to continue sharing demands or experiences. This invitation addressed patients as well as healthcare professionals and affirmed that every person working in the healthcare system, whether they are just entering the field or are experienced, can contribute in multiple ways to raising awareness and engaging in change-making. The overall layout, color, and placement of wording were consciously chosen to grasp and metaphorically hint at the experience of being gaslit.

Limitations

First, most data on sex/gender, racism, and intersectionality in healthcare derives from Anglo-American contexts, and is therefore only partially applicable to German contexts. Further research to illuminate racist, sex/gender-based, and intersecting forms of discrimination in German healthcare contexts is sorely needed. Second, the transdisciplinary and multistep approach proved to be time-consuming and an intensive, multidisciplinary process calling for adaptations that a single disciplinary approach would not have required to the same degree within the project's short timeline. This also accounts for the time given to applied reflexivity, and the decision to inquire with a semi-structured rather than an unstructured interview format, which might have allowed for more in-depth and open conversations. Third, the persons to interview could have been diversified and multiplied to a greater extent, including more dimensions of intersecting identities, languages, social settings, and hence varieties of experiences and psychosocial realities. This is even more relevant with regard to which topics were chosen to be discussed within this paper (sexism, racism). For example, ableism frequently informs healthcare practice, and ability as another layer of social identity must be integrated in an intersectional discourse. We chose to first focus on the core layers of social identity intersectionality as a framework that we as authors brought to this project and then were directed by the participants' narratives. Nevertheless, the aim ought invariably to be to highlight, extensively discuss, and integrate further marginalizing axes and lived realities. The limitations of this project ideally offer avenues for future research and collaborations.

Conclusion

When conventional languages fall short of grasping and portraying complex realities, as Toni Morrison concluded, "this is precisely the time when artists go to work. . . . We speak, we write, we do language. That is how civilizations heal" (2015, 185). Using different tools to communicate complex matters of human existence and observe them from multiple angles can contribute to raising awareness and eventually shifting priorities.

As scientific progress and structural prioritization are a long time coming, this project might serve as a means to reinforce transdisciplinary approaches and draw attention to the significance and urgency of addressing intersectional discrimination in healthcare. As we have learned in our collaboration, these approaches prove to be labor-intensive though indis-

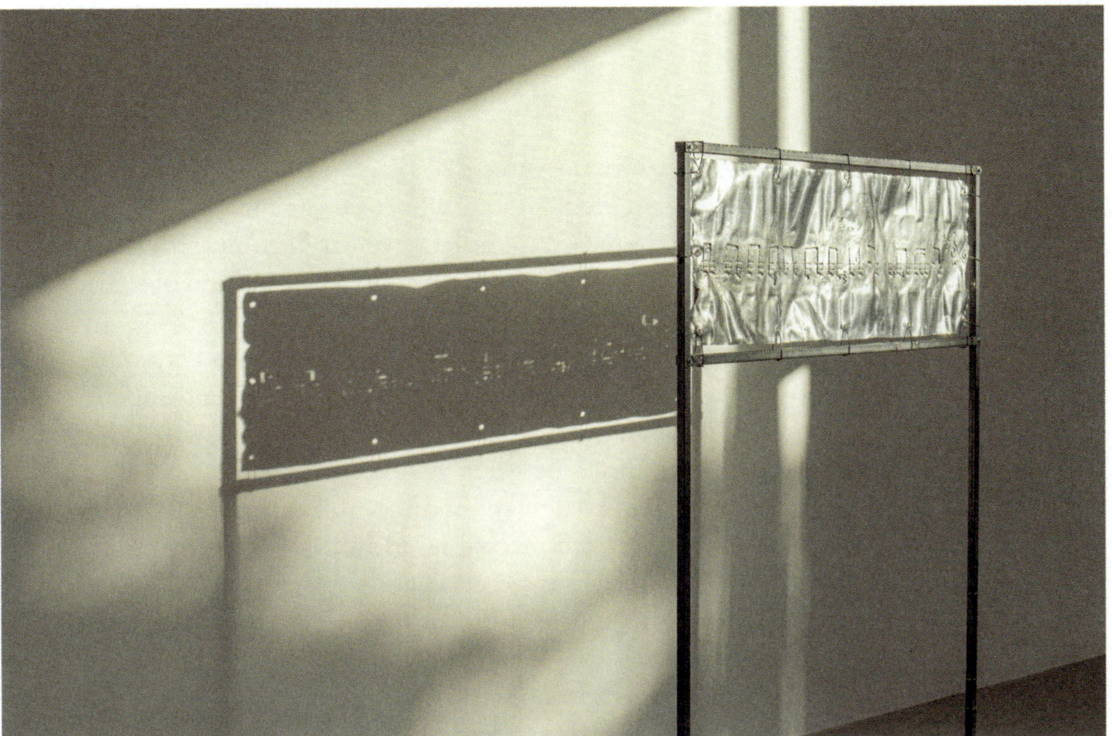

FIG. 2

FIG. 2 Awa Naghipour, Joana Atemengue Owana, Golnar Kat Rahmani, *"Sie haben aber ADHS, Sie können nicht acht Stunden am Tag im Kurs sitzen und zuhören und lernen,"* 2024, lead and steel, 1.8 × 1.3 m. Photo: Joana Atemengue Owona pensable in challenging the intractably unjust status quo.

Artistic Reflections

Joana Atemengue Owona

To engage with the subject of silencing is to listen. It means attempting to democratize whose voices and subjects are given attention. In regard to the labor of carving out this very space, we must acknowledge the emotional toil and toll of sharing our experiences of discrimination.

At the core of our project, we have placed questions of how to render the inherent inequities, the lack of empathy, and gaps in data faced by marginalized individuals within the German healthcare system visible. How can we accentuate this lacking acknowledgment of discomfort and pain, so that it becomes vocal and accessible? How can we fend off the instrumentalization of subjective experiences while employing a participatory approach? How can we combine analytical methods with artistic practices to establish awareness and recognition? How can we listen?

The central foundation of our collaboration is the firsthand accounts of people affected by a plurality of marginalizing practices within the German healthcare system. Out of each interview we conducted, one pivotal statement, highlighted by the participants themselves, has been translated into musical notations. Accordingly, the quotes are embedded in a language that evokes tactility and audibility. Though visible to the eye and tangible by further engagement with the works, the notations and their underlying contents cannot actually be heard. Encapsulated in three sculptures, specifically conceptualized for this project, they are embossed and debossed in three towering sheets of lead, a material that is commonly used in medical practice to shield patients from radiation and that simultaneously holds serious poisonous qualities. All pieces are installed in a steel frame intentionally left with its marks of construction, like surgical wounds or scars and bruises that recall a history of exterior influences. With our project, we intend to center listening and mediation, part of which is the

13 "Unsere Körper werden nie einfach 'nur' gesehen. Sie werden und sind gleichzeitig vergeschlechtlicht und rassifiziert – und zwar auch dann, wenn wir krank sind. Die Konsequenz daraus ist, dass umgekehrt ebenfalls Krankheit als eine Konstruktion zu analysieren ist, in die sich das Ineinandergreifen von 'Rasse,' Geschlecht und Sexualität immer neu einschreibt, die folglich gesellschaftliche Machtfelder wie Rassismus und HeteroSexismus reflektiert und zudem von kolonialen Echos durchzogen ist. . . . Die Unterwerfung Schwarzer Menschen zu passiv und zweckdienlich imaginierten Körpern (Entsubjektivierung) ist dabei eines der zentralen kolonialen Echos, das als Moment Weißer Selbstverständlichkeit auch im heutigen medizinischen Kontext widerhallt" (English translation by the author).

continued offer to share personal experiences regarding the subject matter with us, as portrayed in *How Not to Gaslight*. The following passages will introduce a brief contextualization of the systemic silencing of marginalized bodies within the healthcare system, followed by a more detailed portrayal of the artworks in regard to conceptual, technical, and material aspects.

As introduced in "A Transdisciplinary Approach to Visualizing Intersectional Discrimination in German Healthcare," each conversation with a participant yielded one key moment, chosen by the participants themselves, to employ within the artwork. All quotes appear in their original form in German as the titles of the artwork. Whether a clear personal statement, as in the first quote, or directly echoing the response of a healthcare professional, as in the last two quotes, the inherent violence of these accounts and subsequently the violence of these exposures is evident and an acute representation of the de-subjectification (Hutson 2007) of non-White, non-male bodies. Systemic power relations are drenched in racialized and gendered constructions of sickness, which consequently maintain and (re)produce colonial and patriarchal continuities. In the chapter "Schwarzkrank? Post/koloniale Rassifizierungen von Krankheit in Deutschland," Christiane Hutson examines this issue. Based on her own experiences as a Black woman with a history of sickness, she analyzes how historical and contemporary patterns of power contribute to healthcare that discriminates:

> Our bodies are never simply "just seen." They are simultaneously gendered and racialized—and this is also the case when we are ill. The consequence is that, conversely, illness must also be analyzed as a construct in which the intertwining of "race," gender, and sexuality are constantly reinscribed, one that consequently reflects societal zones of power such as racism and heterosexism and is also permeated by colonial echoes. . . . The subjugation of Black people to passively and expediently imagined bodies (de-subjectification) is one of the central colonial echoes that reverberate as a moment of White self-evidence, included in

14 "Angesichts dieser historischen Verkürzungen oder sogar Enthistorisierungen werden sowohl Kolonialismus als auch strukturell normatives Weißsein nicht als gewaltvolle Kontexte wahrgenommen, die wissenschaftliches Forschen und Arbeiten geformt haben und, in aktualisierten Versionen, noch immer formen" (English translation by the author).

today's medical context. (Hutson 2007, 229–30)[13]

Regarding the medical context, Hutson exposes Western medicine as a White technology of dominance and control and as an exclusionary field of knowledge production. She emphasizes the importance of relating the two to one another, in order to strain toward a space for the articulation of silenced experiences. According to Hutson, this analysis is key for not just enabling a vocalization and a possible overcoming of such silences, but also for deliberately marking the above-mentioned constructions as violent (2007, 230). Her inquiry into how histories of German colonialism have created a basis for racialized biological interpretations demonstrates how the same histories remain disregarded when looking at contemporary linkages between science, politics, and colonial legacies.

> In view of these historical reductions or even de-historicizations, both colonialism and structurally normative Whiteness are not perceived as violent contexts that have shaped and, in updated versions, continue to shape scientific research and work. (2007, 235)[14]

A similar consideration of course can be stated in regard to gendered constructions of illness and legacies of patriarchal junctures. Arguing along kindred scrutiny, May Ayim concludes in the article "White Stress/Black Nerves" (2003) that systemic disregard and bias, more often than not, result in mistrusting the patient, rather than interrogating the precarious legacies of the system.

> Most available cases examining the mental-health situation of immigrants and black Germans are based on medical and symptomatic interpretations. Very seldom do social scientists candidly state their research interests and self-critically reflect upon their own position and assessment methodologies. Nevertheless, if, often, we find reference to differences in the manifestation and handling of illnesses, there remains a lack of guidance and

> examples explaining how such differences can be appropriately incorporated, and where the possibilities and limits of therapeutic efficacy lie. Frequency and characteristics of individual illnesses are the focus of interest, but not the personal and social circumstances within which these illnesses develop. The result is, then, that, instead of pursuing the causal factors for the illness, it is often the patients themselves that become problematized. (2003, 91–92)

These practices of imposing narratives and the systematic deprivation of the right to speak about one's body and its pains exhibit a pattern of silencing individual experiences. Therefore, we have placed the narratives of the affected as the essence of our artistic conceptualization.

The sculptures consist of three pieces of lead, ranging from 1.3 meters to 1.5 meters in width, and 45 centimeters in height. They are each framed by a large steel construction that itself is elevated to a height of 1.8 meters. At the height of the audience's head, the lead is clamped into the frame, punched in with eyelets, held up by wire, and installed like a banner, while evoking barriers, hurdles, or a way to display signs in a public space of sorts. The marks of construction and time are still visible. Seams from welding, scars from sanding, and rust from aging remain an integral part of the material as a marker of its history and reprocessing. Some old and grown over with scabs, some fresh and open, like an exposure of the lower layers of skin. The quotes (see page 10), translated into notations are embossed and debossed on each sheet of lead, naturally appearing mirrored on the opposite side. The malleability of the material allows for it to be bent into shape. Upon further visual investigation, the viewer will be able to decipher that the statements from the medical professionals—directed toward the participants and making a lasting impression on them—emerge outward. The notation translated from a personal statement retracts inward as debossed.

This material translation of the latter topics and

FIG. 3 Awa Naghipour, Joana Atemengue Owana, Golnar Kat Rahmani, *Seen but Not Heard*, installation view, 2024. Photo: Joana Atemengue Owona

FIG. 4 Awa Naghipour, Joana Atemengue Owana, Golnar Kat Rahmani, *"Also ich hab' generell nicht viel Vertrauen, dass mir mit erlebtem Rassismus im medizinischen Kontext geholfen wird, oder dass er als solcher überhaupt anerkannt wird,"* 2024, lead and steel, 1.8 × 1.5 m. Photo: Joana Atemengue Owona

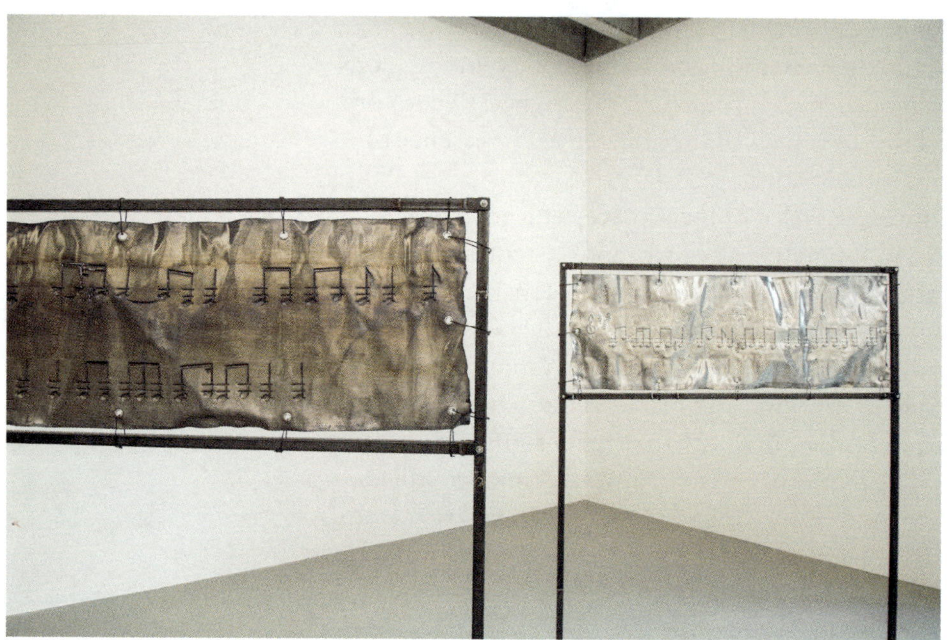

FIG. 3

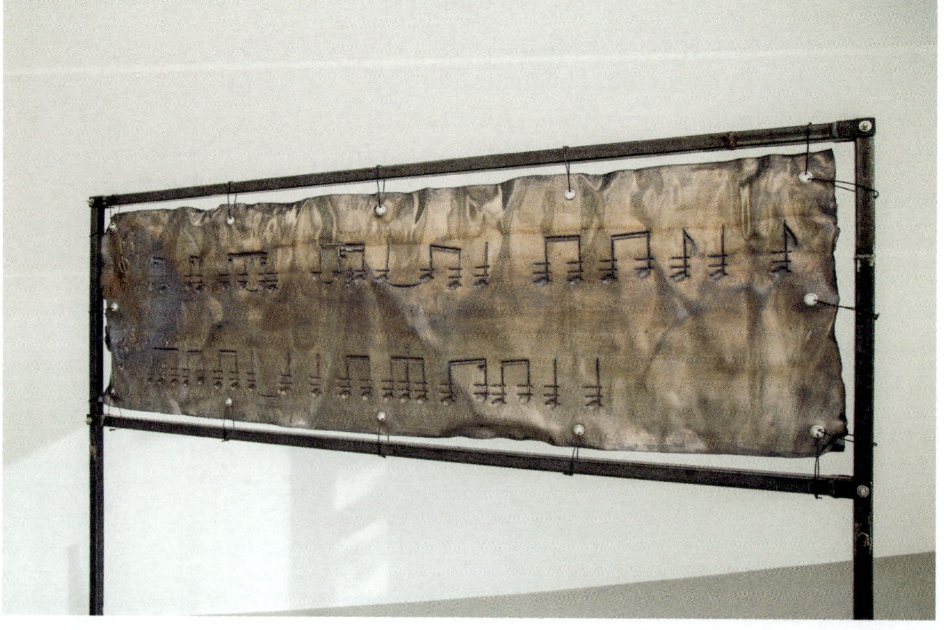

FIG. 4

statements relate to the consideration of embossing and debossing as an intimate technique of laying bare and uncovering the nuances of systemic violent patterns. This amalgamation of the methodological and technical with the physical aspects constitutes a dynamic that becomes visible when looking at the lead as dislocated in its original form. Additionally, the mirroring of the contents both figuratively and metaphorically renders the hegemonic ambivalence of this power dynamic even more prominent. As a conscious, physical action, done by hand and carefully executed, the confrontation with the material is deepened. Pushing, punctuating, dragging, and hammering the lead into shape recalls the way in which words and forms of treatment can inscribe themselves into our bodies, our experiences, and our minds. A lasting impression that leaves its markings, dents, and expansions, sometimes so forceful that it rips small cuts and holes into the metal. These ostensible wounds reflect the distinct micro and macro aggressions of the healthcare system as a whole.

Regarding the lead itself, the most palpable significance it poses for us is its long history in the sciences and medicine to shield and protect a patient from the radiation of X-rays. Contrary to it functioning like an armor, intended to safeguard from harm, it is also heavily toxic. Lead can poison the body, therefore posing a hazardous health risk if ingested. This dooming reality renders it fortuitous and fatal, protective, and devastating at the same time, and transfers a dual and contradictory agency to the installation—a duality of agency that is agonizingly pronounced by the impossibility of promptly translating the musical notations into sound. The works are not simply illustrating the circumstances of discriminatory practices; they are testimonials to the complexity of ramifications that are imposed upon the targeted individuals. On the one hand, not believing a patient, ignoring, stereotyping, or not taking them seriously is an explicit negation of autonomy. Not to be heard, on the other hand, does not mean not being able to speak. On the contrary, it often means having to labor intensely—speak more, louder, repeatedly—in order to be

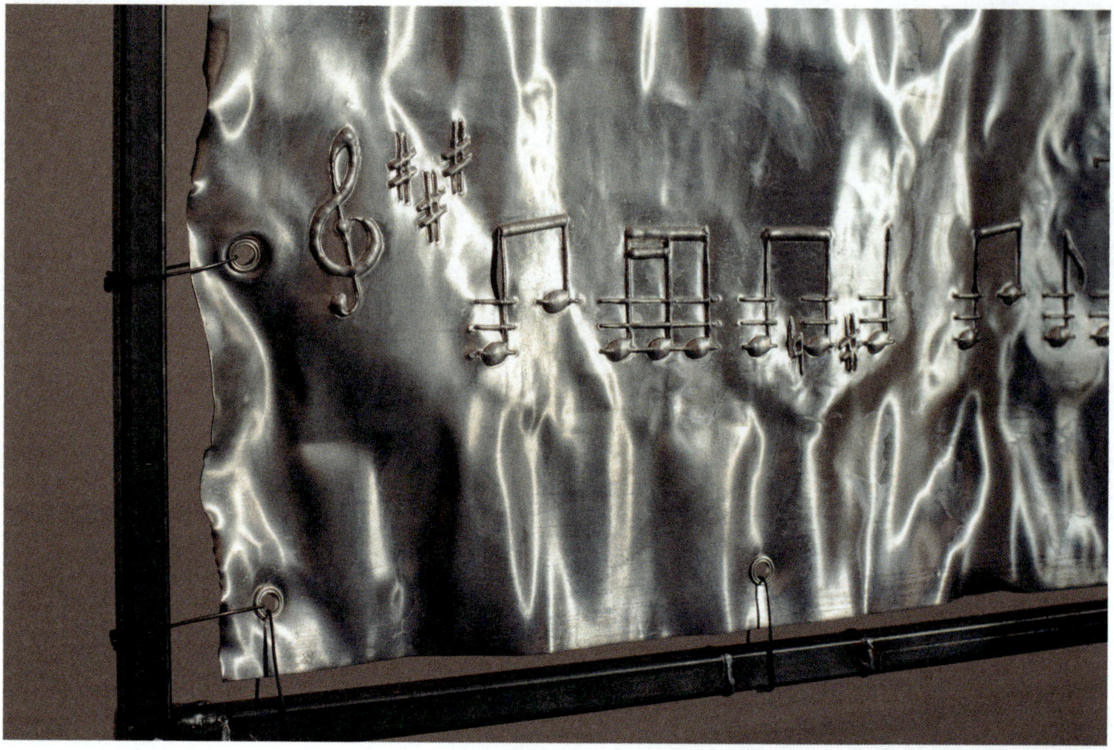

FIG. 5

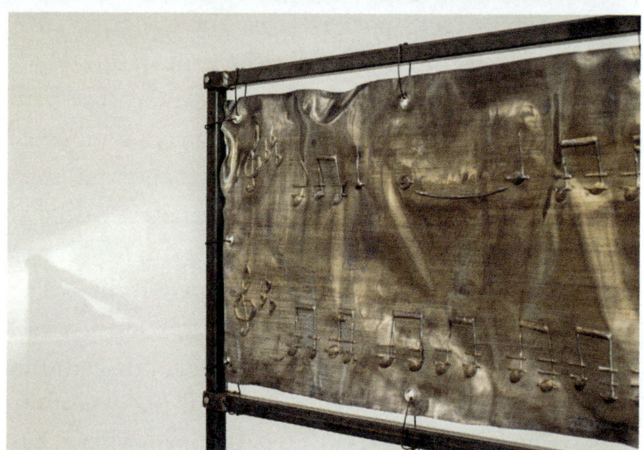

FIG. 6

FIG. 5 Awa Naghipour, Joana Atemengue Owana, Golnar Kat Rahmani, *“Sie haben aber ADHS, Sie können nicht acht Stunden am Tag im Kurs sitzen und zuhören und lernen,”* 2024, lead and steel, 1.8 × 1.3 m. Photo: Joana Atemengue Owona
FIG. 6 Awa Naghipour, Joana Atemengue Owana, Golnar Kat Rahmani, *“So jetzt reicht’s aber, Sie müssen jetzt endlich mit diesem Schmerz lernen zu leben, weil alle Frauen machen das und alle Frauen erleben das,”* 2024, lead and steel, 1.8 × 1.5 m. Photo: Joana Atemengue Owona

noticed. A silent display of sheet music is just that: silent. Only when sitting in this ringing silence are we able to hear the faint clamors of those unheard and disbelieved by the medical system. In some ways, the inaudible notations on the sculptures insist on an engagement with the sound of these voices, especially *because* they are being silenced. The pieces therefore think through the quotes and the meaning they carry. The silence critiques, pokes back, perforates, pinches, and shrieks of absence and presence at the same time. The viewer is thrown back onto themselves, having to deal with a subject that exceeds even spoken words. The evident silencing, then, is juxtaposed by the titles of the works. Directly stating the participants' experiences of bias and uncommonly long for a title, the complete quotes are readable once more.

As mentioned in "A Transdisciplinary Approach to Intersectional Discrimination in German Healthcare," we are extending the offer to anyone affected by these biases to contact us and share their account of their experiences. Contact information can be found on the accompanying leaflet, which includes a representational demand, chosen again by the interview participants themselves and directed toward the hegemonic power structures of the medical system. These demands have their own way of critiquing and disrupting common stereotypical narratives, highlighting social attitudes, and, most importantly, pointing out the absurdity, frustration, intensity, and urgency this project aims to convey. The transdisciplinary approach, but especially the imperative inclusion of individuals with lived experiences of illness, can create a distinct space of attention. It places at its heart the multidimensional perspectives and draws comprehensible links between them, while emphasizing the importance of disrupting imposed silences. Or, in the words of Audre Lorde:

> We can learn to work and speak when we are afraid in the same way we have learned to work and speak when we are tired. For we have been socialized to respect fear more than our own needs for language and definition, and

> while we wait in silence for that final luxury of fearlessness, the weight of that silence will choke us. The fact that we are here and that I speak these words is an attempt to break that silence and bridge some of those differences between us, for it is not difference which immobilizes us, but silence. And there are so many silences to be broken. (2007, 44)

Our collaboration carries with it the intention of political mediation, communication, and exchange so that we can contribute to starting to close the gaps and continuities of a dismissive system and of a broader dialogue about health, illness, and human experience. For being poisoned by a system that should be there to protect us means that this system needs to change drastically.

Contributions

This project was a co-creative collaborative process substantially and collectively carried out by all contributors.
Initiation and first draft of the concept: Awa Naghipour
Concept development and finalization: All
Graphic design: Golnar Kat Rahmani
Interview protocol: All
Interviews: Golnar Kat Rahmani, Awa Naghipour
Musical notations: Awa Naghipour
Lead sculptures: Joana Atemengue Owona
Leaflet content: Interview participants and all
Leaflet design: Golnar Kat Rahmani
"A Transdisciplinary Approach to Visualizing Intersectional Discrimination in German Healthcare": Awa Naghipour
"Artistic Reflections": Joana Atemengue Owona

FIG. 7 Awa Naghipour, Joana Atemengue Owana, Golnar Kat Rahmani, *"So jetzt reicht's aber, Sie müssen jetzt endlich mit diesem Schmerz lernen zu leben, weil alle Frauen machen das und alle Frauen erleben das,"* 2024, lead and steel, 1.8 × 1.5 m. Photo: Joana Atemengue Owona

FIG. 7

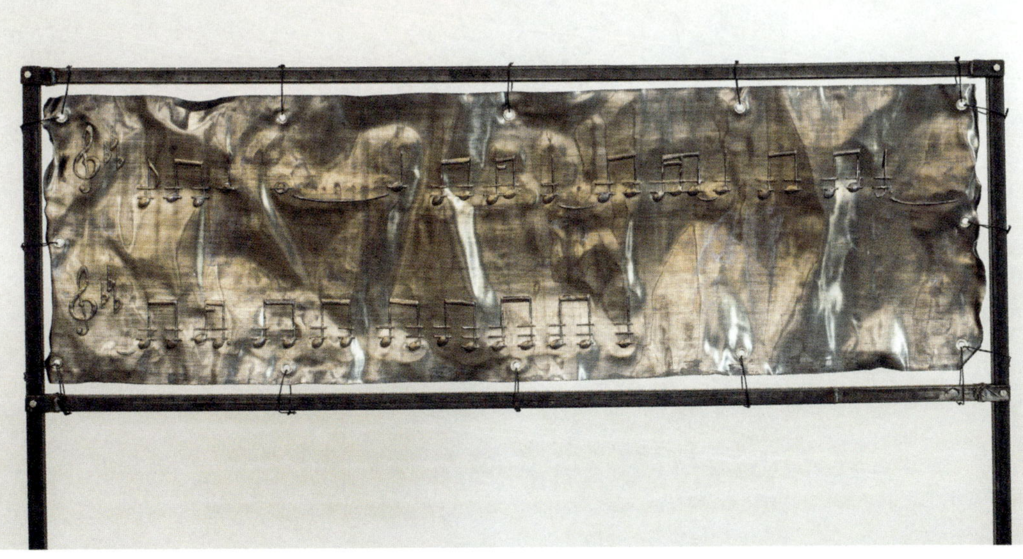

FIG. 8

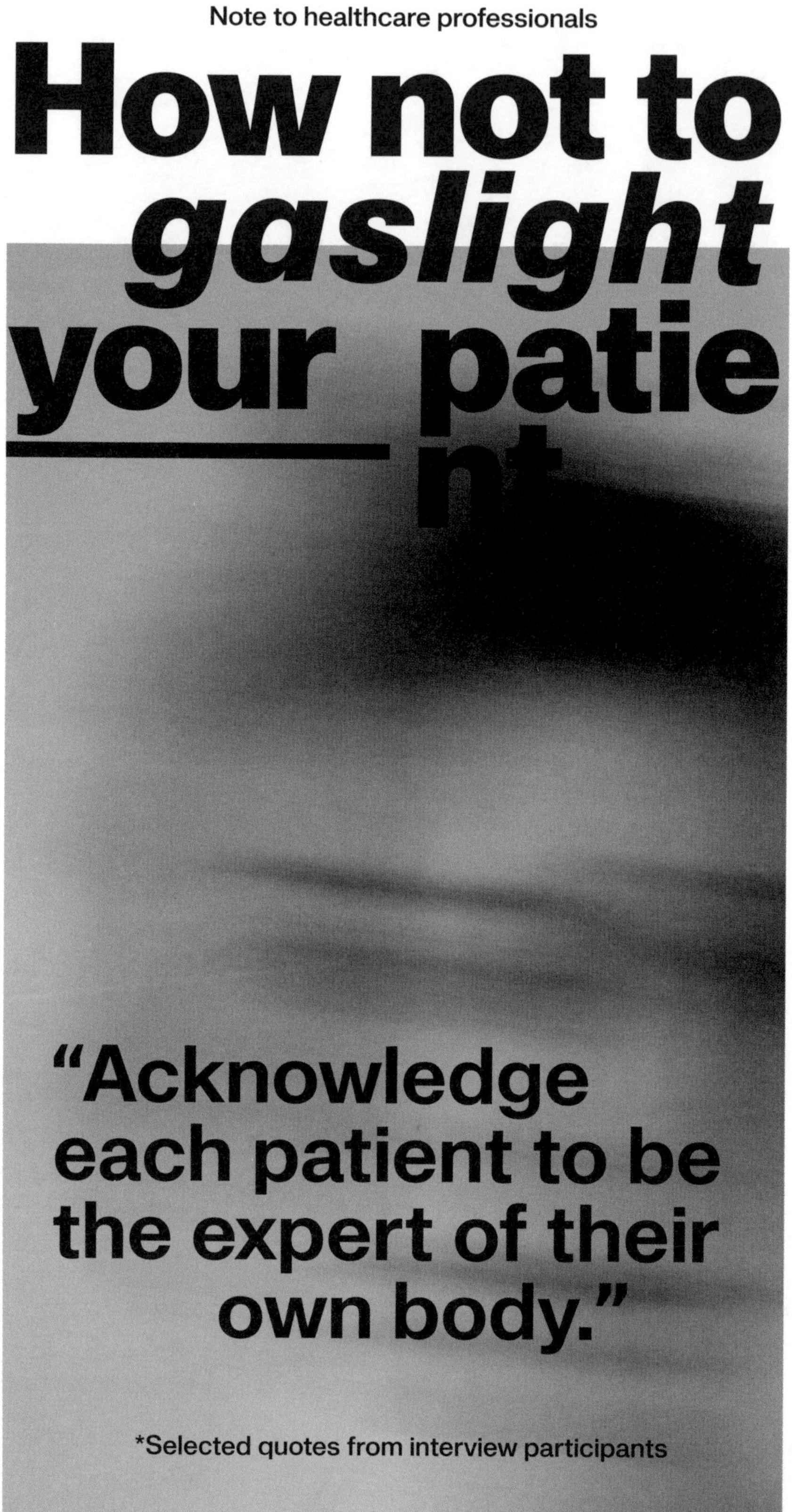

Note to healthcare professionals

How not to *gaslight* your patie nt

“Acknowledge each patient to be the expert of their own body.”

*Selected quotes from interview participants

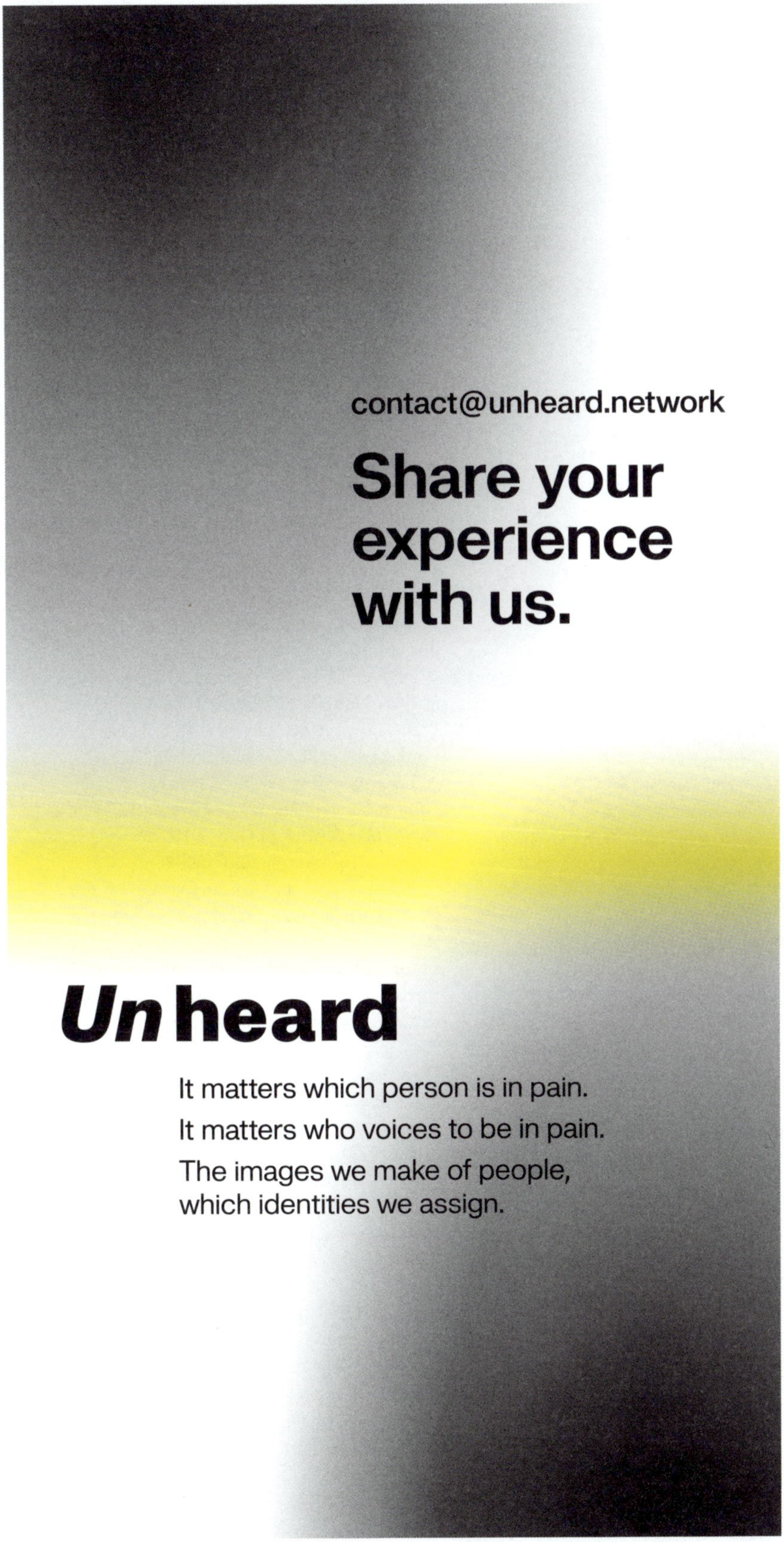

FIG. 8 Awa Naghipour, Joana Atemengue Owana, Golnar Kat Rahmani, *How Not to Gaslight*, 2024, leaflet, 29.7 × 10.5 cm

contact@unheard.network

Share your experience with us.

***Un*heard**

It matters which person is in pain.

It matters who voices to be in pain.

The images we make of people, which identities we assign.

A

Abrams, Jasmine A., Ariella Tabaac, Sarah Jung, and Nicole M. Else-Quest (2020) "Considerations for Employing Intersectionality in Qualitative Health Research." *Social Science & Medicine* 258 (August): 113138. https://doi.org/10.1016/j.socscimed.2020.113138.

Aikins, Muna A., Teresa Bremberger, Joshua K. Aikins, Daniel Gyamerah, and Deniz Yildirim-Caliman (2021) "Afrozensus 2020: Perspektiven, Anti-Schwarze Rassismuserfahrungen und Engagement Schwarzer, Afrikanischer und Afrodiasporischer Menschen in Deutschland, Berlin." EOTO. https://afrozensus.de/reports/2020/.

Akintemi, Olakunle B., and Kenneth B. Roberts (2022) "Race and Urinary Tract Infections in Young Children with Fever." *JAMA Pediatrics* 176 (6): 547–48. https://doi.org/10.1001/jamapediatrics.2022.0693.

Anders, Sari M. van (2015) "Beyond Sexual Orientation: Integrating Gender/Sex and Diverse Sexualities via Sexual Configurations Theory." *Archives of Sexual Behavior* 44 (5): 1177–1213. https://doi.org/10.1007/s10508-015-0490-8.

Andrasfay, Theresa, and Noreen Goldman (2021) "Reductions in 2020 US Life Expectancy Due to COVID-19 and the Disproportionate Impact on the Black and Latino Populations." *Proceedings of the National Academy of Sciences of the United States of America* 118 (5). https://doi.org/10.1073/pnas.2014746118.

Arias, Elizabeth, and Betzaida Tejada-Vera (2023) "Differential Impact of the COVID-19 Pandemic on Excess Mortality and Life Expectancy Loss within the Hispanic Population." *Demographic Research* 48 (12): 339–52. https://doi.org/10.4054/DemRes.2023.48.12.

Ateş, Merih, Kira Bouaoud, Nora Freitag, Matilda M. Gahein-Sama, Tanja Gangarova, Camille Ionescu, Mujtaba A. Isani, Elisabeth Kaneza, Tae J. Kim, and Felicia B. Lazaridou (2023) "Rassismus und seine Symptome: Bericht des Nationalen Diskriminierungs- und Rassismusmonitors." Nationaler Diskriminierungs- und Rassismusmonitor NaDiRa-Bericht.

Ayim, May (2003) "White Stress, Black Nerves: Stress Factor Racism [1995]." In *Blues in Black and White: A Collection of Essays, Poetry and Conversations*. Translated by Anne V. Adams, 73–100. Trenton, NJ: Africa Research & Publications.

B

Bailey, Zinzi D., Nancy Krieger, Madina Agénor, Jasmine Graves, Natalia Linos, and Mary T. Bassett (2017) "Structural Racism and Health Inequities in the USA: Evidence and Interventions." *Lancet* 389 (10077): 1453–63. https://doi.org/10.1016/S0140-6736(17)30569-X.

Bartig, Susanne, Dorina Kalkum, Ha M. Le, and Aleksandra Lewicki (2021) "Diskriminierungsrisiken und Diskriminierungsschutz im Gesundheitswesen – Wissensstand und Forschungsbedarf für die Antidiskriminierungsforschung." Studie im Auftrag der Antidiskriminierungsstelle des Bundes. https://www.antidiskriminierungsstelle.de/SharedDocs/downloads/DE/publikationen/Expertisen/diskrimrisiken_diskrimschutz_gesundheitswesen.html.

Bartram, Isabelle, Laura Schnieder, Nils Ellebrecht, Florian Ruland, Tino Plümecke, and Andrea zur Nieden (2023) "Categorizing People in the German Life Sciences: A Systematic Literature Review of Classifications of Human Diversity." *Discover Social Science and Health* 3 (1): 4. https://doi.org/10.1007/s44155-023-00033-5.

Bauer, Greta R., Siobhan M. Churchill, Mayuri Mahendran, Chantel Walwyn, Daniel Lizotte, and Alma Angelica Villa-Rueda (2021) "Intersectionality in Quantitative Research: A Systematic Review of Its Emergence and Applications of Theory and Methods." *SSM – Population Health* 14 (June): 100798. https://doi.org/10.1016/j.ssmph.2021.100798.

Becher, Eva, and Sabine Oertelt-Prigione (2022) "History and Development of Sex- and Gender Sensitive Medicine (SGSM)." In *International Review of Neurobiology*. Edited by Elena Moro, Gennarina Arabia, Maria Carmela Tartaglia, and Maria Teresa Ferretti, 164: 1–25. "Sex and Gender Differences in Neurological Disease: Sex and Gender Differences in Neurological Disease." In *International Review of Neurobiology* 164: 1–25. https://doi.org/10.1016/bs.irn.2022.06.008.

Bowleg, Lisa (2012) "The Problem with the Phrase Women and Minorities: Intersectionality – An Important Theoretical Framework for Public Health." *American Journal of Public Health* 102 (7): 1267–73. https://doi.org/10.2105/AJPH.2012.300750.

Bowleg, Lisa (2021) "Evolving Intersectionality within Public Health: From Analysis to Action." *American Journal of Public Health* 111 (1): 88–90. https://doi.org/10.2105/AJPH.2020.306031.

Brady, Emer, Mathias Wullum Nielsen, Jens Peter Andersen, and Sabine Oertelt-Prigione (2021) "Lack of Consideration of Sex and Gender in COVID-19 Clinical Studies." *Nature Communications* 12 (1): 4015. https://doi.org/10.1038/s41467-021-24265-8.

C

Collins, Patricia Hill (2015) "Intersectionality's Definitional Dilemmas." *Annual Review of Sociology* 41: 1–20. https://doi.org/10.1146/annurev-soc-073014-112142.

Combahee River Collective (1977) "The Combahee River Collective: A Black Feminist Statement." In *Capitalist Patriarchy and the Case for Socialist Feminism*. Edited by Zillah Eisenstein, 362–72. New York: New York University Press. http://www.jstor.org/stable/jj.17102150.24.

Crear-Perry, Joia, Rosaly Correa-de-Araujo, Tamara Lewis Johnson, Monica R. McLemore, Elizabeth Neilson, and Maeve Wallace (2021) "Social and Structural Determinants of Health Inequities in Maternal Health." *Journal of Women's Health* 30 (2): 230–35. https://doi.org/10.1089/jwh.2020.8882.

Crenshaw, Kimberlé (1989) "Demarginalizing the Intersection of Race and Sex: A Black Feminist Critique of Antidiscrimination Doctrine, Feminist Theory and Antiracist Politics." *University of Chicago Legal Forum* 1: 139–67.

D

Dahlgren, Göran, and Margaret Whitehead (1991) "Policies and Strategies to Promote Social Equity in Health: Background Document to WHO – Strategy Paper for Europe." *Institute for Futures Studies, Arbetsrapport* 14 (January).

Dore, Rebecca A., Kelly M. Hoffman, Angeline S. Lillard, and Sophie Trawalter (2014) "Children's Racial Bias in Perceptions of Others' Pain." *The British Journal of Developmental Psychology* 32 (2): 218–31. https://doi.org/10.1111/bjdp.12038.

DuBois, L. Zachary, and Heather Shattuck-Heidorn (2021) "Challenging the Binary: Gender/Sex and the Bio-Logics of Normalcy." *American Journal of Human Biology: The Official Journal of the Human Biology Council* 33 (5): e23623. https://doi.org/10.1002/ajhb.23623.

Dusenbery, Maya (2017) *Doing Harm: The Truth about How Bad Medicine and Lazy Science Leave Women Dismissed, Misdiagnosed, and Sick*. 1st edition. New York: HarperOne.

E

El-Mafaalani, Aladin (2023) "Diskriminierung von Menschen mit Migrationshintergrund und Migrantisierten." In *Handbuch Diskriminierung*. Edited by Albert Scherr, Anna Cornelia Reinhardt, and Aladin El-Mafaalani, 483–99. Wiesbaden: Springer Fachmedien. https://doi.org/10.1007/978-3-658-42800-6.

F

Foroutan, Naika, Noa Ha, Frank Kalter, Yasemin Shooman, and Cihan Sinanoglu (2022) "Rassistische Realitäten: Wie setzt sich Deutschland mit Rassismus auseinander?" Auftaktstudie zum Nationalen Diskriminierungs- und Rassismusmonitor (NaDiRa). Berlin: Deutsches Zentrum für Integrations- und Migrationsforschung (DeZIM).

Freeman, Lauren, and Heather Stewart (2019) "Epistemic Microaggressions and Epistemic Injustices in Clinical Medicine." In *Overcoming Epistemic Injustice: Social and Psychological Perspectives*. Edited by Benjamin R. Sherman and Stacey Goguen, 95–121. Lanham, MD: Rowman & Littlefield International.

G

GBD 2015 Maternal Mortality Collaborators (2016) "Global, Regional, and National Levels of Maternal Mortality, 1990–2015: A Systematic Analysis for the Global Burden of Disease Study 2015." *Lancet* 388 (10053): 1775–1812. https://doi.org/10.1016/S0140-6736(16)31470-2.

Gkiouleka, Anna, Tim Huijts, Jason Beckfield, and Clare Bambra (2018) "Understanding the Micro and Macro Politics of Health: Inequalities, Intersectionality & Institutions – A Research Agenda." *Social Science & Medicine* 200 (March): 92–98. https://doi.org/10.1016/j.socscimed.2018.01.025.

Guan, Alice, Marilyn Thomas, Eric Vittinghoff, Lisa Bowleg, Christina Mangurian, and Paul Wesson (2021) "An Investigation of Quantitative Methods for Assessing Intersectionality in Health Research: A Systematic Review." *SSM – Population Health* 16 (December): 100977. https://doi.org/10.1016/j.ssmph.2021.100977.

H

Hahne, Alexander (2024) "Trans Und Nichtbinäre Menschen." In *LSBTI* in Pflege Und Medizin: Grundlagen Und Handlungsempfehlungen Zur Versorgung Queerer Menschen*. Edited by Volker Wierz and Michael Nürnberg, 52–59. Stuttgart: Georg Thieme Verlag.

Haider, Ahmed, Susan Bengs, Judy Luu, Elena Osto, Jolanta M. Siller-Matula, Taulant Muka, and Catherine Gebhard (2020) "Sex and Gender in Cardiovascular Medicine: Presentation and Outcomes of Acute Coronary Syndrome." *European Heart Journal* 41 (13): 1328–36. https://doi.org/10.1093/eurheartj/ehz898.

Hankivsky, Olena (2014) *Intersectionality 101*, Vancouver: Institute for Intersectionality Research and Policy, Simon Fraser University.

Hankivsky, Olena, and Ashlee Christoffersen (2008) "Intersectionality and the Determinants of Health: A Canadian Perspective." *Critical Public Health* 18 (September): 271–83. https://doi.org/10.1080/09581590802294296.

Hankivsky, Olena, Colleen Reid, Renee Cormier, Colleen Varcoe, Natalie Clark, Cecilia Benoit, and Shari Brotman (2010) "Exploring the Promises of Intersectionality for Advancing Women's Health Research." *International Journal for Equity in Health* 9 (February): 5. https://doi.org/10.1186/1475-9276-9-5.

Heinz, Andreas, Daniel J. Müller, Sören Krach, Maurice Cabanis, and Ulrike P. Kluge (2014) "The Uncanny Return of the Race Concept." *Frontiers in Human Neuroscience* 8: 836. https://doi.org/10.3389/fnhum.2014.00836.

Heise, Lori, Margaret E. Greene, Neisha Opper, Maria Stavropoulou, Caroline Harper, Marcos Nascimento, Debrework Zewdie, and Gender Equality, Norms, and Health Steering Committee (2019) "Gender Inequality and Restrictive Gender Norms: Framing the Challenges to Health." *Lancet* 393 (10189): 2440–54. https://doi.org/10.1016/S0140-6736(19)30652-X.

Hoffman, Kelly M., Sophie Trawalter, Jordan R. Axt, and M. Norman Oliver (2016) "Racial Bias in Pain Assessment and Treatment Recommendations, and False Beliefs about Biological Differences between Blacks and Whites." *Proceedings of the National Academy of Sciences of the United States of America* 113 (16): 4296–4301. https://doi.org/10.1073/pnas.1516047113.

Hutson, Christiane (2007) "Schwarzkrank? Post/Koloniale Rassifizierungen von Krankheit in Deutschland." In *Re/Visionen: Postkoloniale Perspektiven von People of Color Auf Rassismus, Kulturpolitik und Widerstand in Deutschland*. Edited by Kien Nghi Ha, Nicola Nicola Lauré al-Samarai, and Sheila Mysorekar, 229–41. Münster: Unrast. https://search.library.wisc.edu/catalog/9910055275102121.

Hyde, Janet Shibley, Rebecca S. Bigler, Daphna Joel, Charlotte Chucky Tate, and Sari M. Van Anders (2019) "The Future of Sex and Gender in Psychology: Five Challenges to the Gender Binary." *American Psychologist* 74 (2): 171–93. https://doi.org/10.1037/amp0000307.

L

Lazaridou, Felicia Boma, Andreas Heinz, Daniel Schulze, and Dinesh Bhugra (2023) "Racialised Identity, Racism and the Mental Health of Children and Adolescents." *International Review of Psychiatry* 35 (3–4): 277–88. https://doi.org/10.1080/09540261.2023.2181059.

Lorde, Audre (2007) *Sister Outsider: Essays and Speeches*. Berkeley, CA: Crossing Press.

M

Mathur, Vani A., Jennifer A. Richeson, Judith A. Paice, Michael Muzyka, and Joan Y. Chiao (2014) "Racial Bias in Pain Perception and Response: Experimental Examination of Automatic and Deliberate Processes." *The Journal of Pain* 15 (5): 476–84. https://doi.org/10.1016/j.jpain.2014.01.488.

Mauvais-Jarvis, Franck, Noel Bairey Merz, Peter J. Barnes, Roberta D. Brinton, Juan-Jesus Carrero, Dawn L. DeMeo, Geert J. De Vries, et al. (2020) "Sex and Gender: Modifiers of Health, Disease, and Medicine." *Lancet* 396 (10250): 565–82. https://doi.org/10.1016/S0140-6736(20)31561-0.

McGlothen-Bell, Kelly, Madelyne Z. Greene, Grayson Hunt, and Allison D. Crawford (2023) "Intersectional Examination of Gender-Inclusive Care and Women's Health." *Journal of Obstetric, Gynecologic, and Neonatal Nursing* 52 (6): 442–53. https://doi.org/10.1016/j.jogn.2023.08.007.

Meghani, Salimah H., Eeeseung Byun, and Rollin M. Gallagher (2012) "Time to Take Stock: A Meta-Analysis and Systematic Review of Analgesic Treatment Disparities for Pain in the United States." *Pain Medicine* 13 (2): 150–74. https://doi.org/10.1111/j.1526-4637.2011.01310.x.

Morrison, Toni (2015) "No Place for Self-Pity, No Room for Fear." *The Nation* (March 23): 184–85.

N

Nguyễn, Ann Thúy, and Maya Pendleton (2020) "Recognizing Race in Language: Why We Capitalize 'Black' and 'White.'" Center for the Study of Social Policy. March 23, 2020. https://cssp.org/recognizing-race-in-language-why-we-capitalize-black-and-white/.

O

Oertelt-Prigione, Sabine, and Vera Regitz-Zagrosek, eds. (2012) *Sex and Gender Aspects in Clinical Medicine*. London: Springer. https://doi.org/10.1007/978-0-85729-832-4.

Ogungbe, Oluwabunmi, Amal Mitra, and Joni Roberts (2019) "A Systematic Review of Implicit Bias in Health Care: A Call for Intersectionality." *IMC Journal of Medical Science* 13 (1): 5. https://doi.org/10.3329/imcjms.v13i1.42050.

OHCHR and WHO (2008) "Fact Sheet No. 31: The Right to Health." United Nations Geneva. https://www.ohchr.org/en/publications/fact-sheets/fact-sheet-no-31-right-health.

P

Painter, Nell Irvin (2020) "Why 'White' Should Be Capitalized, Too." *Washington Post* (July 22). https://www.washingtonpost.com/opinions/2020/07/22/why-white-should-be-capitalized/.

Pascoe, Elizabeth A., and Laura Smart Richman (2009) "Perceived Discrimination and Health: A Meta-Analytic Review." *Psychological Bulletin* 135 (4): 531–54. https://doi.org/10.1037/a0016059.

Peters, Sanne A. E., and Mark Woodward (2023) "A Roadmap for Sex- and Gender-Disaggregated Health Research." *BMC Medicine* 21 (1): 354. https://doi.org/10.1186/s12916-023-03060-w.

Poteat, Tonia (2021) "Navigating the Storm: How to Apply Intersectionality to Public Health in Times of Crisis." *American Journal of Public Health* 111 (1): 91–92. https://doi.org/10.2105/AJPH.2020.305944.

Puca, Antonella (1997) "Steve Reich and Hebrew Cantillation." *The Musical Quarterly* 81 (4): 537–55.

R

Reimer, Franz (2021) "Das Recht auf Gesundheit, eine rechtsvergleichende Perspektive: Deutschland." EPRS: Wissenschaftlicher Dienst des Europäischen Parlaments.

Rosser, Sue V. (1994) *Women's Health – Missing from U.S. Medicine*. Bloomington: Indiana University Press. https://iupress.org/9780253114976/womens-healthmissing-from-u-s-medicine/.

S

Samulowitz, Anke, Ida Gremyr, Erik Eriksson, and Gunnel Hensing (2018) "'Brave Men' and 'Emotional Women': A Theory-Guided Literature Review on Gender Bias in Health Care and Gendered Norms towards Patients with Chronic Pain." *Pain Research & Management*. https://doi.org/10.1155/2018/6358624.

Schiebinger, Londa (2000) "Has Feminism Changed Science?" *Signs: Journal of Women in Culture and Society* 25 (4): 1171–75.

Sebring, Jennifer C. H. (2021) "Towards a Sociological Understanding of Medical Gaslighting in Western Health Care." *Sociology of Health & Illness* 43 (9): 1951–64. https://doi.org/10.1111/1467-9566.13367.

Shildrick, Margrit (1997) *Leaky Bodies and Boundaries: Feminism, Postmodernism and (Bio) Ethics*. 1st edition. London: Routledge.

Sjoding, Michael W., Dickson Robert P., Iwashyna Theodore J., Gay Steven E., and Valley Thomas S. (2020) "Racial Bias in Pulse Oximetry Measurement." *The New England Journal of Medicine* 383 (25): 2477–78. https://doi.org/10.1056/NEJMc2029240.

Statistisches Bundesamt (2024) "Migration und Integration: Migrationshintergrund." Statistisches Bundesamt. 2024. https://www.destatis.de/DE/Themen/Gesellschaft-Umwelt/Bevoelkerung/Migration-Integration/Glossar/migrationshintergrund.html.

Staton, Lisa J., Mukta Panda, Ian Chen, Inginia Genao, James Kurz, Mark Pasanen, Alex J. Mechaber, Madhusudan Menon, Jane O'Rorke, JoAnn Wood, Eric Rosenberg, Charles Faeslis, Tim Carey, Diane Calleson, and Sam Cykert (2007) "When Race Matters: Disagreement in Pain Perception between Patients and Their Physicians in Primary Care." *Journal of the National Medical Association* 99 (5): 532–38.

Stefanick, Marcia L., and Londa Schiebinger (2020) "Analysing How Sex and Gender Interact." *Lancet* 396 (10262): 1553–54. https://doi.org/10.1016/S0140-6736(20)32346-1.

T

Tannenbaum, Cara, Robert P. Ellis, Friederike Eyssel, James Zou, and Londa Schiebinger (2019) "Sex and Gender Analysis Improves Science and Engineering." *Nature* 575 (7781): 137–46. https://doi.org/10.1038/s41586-019-1657-6.

Tasca, Cecilia, Mariangela Rapetti, Mauro Giovanni Carta, and Bianca Fadda (2012) "Women and Hysteria in the History of Mental Health." *Clinical Practice and Epidemiology in Mental Health: CP & EMH* 8: 110–19. https://doi.org/10.2174/1745017901208010110.

Truth, Sojourner. 1851. "'Ain't I a Woman.'" The Sojourner Truth Project. 1851. https://www.thesojournertruthproject.com/compare-the-speeches.

V

Vyas, Darshali A., Leo G. Eisenstein, and David S. Jones (2020) "Hidden in Plain Sight – Reconsidering the Use of Race Correction in Clinical Algorithms." *The New England Journal of Medicine* 383 (9): 874–82. https://doi.org/10.1056/NEJMms2004740.

W

Waytz, Adam, Kelly Marie Hoffman, and Sophie Trawalter (2015) "A Superhumanization Bias in Whites' Perceptions of Blacks." *Social Psychological and Personality Science* 6 (3): 352–59. https://doi.org/10.1177/1948550614553642.

Weiss, Robert S (1994) *Learning from Strangers: The Art and Method of Qualitative Interview Studies*. New York: Free Press.

Wingfield, Paul (1992) "Janáček's Speech-Melody Theory in Concept and Practice." *Cambridge Opera Journal* 4 (3): 281–301.

Y

Yeboah, Amma (2017) "Rassismus und psychische Gesundheit in Deutschland." In *Rassismuskritik und Widerstandsformen*. Edited by Karim Fereidooni and Meral El, 143–61. Wiesbaden: Springer Fachmedien. https://doi.org/10.1007/978-3-658-14721-1_9.

Z

Zhang, Bin, Bo Chang, and Wenqian Du (2021) "Employing Intersectionality as a Data Generation Tool: Suggestions for Qualitative Researchers on Conducting Interviews of Intersectionality Study." *International Journal of Qualitative Methods* 20 (January): 16094069211064672. https://doi.org/10.1177/16094069211064672.

Taking and Making Pictures: The Art of Science and Science of Art

Cat Dawson

In 1986, the historian of science Londa Schiebinger made a somewhat radical claim: attempts to "define the position of women in European society" significantly impacted early European anatomical drawings of what was then generally categorized as the "female" skeleton (1986, 42). Over the eighteenth and nineteenth centuries, Schiebinger argued, a "tendency to look to science as an arbiter of social questions" had increased apace of a similar tendency to use the concept of nature as a way of explaining and reinforcing social orders along lines drawn to define race, sex, and class (1986, 43). In anatomy, this manifested as an effort to locate a single physiological origin for gendered difference that routinely turned up different answers, such that the topography of sex in the body was—and remains—in ongoing flux. The greater the credibility that science gained, the greater the barriers became for minoritized subjects to participate in authorized discourse, and mount credible challenges to it.

Schiebinger's essay, "Skeletons in the Closet: The First Illustrations of the Female Skeleton in Eighteenth-Century Anatomy," is a key early example of how scholarship in the history of science, feminist science and technology studies (STS), and related fields have, over the last several decades, laid increasingly bare the ways in which bodies have long been sorted by biomedical science into categories both according to the dictates of the social order and despite abounding evidence of the fundamental instability of those categories. It is also an early interrogation of the relationship between the production of images and the production of knowledge. Schiebinger describes a process through which the production of knowledge relies on the production of images to confirm and even confer expertise, at times ahead of the actual information that the image purports to contain. Each image that Schiebinger includes was crafted by anatomists to perform a very specific kind of illustrative labor relative in the service of articulating distinctions between two ostensible categories for sex—one that at times even transcends the human/non-human divide. But removed from the historical contexts in which they were put forth as expert knowledge and recontextualized among other contemporaneous anatomical drawings, they constitute a parallel and distinct argument from Schiebinger's about the centrality of images to the accumulation of the power of knowledge.

This volume, in both premise and promise, investigates the relationship between vision and biomedicine. Conceived of as both the production and consumption of images, vision is not just about the act of viewing, and so the study of vision can reveal how knowledge is produced; how images echo, enhance, or impact not only how we see, but also what we see. The chapters in this book explore how interdisciplinary collaboration and coproduction can inflect the limits and limitations of biomedical vision. In the call for papers for the Biomedical Visions project, the editors sought to foster interdisciplinary dialogue that would elucidate how the visual orders, perpetuates, or challenges norms in medicine, and how that ordering might result in differential access to knowledge about disease. Central to the resulting contributions are thus images themselves, which loosely coalesce around three representational principles: making epistemic things accessible *within* biomedicine, making expert knowledge intelligible *beyond* biomedicine, and making art objects *from* biomedicine. Images produced by those in biomedicine for the purpose of sharing information with other specialists, which appear in chapters 7 and 8, appear in this volume to interrogate the promise and pitfalls of that particular kind of image. Images such as those that appear in chapters 1, 5, and 9 endeavor to translate biomedical forms and facts of knowing into something that can be consumed or processed by the public. Finally, images that appear in the other chapters make use of biomedical resources both formally and conceptually in the service of producing art.

Biomedical Visions exposes two fundamental problems at the heart of many biomedical projects. The first is that biomedical conversations are nearly impossible to deracinate from a binary of problem and cure—something that manifests well beyond traditionally biomedical contexts, for example in "wellness" space conversations around how to optimize bodies. The second is that, though they are often staged as a form of information that can complete an otherwise invisible loop in biomedical contexts, images participate in their own semantic economies that exceed and are therefore never wholly assimilable to (or explainable through) the contexts that produce them.

Most of the essays in this volume trouble the coproduction of visualization and knowledge by describing the opacities between scientific images and the processes from which they stem. Among them, Jaipreet Virdi's essay stands out for its clarion explication of how that opacity both stems from and contributes to the ways in which bodies are ordered and othered. Virdi describes the convoluted process through which people living with endometriosis have to convince an often skeptical medical-industrial system of the presence of their pain and necessity for treatment. Using her own experience with the disease as an example—Virdi is an historian of medicine and self-described "endo sufferer" who has experienced the dismissal of expert practitioners in spite of herself possessing substantial relevant expertise both sanctioned (professional) and unsanctioned (somatic) by the biomedical fields—the author describes the particular ways in which endo sufferers are doubly impacted by gendered and imaging bias in biomedicine: because the disease is primarily associated with the uterus, it is one most often experienced by people who are assigned female, a population often given less credibility in medical contexts, which also often gives more credence to images than to patients.

The reliance by the medical establishment on images for the kinds of "confirmation" that Virdi describes both indicates and names the degree to which the experiences of individuals who encounter the medical-industrial complex are not taken into account until medical science has produced an image through which something can be confirmed. Yet, just as visualizations "can legitimize patient experiences," as Freeborn notes in the introduction, they are most often "only legible to trained specialists" and even in those contexts—and this is key—are of limited epistemic worth.[1] Manning and Geller describe in their chapter how the eye has to be trained, the conditions in the image and the body just right, for an inference—usually a diagnosis of illness or health—to be made. In other words, as much conditioning and training goes into recognizing an image as one of illness or health as goes into other forms of looking. Though that kind of highly specialized looking is not native to the body—we learn to experience pain before we learn to read images, never mind medical ones for those trained to do so—it nevertheless supersedes the experiential in biomedical contexts. In the example offered by Manning and Geller, the image takes on its own life beyond the body: the object has to be perfectly prepared for examination to conform to the ways in which a practitioner has been trained on visual materials about an illness or procedure for the correct assessment to be made. The body, in other words, is being asked to conform to secondary source material on itself.

That highly specialized form of looking often comes from and contributes to the fabrication of expertise that is in turn premised on the idea that the passage of time, accumulation of knowledge, and ever-better imaging technology will finally realize a still-held belief in the promise of totalizing knowledge. Virdi also raises and critiques this premise by describing the biomedical reliance on imaging technology ahead of the patient's experience of pain for evidentiary support for the need for treatment. However, as demonstrated in this volume by Bhanot and Virdi, Borck and Meunier, and Keuck and van der Beugel, the proliferation of imaging technologies

1 Freeborn, this volume, 8.

does not itself redress the fundamental problem that images will always fail along multiple axes to describe the processes of the body. Furthermore, as suggested as early as 1981 by Schiebinger and countless times since by scholars in the fields of the history of science and STS, the ongoing production of knowledge, though frequently indexed to progress, does not necessarily mean the production of progressively better knowledge. It may be that evolution in scientific knowledge production is, by some measures, most accurate as a representation of social norms and expectations for the organisms in question. As in Schiebinger's essay—which is fundamentally about the ways in which binary sex in science is concocted out of thickly gendered social air—these articles demonstrate that there is far more complexity at the juncture of art and science than is often acknowledged.

Among the myriad ways in which images are deployed in this book, three particular instances serve as limit cases for biomedical vision.

The first, drawn from chapter 1, relates to the exportation of scientific imagery into fine art contexts. In a discussion of the "use, reuse, and misuse" of scientific images in art, Marano, Matter, and Valterio argue that recontextualizing medical images "open[s] up the possibility to reconsider conceptions of use and value."[2] Among the various images and apparatuses that either derive from or gesture toward the intersections of bodies and medical technologies is a series of X-rays of a skull—perhaps the most recognizable form of medical imaging—with similarly translucent photos of a hand or finger superimposed on top of it, and the word "you" written on top of the image along the visible edges of the objects in the frame. Like other forms of medical imaging, X-rays are used in the process of repairing a body to a medical norm of healthful wholeness to identify either a corporeal cause or its absence. Here, the utility of the image is disrupted not only by its recategorization as art, but also by the digits, photographs desaturated to a degree that they have a similar aesthetic quality as the medium of X-ray that also literalizes the projective visual

2 Marano, Matter, and Valterio, this volume, 45.

3 Beugel and Keuck, this volume, 50.

excavation of the technology of the X-ray. The repetitious deictic and its aesthetic description of the bounds of the body, then, gives form to the profound othering of the processes and effects of biomedical visions, while also demonstrating the degree to which biomedical imagery and the systems of knowledge production from which they stem and to which they contribute are readily available to disruption.

In biomedical contexts whether as the patient or the provider, images, as this volume bears out, offer the possibility of reflection, if not also relief or repair. A second limit case is Keuck and van de Beugel's chapter, which addresses how biomedical imagery is used as a point of departure to create a work of art—decidedly not for traditionally scientific purposes—but one that was supposed to "disentangle this notion of Alzheimer's so that the public perceive it as a disease that needs to be tackled in certain ways."[3] Famously a disease of forgetting—Alzheimer's gradually destroys the key memory and thinking functionalities of the brain—there is a particular richness to using abstract art to represent something about it to the public. Comprised of a gradient of tiles, the work is an artistic rendering of a biomedical representational convention that takes up not only that convention and its utility to efforts to give nonspecialists a way of visualizing what cannot be seen—something perhaps as important affectively as it is intellectually—but is also the distinction between art and science by pointing to the substantial overlaps between, and subjectivities shared by, the two arenas. This work, in other words, is an elegant distillation of the fundamental subjectivity of image cultures; it is no more or less representational of Alzheimer's imaging than the biomedical images that are accepted as the representational convention in a scientific context.

The final limit case in this volume also takes up the mantle in the editors' original call in the most traditional sense of commissioning a work of art to accompany an exploration of the production of research. The introduction to this volume asserts that "Human beings are complex biopsychosocial systems with individual life histories that are not epistemologically exhausted by quantitative definitions of normality and abnormality."[4] In a departure from the majority of essays in this volume that take a critical eye to the relationship between biomedical images, chapter 9, by Christianson, Hanemaayer, Martineck, Hamann, Friedman, and Elliot, focuses instead on refining an existing set of images that serve as tools to share scientific knowledge with nonspecialists. In some ways their project can be understood as a practical solution to the problematic that other authors in this volume describe; after all, if the best way we currently have for sharing biomedical knowledge is through a visual medium that will never be wholly representative, then it makes sense to refine the use of that medium.

4 Freeborn, this volume, 11.

At the same time, most essays in this volume explicitly understand the relationship between knowledge and visualization as inherently problematic or suspect, while Christianson, Hanemaayer, Martineck, Hamann, Friedman, and Elliot implicitly suggest that the visual communication of biomedical knowledge can be perfected. Furthermore, implicit in the topic they take up—the field of genetic counseling, which has routinely been motivated by and tainted with eugenic thought—is an anachronistic positivism that presumes, echoing nineteenth-century scientists, that the body is, as trans studies scholar Hil Malatino puts it, "an epistemological object with its own truth to tell" (2019, 133). The insistence that the body both can and should be cured toward an ideal, and that biomedicine in general and the genome in particular are a path to a prediscursive truth that will unlock that path toward cure, is staked on a range of assumptions that scholars in a host of disciplines might understand to have long ago been vanquished. For example, there is no way to use genetic profiling to identify the trans subject, no way of looking within the body to predict the eventuality of that often-medicalized experience. The word *medicalization* is also telling: the promise of looking within the body is often and incorrectly related to that of looking at the body because science, like vision, is so rigorously a product of the social, and meant to communicate things about the social. Malatino also points to this when they argue that that such images of the body are not only far from the claims to detached objectivity on which biomedical authority is staked but may indeed be deeply motivated through the psychosocial conditions of so-called objective practitioners (2019, 142–143).

As the study of the intersection of minoritized experience and medical science has demonstrated time and again—and as the authors in this volume mostly also hold—there is no way of fully pictorially representing the lived experience of embodiment, whether heathy or sick or some place in between or even beyond that binary. The theorist and poet Cameron Awkward-Rich has proposed a way beyond (or between or whatever other adverbial is appropriate to a project's politics, investments, and aims) the dyad of pain and cure, difference and its "correction" by "taking feeling bad as a mundane fact": "There will always be a residue of bad feeling, an unavoidable fact of being embodied, of being a self in a world inevitably split by difference" (2017, 826). Awkward-Rich works against what he calls the "affirmative project of trans studies," but his argument applies to the positivist project of genetics, too (2017, 823). There is little that links biomedical ways of seeing to the production of knowledge that does not descend from or perpetuate systems of knowing that turn on the repetitious privileging of certain ways of being embodied over others. The truth one can discern may be that it is those of us who eschew the pre-discursive in favor of an understanding of the body as a complex biopsychosocial system who remain in the minority.

Where do these leave us? If we can understand our present moment of biomedical vision as one in which the boundaries between what is authorized and not are historically specific and constituted through the terms of capture, which Malatino describes as a way to "fix the meaning of the image so as to confirm . . . diagnosis of pathology," it is not only possible but indeed imperative to understand that there is both value and a cost to the fabrication and sustenance of both biomedical image cultures, and the underlying claims and assumptions that motivate both that and how they are produced (2019, 139).

Rhetorics of repair, as Jasbir Puar reminds us, often stem from an understanding of the healthful subject as one not only recoverable to the operations of capitalist production, but also incompatible with debility, non-whiteness, and other subject positions already minoritized within neoliberal and nationalist projects (2017, 35–36). The pain-free body is often a productive body, a means of production, a well-oiled cog in the machine. Pain, then, is not only something to be repaired; its repair—whether in promise or substance—is highly prized in part because it is staged as a step toward the recovery of the productive subject. To leave aside the productive dictates of capitalism for a moment—providing such a thing is even possible—enables us to rethink the embodied condition of pain and other ways of nonconformity to a capitalist subject. There are myriad subjects for whom pain is ineradicable, or whose journey through the medical-industrial complex at best is fruitless and at worst makes matters worse. Awkward-Rich asks what would become possible if we were to eschew the age-old construction of illness and health and develop instead a "different kind of orientation to bad feelings" (2017, 825). This is neither to conflate bad (affective) feelings and physical pain, nor to obscure the sites at which those two conditions are co-constitutive and difficult at best to disentangle, but to ask what becomes possible when biomedical visions of both one's ontological norm and deviations from it exceed or escape the biomedical context. This inquiry might be carried over into the diagnostic imaging realm: what would become possible were we to construct a world of biomedical images that is not premised on expertise and its severance from the rest of the world—something that, as Borck and Meunier note, is already a tenuous connection—but rather on a set of principles of envisioning bodies and processes that partake of a broader legibility? In such a scenario, biomedical images might become a substrate across which patients and doctors could communicate through co-creation, and biomedical visions one in which a broad swath of us might be able to partake. This is, as the introduction to this volume demonstrates, already happening as medical images precipitate out into visual culture beyond not only their use cases but beyond the realm of their delimited utility; what remains to be seen is how and in what ways communication cultures beyond the biomedical will continue to do what they have long done: to shape the biomedicine itself.

A

Awkward-Rich, Cameron (2017) "Trans Feminism: Or, Reading like a Depressed Transsexual." *Signs: Journal of Women in Culture and Society* 42, no. 2: 819–841.

M

Malatino, Hil (2019) *Queer Embodiment: Monstrosity, Medical Violence, and Intersex Experience*. Lincoln: University of Nebraska Press.

P

Puar, Jasbir (2017) *The Right to Maim: Debility, Capacity, Disability*. Durham, NC: Duke University Press, 2017.

S

Schiebinger, Londa (1986) "Skeletons in the Closet: The First Illustrations of the Female Skeleton in Eighteenth Century Anatomy." *Representations* 14: 42–82.

Acknowledgments

This book was made possible by the generous support of the Max Planck Institute for the History of Science (MPIWG), Berlin.

Elizabeth Hughes and Alfred Freeborn

We would like to express our deepest gratitude to Lara Keuck as the leader of the Max Planck Research Group (RG) Practices of Validation in the Biomedical Sciences, who offered unwavering encouragement and valuable feedback from the very beginning.

From concept to workshop to publication, there have been so many people who have helped to shape this book. Many thanks are due to the members of the RG's Research Therapy for their helpful advice from the start. We are so very grateful to the people who agreed to take on this art-science experiment with us. At the authors' workshop on September 28 and 29, 2023, the contributors to this volume met in Berlin and online to present works-in-progress and exchange thoughts on interdisciplinary methods. We were also joined by Nate Lewis, Niama Safia Sandy, and Mae Eskenazi at the workshop, and we would like to thank them for their stimulating presentations and insightful comments.

We'd also like to extend our thanks to Birgitta von Mallinckrodt for her incredible administrative support, and also to Maren Nie and Emma Sevink for their excellent editorial support in bringing this volume to life. Lastly, we'd like to mention that the group welcomed four babies into the world over the course of this project. A round of thanks to these unwitting participants who allowed their parents just enough time and energy to finish their work!

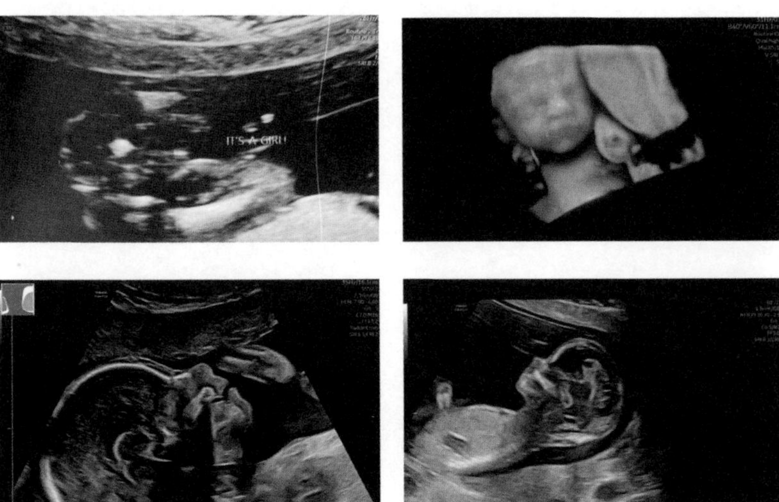

Jacob van der Beugel

I would like to thank University of Cambridge for commissioning *Matter in Grey*, and professor Sabina Leonelli and Egenis at the University of Exeter for introducing me to Lara Keuck and her work.

Milton Fernando Gonzalez Rodriguez and Paula Muhr

We extend our sincere gratitude to Cornelius Borck, Robert Meunier, and Flora Lysen for their generous feedback on the chapter and their insightful suggestions, which not only enhanced our analysis of the case studies but also provided essential new perspectives. The unwavering support offered by Alfred Freeborn and Elizabeth Hughes from the outset was crucial in drafting the final version, as was the valuable input we received from all the project participants throughout. We deeply appreciate the organizers' efforts in creating such a remarkable collaborative project, a truly unforgettable experience—thank you. This chapter has received funding from the European Union's Horizon 2020 research and innovation program under the Marie Skłodowska Curie grant agreement no. 101026198.

Flora Lysen

I would like to express my gratitude to Alfred Freeborn and Elizabeth Hughes for the invitation to contribute to this volume, their patience, their insightful reviews, and, most importantly, for initiating a highly fruitful collaboration with the artist Marlene Bart. Many, many thanks to Marlene Bart for being such a warm, engaging, and perceptive conversation partner and collaborator from the very beginning. I am also deeply appreciative of Cornelius Borck for his invaluable feedback on this chapter, which provided me with more insights than I could incorporate. This article has further benefitted from generous responses to a draft by participants of the symposium Forgotten by Design: Foundational Limits and Dysfunctionalities in Computational Cognitive-Behavioral Environments, organized by Christina Vagt and Florian Sprenger at the College for Social Sciences and Humanities in Essen. I would also like to thank my colleagues in the Science, Technology, and Society Studies research group at Maastricht University for their feedback, particularly Jo Wachelder and Sally Wyatt. My research was generously supported by the Dutch Research Council (NWO) as part of the RAIDIO research project grant (number 406.DI.19.089).

Marlene Bart

I would like to thank my coproducers on the AR piece, Ikonospace, Joris Demnard, and Manuel Farré.

Robert Meunier and Cornelius Borck

The authors would like to thank Johannes Richers for his generous insights into his work. Robert Meunier's work was funded by the Deutsche Forschungsgemeinschaft (DFG) within the Cluster of Excellence "Precision Medicine in Chronic Inflammation" (EXC 2167), project no. 390884018.

Adam Christianson, Ariane Hanemaayer, Sophia Martineck, Alexandra Hamann, Jan M. Friedman, and Alison Elliott

The authors would like to thank Shelin Adam and Barney P. for their assistance with this project, as well as Elizabeth Hughes, Alfred Freeborn, and the members of the 2023 Visualizing Disease Workshop in Berlin. Ariane Hanemaayer is supported in part by funding from the Social Sciences and Humanities Research Council of Canada. The DECIDE tool was created with funding from the project "Paediatric Epilepsy: Using Genomics to Improve Patient Care and Outcomes," which was supported by the Canada Excellence Research Chair (MF) and the Alva Foundation (MC). The DECIDE research was funded by a Canadian Institutes of Health Research grant to Jan Friedman and a Canadian Institutes of Health Research New Investigator Award. Adam Christianson is supported by the Wellcome Trust and Social Sciences and Humanities Research Council of Canada.

Awa Naghipour, Joana Atemengue Owona, and Golnar Kat Rahmani

We dearly thank Lara Keuck for introducing us to this project and her support as head of the Max Planck Research Group Practices of Validation in the Biomedical Sciences. We are especially grateful to Elizabeth Hughes and Alfred Freeborn for their initiation and organization of this transdisciplinary volume, for providing the opportunity to contribute, and for their exemplary balance of constructive criticism, fruitful ideas, and enthusiastic encouragement. We would like to thank all other authors of this volume for their incredibly valuable input throughout the process, and also Marie Séférian and Dr. Astrid Mania for their expertise, external review, and feedback. We sincerely appreciate Josianne Owona, Dejvi Haxhi, Lucia Mair, and the anonymous reviewers for their contributions to the manuscript revision. Finally, we acknowledge the three interview participants without whom this project would not have been possible in its current form.

Cat Dawson

I would like to thank Banu Subramaniam and Beans Velocci.

List of Contributors

Elizabeth W. Hughes, Max Planck Institute for the History of Science, elizabeth-hughes.com
Alfred Freeborn, Max Planck Institute for the History of Science
Virginia Marano, Kunsthistorisches Institut in Florenz (Max Planck Institute) and University of Zurich, disability-arthist.net
Charlotte Matter, University of Basel, disability-arthist.net
Laura Valterio, University of Zurich, disability-arthist.net
Jacob van der Beugel, jacobvanderbeugel.com
Lara Keuck, Bielefeld University
Jaipreet Virdi, University of Victoria, jaivirdi.com
Nimisha Bhanot, nimishabhanot.com
Paula Muhr, Brand University of Applied Sciences Hamburg, University of Zurich, paulamuhr.de
Milton Fernando Gonzalez Rodriguez, KU Leuven
Stephen A. Geller
Gideon Manning, Cedars-Sinai Program in the History of Medicine, researchers.cedars-sinai.edu/Gideon.Manning
Flora Lysen, Maastricht University, floralysen.net
Marlene Bart, marlenebart.com
Cornelius Borck, University of Lübeck, imgwf.uni-luebeck.de/mitarbeiter/borck.html
Robert Meunier, University of Lübeck, uni-luebeck.academia.edu/RobertMeunier
Adam Christianson, Goldsmiths, University of London
Ariane Hanemaayer, Brandon University
Sophia Martineck, martineck.com
Alexandra Hamann, mintwissen.com
Jan M. Friedman, University of British Columbia, friedmanlab.org
Alison Elliott, University of British Columbia, bcchr.ca/GenCOUNSEL
Awa Naghipour, unheard.network
Joana Atemengue Owona, unheard.network
Golnar Kat Rahmani, unheard.network
Cat Dawson, Smith College, catvdawson.com

Editors
Elizabeth W. Hughes and Alfred Freeborn

Editorial management
Juliane Eisele, Hatje Cantz

Copyediting
Elizabeth W. Hughes, Aaron Bogart, Maren Nie, Emma Sevink

Graphic design and typesetting
Studio Thomas Spallek

Typeface
Stempel Garamond LT Pro

Reproductions
DLG Graphic, Paris

Production
Alise Ausmane, Hatje Cantz

Paper
Munken Print White 1.5, 90g/m²

Printed by
Livonia Print, Riga

Published by
Hatje Cantz Verlag GmbH
Mommsenstraße 27
10629 Berlin
Germany
contact@hatjecantz.de
www.hatjecantz.com
A Ganske Publishing Group Company

ISBN: 978-3-7757-6085-0 [PRINT]
ISBN: 978-3-7757-6110-9 [PDF]
ISBN: 978-3-7757-6160-4 (EPUB)

Printed in Latvia

Cover illustration
Ketty La Rocca, *Craniologia 12*, 1973, lightbox, handwriting on X-ray, 70 × 50 × 15 cm
© Courtesy of Archive Ketty La Rocca | Michelangelo Vasta and Kadel Willborn, Düsseldorf

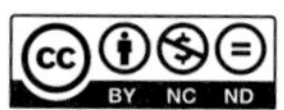